HANDBOOK *of* CARDIOVASCULAR CELL TRANSPLANTATION

HANDBOOK *of* CARDIOVASCULAR CELL TRANSPLANTATION

Edited by

Nicholas N Kipshidze MD PhD FACC FSCAI
Professor and Director
Experimental Pharmacology and Physiology
Lenox Hill Heart and Vascular Institute and the
Cardiovascular Research Foundation of New York
New York
USA

and

Patrick W Serruys MD PhD FACC FESC
Head of Interventional Cardiology
Thoraxcenter
Erasmus University
Rotterdam
The Netherlands

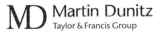

Martin Dunitz
Taylor & Francis Group

© 2004 Martin Dunitz, an imprint of the Taylor & Francis Group

First published in the United Kingdom in 2004
by Martin Dunitz, an imprint of the Taylor and Francis Group, 11 New Fetter Lane,
London EC4P 4EE

Tel.:   +44 (0) 20 7583 9855
Fax.:   +44 (0) 20 7842 2298
E-mail: info@dunitz.co.uk
Website: http://www.dunitz.co.uk

Although every effort has been made to ensure that all owners of copyright material have
been acknowledged in this publication, we would be glad to acknowledge in subsequent
reprints or editions any omissions brought to our attention.

A CIP record for this book is available from the British Library.

ISBN 1–84184–214–1

Distributed in the USA by
Fulfilment Center
Taylor & Francis
10650 Tobben Drive
Independence, KY 41051, USA
Toll Free Tel: +1 800 634 7064
E-mail: taylorandfrancis@thomsonlearning.com

Distributed in Canada by
Taylor & Francis
74 Rolark Drive
Scarborough, Ontario M1R 4G2, Canada
Toll Free Tel: +1 877 226 2237
E-mail: tal_fran@istar.ca

Distributed in the rest of the world by
Thomson Publishing Services
Cheriton House
North Way
Andover, Hampshire SP10 5BE, UK
Tel: +44 (0)1264 332424
E-mail: salesorder.tandf@thomsonpublishingservices.co.uk

Composition by 🅣 Tek-Art, Croydon, UK

Printed and bound in Singapore by Kyodo Printing Co (S'pore) Pte Ltd

CONTENTS

CONTRIBUTORS

Takayuki Asahara MD
Department of Regenerative Medicine
Kobe Institute of Biomedical
Research and Innovation
Chou-ku
Kobe
Japan

Richard Baffour PhD
Cardiovascular Research Institute
Division of Cardiology
Washington Hospital Center
Washington, DC
USA

Leo A Bockeria MD
Bakoulev Scientific Center for
Cardiovascular Surgery
Russian Academy of Medical Sciences
Moscow
Russia

Michael Brehm MD
Department of Internal Medicine
Division of Cardiology/Pneumology
and Angiology
Heinrich-Heine-University
Düsseldorf
Germany

Valeri Chekanov MD PhD
Clinical Professor of Medicine
University of Wisconsin Medical School
Director, Cardiology Basic Research
Milwaukee Heart Institute/Heart
Care Foundation
Wisconsin, WI
USA

Thomas K Chin
Department of Pediatrics
JH Quillen College of Medicine
East Tennessee State University
Johnson City, TN
USA

Ray C-J Chiu MD PhD FRCSC
Professor
Division of Cardiothoracic Surgery
McGill University
Montreal, Quebec
Canada

Florence Chua PhD
Cell Transplants International
LLC
Memphis, TN
USA

Joan Dow BS
Heart Institute
Good Samaritan Hospital
Los Angeles, CA
USA

Elazer R Edelman MD PhD
Harvard-MIT Division of Health
Sciences and Technology
Massachusetts Institute of Technology
Cambridge, MA
USA

Mahboubeh Eghbali-Webb PhD
Alexcell, LLC
Biotechnology and Biomedical
Consulting
Woodbridge, CT
USA

Sharon Etzion PhD
Neufeld Cardiac Research Institute
Sheba Medical Center
Tel-Aviv University
Tel-Hashomer
Israel

Gwendolyn Fang MD
Cell Transplants International
LLC
Memphis, TN
USA

Paul W M Fedak MD
Department of Cardiovascular
Surgery
University of Toronto
Toronto, Ontario
Canada

Peter J Fitzgerald MD PhD
Cardiovascular Medicine
Stanford University Medical Center
Stanford, CA
USA

Shmuel Fuchs MD
Head, Catheterization Laboratory
Rabin Medical Center
Petach Tikva
Israel

Charles E Ganote
Department of Surgery
JH Quillen College of Medicine
East Tennessee State University
Johnson City, TN
USA

Lior Gepstein MD PhD
Head, Cardiovascular Research
Laboratory/Department of
Biophysics and Physiology
The Bruce Rappaport Faculty of
Medicine
Technion-Israel Institute of Technology
Haifa
Israel

James L Greene
Global Vice President
Bioheart Inc
Weston
Florida FL
USA

Husnian Kh Haider PhD
Department of Cardiac Thoracic &
Vascular Surgery
National University Hospital
Singapore

Howard B Haimes PhD
Executive Director Preclinical Studies
Bioheart Inc
Weston
Florida FL
USA

Sharon Hale BS
Heart Institute
Good Samaritan Hospital
Los Angeles, CA
USA

Jack Harvey MPH
Vice President
MyoCell (TM) Operations
Bioheart Inc
Weston
Florida FL
USA

Christian C Haudenschild MD
Professor of Pathology
Head, Department of Experimental
Pathology
American Red Cross
Rockville, MD
USA

Silviu Itescu MD
Departments of Medicine and
Surgery
Columbia University
New York, NY
USA

Tea Kakuchaya MD
Bakoulev Scientific Center for
Cardiovascular Surgery
Russian Academy of Medical Sciences
Moscow
Russia

Race L Kao PhD
Department of Surgery
JH Quillen College of Medicine
East Tennessee State University
Johnson City, TN
USA

Atsuhiko Kawamoto MD
Department of Regenerative Medicine
Kobe Institute of Biomedical Research
and Innovation
Chou-ku
Kobe
Japan

Larry Kedes MD
Institute of Genetic Medicine
University of Southern California
Los Angeles, CA
USA

Michael H Keelan MD
Department of Cardiology
Division of Cardiovascular Medicine
Medical College of Wisconsin
Milwaukee, WI
USA

Izhak Kehat
Cardiovascular Research Laboratory
Department of Physiology
The Bruce Rappaport Faculty of
Medicine
Technion-Israel Institute of
Technology and Rambam Medical
Center
Haifa
Israel

Tim Kinnaird MD
The Cardiovascular Research Institute
MedStar Research Institute
Washington Hospital Center
Washington, DC
USA

Nicholas Kipshidze MD PhD FACC FESC
Director, Experimental Pharmacology
and Physiology
Lenox Hill Heart and Vascular
Institute of New York
Lenox Hill Hospital
New York, NY
USA

Robert A Kloner MD PhD
Heart Institute
Good Samaritan Hospital
Keck School of Medicine
Cardiovascular Division
University of Southern California
Los Angeles, CA
USA

Alfred A Kocher MD
Department of Surgery
Columbia University
New York, NY
USA

Ran Kornowski MD FACC
Rabin Medical Center
Cardiology Department
Petach-Tikva and Sackler Faculty of
Medicine
Tel Aviv University
Tel Aviv
Israel

John J Laffan
Department of Microbiology
JH Quillen College of Medicine
East Tennessee State University
Johnson City, TN
USA

Peter K Law PhD
Cell Transplants International
LLC
Memphis, TN
USA

Martin B Leon MD FACC
Director and CEO
Cardiovascular Research Foundation
Lenox Hill Heart and Vascular
Institute
New York, NY
USA

Jonathan Leor MD
Neufeld Cardiac Research Institute
Sheba Medical Center
Tel-Hashomer
Israel

Ren-Ke Li MD PhD
Professor of Surgery
Division of Cardiovascular Surgery
University of Toronto
Toronto General Hospital
Ontario
Canada

Douglas W Losordo MD
Division of Cardiovascular Research
St. Elizabeth's Medical Center
Tufts University School of Medicine
Boston, MA
USA

Briain D MacNeill MB BCh MSc
BAO MRCPI
Department of Interventional
Cardiology
Massachusetts General Hospital and
Harvard Medical School
Boston, MA
USA

Patrick M McCarthy MD
Departments of Cardiovascular
Medicine and Thoracic and
Cardiothoracic Surgery
The Heart Center/Cleveland Clinic
Foundation
Cleveland, OH
USA

Keith L March MD PhD
Indiana Center for Vascular Biology
and Medicine/
Krannert Institute of Cardiology
Indiana University School of
Medicine
Indianapolis, IN
USA

Hiroaki Matsubara MD PhD
Department of Cardiovascular Medicine
Kyoto Prefectural University School
of Medicine
Kyoto
Japan

Philippe Menasché MD PhD
Department of Cardiovascular Surgery
Hôpital Européen Georges Pompidou
Paris
France

Katsumi Miyauchi MD
Minneapolis Heart Institute Foundation
Minnesota Cardiovascular Research
Institute
Minneapolis, MN
USA

E Michael Molnar MD
Bio-Cellular Research Organization
Newark, NJ
USA

Jeffrey W Moses MD FACC
Chief, Interventional Cardiology
Lenox Hill Heart Hospital and
Vascular Institute
New York, NY
USA

Jochen Müller-Ehmsen MD
Heart Institute
Good Samaritan Hospital
Los Angeles
USA

Bari Murtuza MA FRCS
Harefield Heart Science Centre
Imperial College Faculty of Medicine
Middlesex
UK

Victor Nikolaychik MD PhD
Clinical Professor of Medicine
Chemistry Department
University of Wisconsin
Milwaukee, WI
USA

Helen M Nugent PhD
Harvard-MIT Division of Health
Sciences and Technology
Massachusetts Institute of Technology
Cambridge, MA
USA

Stephen N Oesterle MD FACC
Division of Cardiology
Massachusetts General Hospital
Boston, MA
USA

Marc S Penn MD PhD
Departments of Cardiovascular
Medicine and Thoracic and
Cardiothoracic Surgery
The Heart Center/Cleveland Clinic
Foundation
Cleveland, OH
USA

D Glenn Pennington
Department of Surgery
JH Quillen College of Medicine
East Tennessee State University
Johnson City, TN
USA

Kirk L Peterson MD
Heart Institute
Good Samaritan Hospital
Los Angeles, CA
USA

Eric T Price MD
Cardiovascular Medicine
Stanford University Medical Center
Stanford, CA
USA

Thorsten Reffelmann MD
Heart Institute
Good Samaritan Hospital
Los Angeles
USA

Jalees Rehman MD
Indiana Center for Vascular Biology
and Medicine/
Krannert Institute of Cardiology
Indiana University School of Medicine
Indianapolis, IN
USA

Vadim S Repin MD
Bakoulev Scientific Center for
Cardiovascular Surgery
Russian Academy of Medical Sciences
Moscow
Russia

Mehrdad Rezaee MD PhD
Cardiovascular Medicine
Stanford University Medical Center
Stanford, CA
USA

Patrick W Serruys MD PhD FACC FESC
Thoraxcenter
Erasmus Medical Center
Rotterdam
The Netherlands

Michael D Schuster MS
Department of Surgery
Columbia University
New York, NY
USA

Robert S Schwartz MD FACC FAHA
Medical Director
Minnesota Cardiovascular Research
Institute
Minneapolis Heart Institute Foundation
Minneapolis, MN
USA

Eugene KW Sim MD
Department of Cardiac Thoracic &
Vascular Surgery
National University Hospital
Singapore

Boris Simkhovich MD PhD
Heart Institute
Good Samaritan Hospital
Keck School of Medicine
Cardiovascular Division
University of Southern California
Los Angeles, CA
USA

Pieter C Smits MD PhD
Thoraxcenter
Erasmus Medical Center
Rotterdam
The Netherlands

Eugenio Stabile MD
The Cardiovascular Research Institute
MedStar Research Institute,
Washington Hospital Center
Washington, DC
USA

Bodo E Strauer MD FRCP
Department of Internal Medicine/
Division of Cardiology Pneumology
and Angiology
Heinrich-Heine-University
Düsseldorf
Germany

Ken Suzuki MD PhD
Harefield Heart Science Centre
Imperial College Faculty of Medicine
Middlesex
UK

Doris A Taylor PhD
Department of Cardiology
Duke University Medical Center
Durham, NC
USA

CA Thompson
Massachusetts General Hospital
Boston, MA
USA

Mykola Tsapenko MD PhD
Department of Medicine
Bronx VA Medical Center
Bronx, NY
USA

Ewout J van den Bos MD
Department of Experimental
Cardiology, Thoraxcenter
Erasmus Medical Center
Rotterdam
The Netherlands

WJ van der Giessen MD PhD
Thoraxcenter
Erasmus Medical Center
Rotterdam
The Netherlands

Ron Waksman MD
Cardiovascular Research Institute
Division of Cardiology
Washington Hospital Center
Washington, DC
USA

Jih-Shiuan Wang MD
Assistant Professor
Division of Cardiovascular Surgery
Yang-Ming University/Veterans
General Hospital-Taipei
Taipei
Taiwan

Magdi H Yacoub FRS
Royal Brompton & Harefield NHS Trust
Royal Brompton Hospital
London
UK

Lior Yankelson
Cardiovascular Research Laboratory
Department of Physiology
The Bruce Rappaport Faculty of
Medicine
Technion- Israel Institute of
Technology and Rambam Medical
Center
Haifa
Israel

Mu Yao MD PhD
Heart Institute
Good Samaritan Hospital
Los Angeles, CA
USA

Alan C Yeung MD
Cardiovascular Medicine
Stanford University Medical Center
Stanford, CA
USA

Paul G Yock MD
Cardiovascular Medicine
Stanford University Medical Center
Stanford, CA
USA

Tobias Zeus MD
Department of Internal Medicine
Division of Cardiology/Pneumology
and Angiology
Heinrich-Heine-University
Düsseldorf
Germany

Hao Zhang MD
Division of Cardiovascular Surgery
University of Toronto
Toronto, Ontario
Canada

PREFACE

Over the past three decades enormous progress has been made in the medical, surgical, and catheter-based therapy of acute and chronic heart disease. The concerted efforts of basic scientists, cardiologists, and cardiothoracic surgeons have advanced our understanding of the pathophysiology of ischemic and hypertensive heart pathologies, as well as viral myocarditis and cardiomyopathies, all characterized by irreversible loss of cardiomyocytes. These conditions may lead to progressive impairment of ventricular function and development of end-stage heart failure.

Congestive heart failure is a growing epidemic that affects more than 5 million Americans. The prognosis for these patients remains poor. Accordingly, the development of new therapeutic paradigms for these patients has become imperative. At present, the only definitive treatment option for end-stage heart failure is heart transplantation. However, given the chronic lack of donors limiting the number of end-stage heart failure patients that could benefit from heart transplantation, permanently implanted left ventricular assist devices are gaining in prominence.

Cell transplantation for treating cardiac disease represents one intriguing approach for developing new therapeutic strategies for the treatment of end-stage cardiac disease. Additionally, there is a significant number of patients who are not optimal candidates for standard forms of therapy including surgical revascularization and interventional procedures due to extent and/or anatomy of disease. Promotion of new vessel growth by cell therapy may offer promising approaches for the treatment of these non-option (non-operable) patients. Finally cell transplantation may have a role in vascular tissue engineering: from tissue engineered small vessel grafts to vascular reconstruction and new vessel formation.

Evidence from a number of preclinical and clinical studies suggests that myocardial function is improved after cell transplantation. In this handbook, updated experimental studies and first clinical trials will explore the use of a number of different cell types including embryonic stem cells, cardiac myocytes, fetal and neonatal cardiomyocytes, skeletal myoblasts, fibroblast stem cells, endothelial, progenitor endothelial cells, and smooth muscle cells to repair damaged myocardium and/or coronary vessels and to induce angiogenesis. These studies showed that cell transplantation was associated with smaller infarcts, prevented ventricular dilatation and even improved the ventricular systolic function in some of these studies.

This handbook seeks to strike a balance between the basic and clinical science of cell transplantation and is interdisciplinary in approach. It brings together pioneers in this field including vascular biologists, molecular cardiologists, physiologists, cardiothoracic surgeons, interventional cardiologists and others.

ACKNOWLEDGMENTS

The editors are much indebted to the contributing authors. They are each leading authorities in their fields and have made extraordinary efforts in synchronizing basic science and clinical data to provide information on this topic. The editors would also like to thank Mr. Alan Burgess, our Commissioning Editor at Martin Dunitz, Ltd. for his patience, encouragement and guidance, and lastly, Ms. Cathy Kennedy, Project Editor at Lenox Hill Heart & Vascular Institute who deserves special recognition for her expert coordination, management and assistance in putting this book together.

Nicholas Kipshidze and Patrick W Serruys

1. NOVEL APPROACHES TO CARDIAC REGENERATION – THE (PRECLINICAL) REALITY OF MYOBLAST TRANSPLANTATION

Doris A Taylor and Ewout J van den Bos

Introduction

As patients survive acute myocardial infarction (MI), many are progressing to heart failure, which subsequently has become the most prevalent cardiovascular disease in this century. This high prevalence is due in large part to the inability of the heart to repair damaged or dying cardiomyocytes. At present, the only definitive treatment option for end-stage heart failure is heart transplantation, although 'destination therapies' such as permanently implanted left ventricular assist devices are gaining in prominence.

An exciting new treatment modality to combat or reverse the underlying loss of cells and the accompanying functional decline is transplantation of myogenic cells into the infarct scar.[1-4] The premise of cell-based cardiac repair is that immature or undifferentiated cells will mature in the cardiac microenvironment, adapt their phenotype to the conditions present in the damaged area of the heart, engraft, take over the role of lost cardiomyocytes and restore the loss in functional tissue. Yet, this requires several things: first, that immature or undifferentiated cells can survive transplantation into ischemic or infarcted tissue; next, that surviving cells can differentiate appropriately in this scarred environment; and finally, that the resulting cells can electromechanically integrate into the beating heart and contribute to function. Accomplishing this is the current goal of most investigators.

Cell transplantation began as an active area of investigation with the introduction of exogenous myoblasts into the canine heart.[1] Some time later, our group reported the first functional repair of myocardium.[2] Since that time, a number of cell types, ranging from embryonic stem cells[5] and fetal cardiomyocytes[6] to adult bone marrow-derived progenitors[7] have been proposed for cardiac repair. Although many cell types have been proposed for repair of injured or damaged heart, myoblasts remain the most well studied. Thus we will discuss the lessons learned, the progress to date and the outstanding questions of myoblast transplantation as a template for all cell-based cardiac repair.

1

Several factors must be considered in choosing a cell for cardiac repair. These include ease of obtaining the cells, risk of cell rejection, safety and compatibility of the cells after transplantation and functional effectiveness. The risk of rejection is primarily dependent upon whether the cells are autologous or allogeneic. Although allogeneic cells offer advantages to commercial entities (batch release, off-the-shelf capability), autologous cells have benefits for patients that include no need for immunosuppression and no risk of graft-versus-host disease. Ease of obtaining the large number of cells needed to improve cardiac function is important in determining the requirement for the size of the initial donor tissue, be it muscle, marrow or blood. Muscle offers the advantage that a large number of autologous myoblasts can be obtained via a relatively small biopsy. Safety and compatibility are also of concern, as is efficacy. Again, myoblasts are the only progenitor cells in the human body that normally develop a striated muscle contractile apparatus, which makes them more likely to restore contractile function in the damaged fibrous region of the heart.

The goal of cellular cardiomyoplasty is to find a cell that responds appropriately to the surrounding cardiomyocytes and non-cardiomyocyte cells to perform cardiac work. Clearly, because of the complexity of end-stage heart failure, this is not a trivial task. Instead, it is one that is likely to depend critically on cell phenotype or differentiation state, dosage, delivery method, timing post-injury and comorbidities. We will examine and discuss the impact of these factors.

Myoblast physiology in skeletal and cardiac muscle

In attempts to regenerate functional myocardium, the most widely used cells to date are skeletal muscle-derived progenitor cells or myoblasts. These cells are located under the basal lamina of muscle fibers and are the undifferentiated precursors of myotubes that comprise and repair the adult muscle.[8] Myoblasts were initially chosen for cardiac repair by our group because: (1) they normally develop into striated muscle; (2) as they mature, myoblasts express many of the same genes expressed in cardiomyocytes; (3) their prominence in skeletal muscle makes myoblasts relatively easy to obtain; (4) myoblasts are more resistant to ischemia than cardiomyocytes and thus more likely to survive in an infarct; and (5) muscle progenitors, by their very nature, respond to injury by proliferating and forming muscle fibers.

Developmentally, myoblasts arise from somites and first appear as a distinct myoblast cell type well before birth. Even though different types of skeletal muscle exist, the populations of myoblasts from each muscle appear very similar and seem able to differentiate into multiple muscle fiber types, regardless of their origin. In the adult muscle under normal conditions, myoblasts are in a quiescent state. They become activated and start proliferating after growth stimuli or tissue injury and are able to totally regenerate damaged muscle. In both development and repair, myonuclear accretion is accomplished by mitotic divisions of myoblasts throughout the growth period and fusion of the daughter cells into multinucleated myotubes. This process is readily reproduced in vitro (Figure 1.1).

Until recently, there was no evidence for multilineage plasticity in adult muscle; instead, myoblasts were thought to differentiate exclusively to the muscle phenotype. Although myoblasts primarily contribute to peripheral muscle repair, cells isolated from muscle have been more recently shown to possess multilineage potential. In the literature, these cells are termed muscle-derived stem cells (MDSCs). It is generally agreed that stem cells share the property of plasticity, are capable of self-renewal and have multilineage potential. Recent reports have suggested that MDSCs can commit to multiple lineages and differentiate into non-muscle cells, given the right environmental clues or when certain inducers of differentiation are present in vitro.[9] For example, sca-1[pos] and CD45[neg] progenitor cells in the muscle compartment were shown to repopulate the hematopoietic system.[10,11] Other studies have shown that muscle-derived progenitor cells can give rise to cells of the adipogenic lineage[12] and to neuronal cells.[13]

Beyond MDSCs, two distinct groups of myoblasts have been discerned.

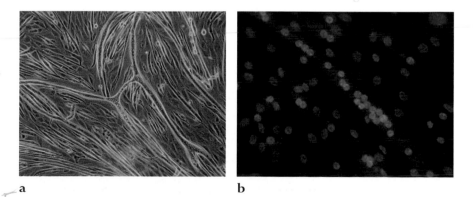

a   b

Figure 1.1 *(a) Light micrograph of primary mouse myoblasts after 6 days of exposure to differentiation conditions. This picture depicts both single mononuclear cells and multinucleated myotubes generated by the fusion of single cells. (b) The same cells after staining with the DNA marker diamidino-phenylindole (DAPI). Multiple nuclei are visible within a single myotube.*

3

The first group, a majority of myoblasts, is rapidly dividing, involved in muscle regeneration and muscle growth and readily available for incorporation into myotubes and muscle. A small subset of more slowly dividing cells potentially comprises a highly proliferative reserve population, which is involved in the generation of the former population and in self-renewal. This group of cells remains undifferentiated in vitro under conditions that normally induce terminal myoblast differentiation.[14]

These studies raise the exciting possibility that myoblasts or other muscle-derived cells are progenitors with multilineage potential that are suitable for multi-tissue repair, including that of myocardium. However, several cautions should be raised. It is possible that the lineage plasticity described here could be accounted for by contaminating circulating bone marrow-derived stem cells. Equally, it is not clear whether the differences between myoblast populations represent two distinct subpopulations of cells or whether they reflect stochastic differences within one population. Finally, the apparent conversion of myoblasts or muscle-derived progenitors into different lineages could represent transdifferentiation or even fusion between different cell types as much as it proves the plastic characteristics of a true stem cell. Clearly, this field requires extensive future research to resolve these issues.

Practical considerations of myoblast transplantation

Several practical considerations arise when discussing myoblast transplantation. They include harvesting and processing of a muscle biopsy, preparation and delivery of the resulting cells and status and effect of the cells in vivo. Typically, myoblasts are isolated from a peripheral skeletal muscle biopsy of a few grams, usually from a muscle rich in slow-twitch fibers. Preclinically, tibialis anterior, extensor digitorum longus or soleus is used, whereas vastus lateralis is used clinically. The muscle is then minced or enzymatically dissociated, and the resulting cells are expanded in vitro, typically for 2 weeks, to grow a sufficient number of cells necessary for transplantation.

The transplantation method is relatively easy; cells are harvested, resuspended in saline or medium and injected with a small needle into multiple locations within the infarct area under direct vision via thoracotomy, median sternotomy or thoracoscopic approach. Successful delivery and engraftment of cells has been noted both after intramural injection and after intracoronary injection, confirming the idea that myoblasts can adhere to and cross the vascular endothelium.[15] A possible factor that mediates translocation of the myoblasts is the transient ischemia that results from capillary plugging. Alternatively, cells can be delivered percutaneously via endoventricular

4

injection catheters. Especially in severely ill patients, this non-surgical approach is attractive. In a porcine model of MI, successful endoventricular delivery of myoblasts has been reported.[16] One potential limitation of catheter-based approaches, besides the obvious lack of visualization, is the limited angle of cell delivery. Use of catheter-based techniques implies delivery of cells perpendicular to the surface of the left ventricle, which limits the delivery of cells to several small pockets within an infarct. In contrast, with the surgical approaches used to date, injections were made parallel to the surface of the heart, along a long needle track, traversing the whole infarct area. This could obviously yield different results. A method being investigated to provide catheter-based parallel delivery includes use of a transvascular injection catheter, through which cells can be injected directly into the myocardium via access obtained through the coronary sinus.

The timing of the injection may be critical. Preclinically, most, if not all, data have been gathered in relatively early injury, several weeks to months post-injury. Clinically, the scenario may ultimately be very different. Regardless of the injury, cell injections usually occur 2 or 3 weeks after the biopsy, because of the time needed to obtain a sufficient cell number. Our data show that injecting cells directly after injury does not result in sufficient engraftment to improve function. This is probably due to the inflammatory process in the infarct area. As cell therapy continues to be considered for end-stage disease, longer time periods between injury and transplantation should be investigated and adequately compared to determine the ideal time for injection.

Outcomes

The initial focus of cell transplantation is efficient engraftment and differentiation of cells in infarcted or myopathic myocardium. Histologic data suggest that the events taking place after cell injection into the infarct and peri-infarct regions of the myocardium parallel the normal muscle developmental pathway for myoblasts. That is, injected myoblasts appear to have several fates. Either they remain as undifferentiated proliferating cells or they exit the proliferation state and remain as single cells or start forming myotubes. In the ideal case, they are capable of regenerating almost transmurally the infarcted area with a decrease in fibrosis and wall thinning (Figure 1.2).[2] More often though, small islands of cells are found within the scar. As they engraft, cells are expected to impact on remodeling or contractility.

One striking finding is that on histologic examination a day after injection,

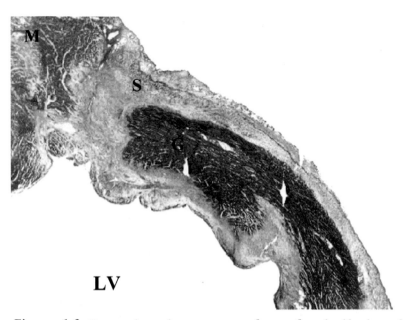

Figure 1.2 *Hematoxylin and eosin staining of cryo-infarcted rabbit heart 3 weeks after transplantation of autologous skeletal muscle cells shows engrafted striated muscle cells in elongated fiber-type orientations (G) which replace approximately 75% of the infarcted scar (S). Healthy myocardium is visible on the left (M). LV represents the left ventricular cavity. Note that the transplanted cells comprising undifferentiated cells and differentiated striated muscle remain surrounded by scar. (With permission, Nature Medicine.)*

generally, a lower number of cells is found than would be expected based on the number of injected cells. This implies that a significant number of myoblasts either do not survive the first 24 h after injection or that cell retention in the infarct region is very low. Studies of 'classic' myoblast transfer therapy, performed in Duchenne muscular dystrophy (DMD) patients, showed that cell death can be as high as 90% during the first hour after injection.[17] However, the cells used for DMD patients are all allogeneic, so results cannot be directly translated to autologous transplantation.

Once cells engraft and differentiate, some express muscle markers. For example, expression of both the fast-twitch as well as the more cardiac-compatible slow-twitch myosin heavy chain is observed in the engrafted muscle after several weeks, the latter suggesting that in the cardiac milieu the developmental program of the implanted cells was altered to induce contractile proteins more capable of cardiac workload.[18]

The location of cells varies. With direct injection into the center of the infarct area, the regenerated tissue is mostly central and surrounded by dense scar tissue, probably because the injected cells have difficulties migrating through the infarct area. This essentially prevents the cells from making contact with healthy cardiomyocytes, and makes electrical integration very remote. Since the scar tissue does not transfer electrical conduction through the heart muscle, action potential propagation into the grafted area is unlikely.

A potential disadavantage of myoblasts for cardiac regencration is that they are too committed to skeletal muscle and cannot adapt sufficiently to perform cardiac workload and respond to cardiac rhythmicity. In the myocardium, action potentials are propagated via intercellular gap junctions, whereas in skeletal muscle each myofibril is activated by its own motor unit, and few gap junctions are present.[19] This gives rise to the questions of whether myoblasts are indeed capable of synchronous contraction with the myocardium and whether or not arrhythmicity might be induced by their differing electrical properties. However, contractility does not necessarily require connections between cells, since a simple stretch may initiate contraction. In all reports studying direct injection of myoblasts into the heart, no expression of the gap junction marker connexin 43 was observed between graft and host myocardium. However, when myoblasts were delivered via the coronary circulation, connexin 43 was immunolocalized to some sites of donor and host cell contact, implying that this method conserves the possibility of myoblasts indeed forming gap junctions even after 6 months.[20]

Over the last few years, several investigators have reported the possible transdifferentiation of myoblasts into cardiac muscle after grafting; the main criterion used was that the transplanted cells showed a distinct cardiac-like morphology and formed junctions with the surrounding myocardium.[21,22] Strictly speaking, transdifferentiation describes the process of conversion of a committed cell into another cell type with a distinct phenotype. Proof of myoblast transdifferentiation requires evidence that the cells studied are derived from the transplanted cells and convert into a cardiac phenotype based on expression of molecular markers. Second, it should be ruled out that the cardiac-like cell studied arose from any uncommitted progenitor cell type(s) that contaminated the transplanted cell population. All reports of transdifferentiation have failed to do this thus far. Murry et al showed that there was no expression of cardiac-specific markers, such as cardiac troponin I, or α-MHC, in engrafted myoblasts.[18]

To demonstrate transdifferentiation also requires ruling out fusion between transplanted cells and cardiomyocytes. Although recent reports suggest that there may be a significant amount of fusion between stem cells and more committed cell types,[23] the ability of myoblasts to fuse with cardiomyocytes has not been rigorously investigated. Although it is unlikely that heterokaryons are formed between cardiac and skeletal muscle, it is possible and could account for some of the reports of transdifferentiation.

Taken together, these data suggest that myoblast therapy in the injured heart is feasible, but that, for it to succeed, engraftment potential has to be increased, which could possibly be accomplished by altering dose, concentration or timing of delivery.

As discussed below, the functional improvement of cell therapy is strongly correlated with the number of injected cells. It might be possible, however, that there is a critical limit to this.

Functional improvement

The ultimate goal of cell therapy is functional improvement in infarcted myocardium. Accomplishing this seems fairly straightforward, although the mechanisms remain obscure. In all animal models of MI studied, myoblast transplantation has been shown to be able to improve cardiac function, irrespective of the method used for measuring function. This is seen in both in vivo and in vitro studies, with increased ejection fractions and increased dP/dt,[24,25] as well as an increase in regional function as measured by sonomicrometry[2] or color kinesis echocardiography.[3] This increase in function is accompanied by a decrease in cavity dilatation. The beneficial effect of transplantation is more marked in animals with low ejection fractions[24] and is highly correlated with the number of injected cells.[26] It has long been questioned whether the improvement in myocardial performance is a direct effect of synchronous contraction of the graft with the surrounding cardiomyocytes or simply an effect on remodeling. In vitro data show that isolated strips of infarct area containing transplanted cells can be electrically stimulated to contract simultaneously with beating cardiomyocytes.[4,27] Until now, the only in vivo data that support synchronous contraction of the transplanted cells are the data obtained by sonomicrometry[2] and color kinesis echocardiography.[3,28] However, so far no study has shown improved wall thickening at the infarct site after myoblast transplantation. Regional stroke work analysis by sonomicrometry showed a significant increase in systolic functioning. Furthermore, this study showed that diastolic properties of the infarct improved as well, with a reduction in diastolic creep (Figure 1.3).[29] This suggests that implanting cells not only contributes to increased contractility but that it also changes the compliance of the scar area. These data are further supported by the fact that, after the implantation of only

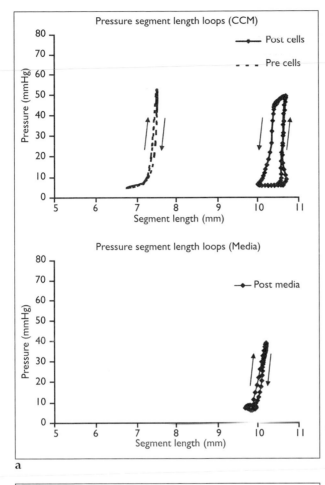

a

Figure 1.3 Pressure *segment loops generated by sonomicrometry and micromanometry 3 weeks after myoblast transplantation into a rabbit cryo-infarct.* (a) *Improved regional cardiac function after myoblast transplantation, as evidenced by reversal of the clockwise negative loop direction before cell transplantation to a counterclockwise positive one 3 weeks after cells.* (b) *In contrast, this shows improved strain or compliance within the infarct area after injection of either myoblasts or fibroblasts more like that seen in control normal hearts. Compliance is derived from the exponential relationship between left ventricular pressure and strain.*

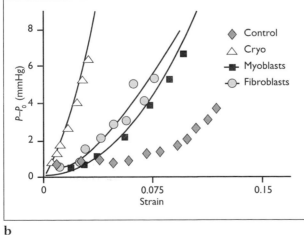

b

fibroblasts, contractility did not improve, but instead declined, even though diastolic function was improved.[30]

The effect of myoblast transplantation on contraction remains controversial. It is possible, for example, that the beneficial effect of transplantation results from a passive effect of increased wall thickness with a resultant decrease in wall stress and functional improval, limiting infarct size. Furthermore, it could be that the decrease in cavity dilatation prevents a decrease in pump function. It has also been suggested that secretion of angiogenic or growth factors by the transplanted cells may improve systolic functioning of the heart, as supported by an increase in global function after heart transplantation.

Suzuki et al showed that good functional results can also be obtained by directly injecting muscle fibrils into the heart.[31] However, injection of minced muscle did not have any beneficial effect.[32]

Apart from the study mentioned above, which compared the functional effects of myoblasts and fibroblasts,[30] few studies have been undertaken to date to directly compare the effects of different cell types on functional improvement. One could argue that the best cell type for improving contractility in the infarcted region without any side-effects would be the most suitable one for cell transplantation into the heart. It might seem that cardiomyocytes would be the ideal cell type. However, cardiomyocytes do not appear to be able to engraft sufficiently to alter function and they are much less ischemia resistant. Myoblasts and bone marrow-derived cells are the next obvious choices. It appears that bone marrow-derived stem cells are capable of differentiation into the cardiac phenotype. Both populations of bone marrow-derived enriched hematopoietic cells, the so-called 'side-population', as well as mesenchymal cells were shown to be able to express cardiac lineage markers after transplantation into the heart.[33,34] However, the data further suggest, as shown by Wang et al, that after injection, bone marrow-derived cells will also develop characteristics of the scar, such as a fibroblast phenotype, which is potentially deleterious for functional improvement.

Questions to be answered

Although myoblast transplantation into the heart has been proven to be feasible in animal models of cardiovascular disease, many questions remain to be answered. These include, but are not limited to, questions of the best cell type, best timing and site of injection, optimal dose and best delivery method. For optimization of myoblast transplantation into the heart, the criteria that are limiting the effectiveness of myoblast engraftment should be clearly defined. The relationship between number of injected cells and engraftment remains unclear, as does the optimal time of cell delivery after infarction. Defining what limits both cell engraftment and function is also critical. Improvement of function is strongly correlated with the number of injected cells. Improving cell survival, especially during the first 24h after injection, could then be a very valuable tool. One of the solutions would be to make the cells more resistant to hypoxic and low-serum conditions, or to select the proportion of myoblasts that are genetically protected from such an environment. Function could be improved by optimizing the injection technique and location of the injection sites. Further exploration of clinical-based catheter-based techniques could move myoblast transplantation further in the direction of clinical practice.

Most of the problems encountered are complicated by the heterogeneity of cardiovascular disease; for example, the criteria for reproducible engraftment of large numbers of cells may be very different in the early postmyocardial infarction state versus the end-stage cardiac dysfunction in the failing and fully remodeled left ventricle. The optimal timing of the myoblast injection should therefore be investigated to determine when to inject the cells and whether myoblast injection is also favorable in the end-stage failing heart and is still beneficial even years after injection.

The improvement of electromechanical integration of the grafted cells is the next preclinical frontier. A potential threat for heart function is the arrhythmic potential of the injected cells. The injected cells are mostly isolated by scar tissue from the surrounding myocardium this is partly caused by reactive scar formation at the needle injection site. The injected cells could in this way create re-entry circuits and cause dysrhythmicity, such as ventricular tachycardia or fibrillation. This could be an explanation for the modest rate of sudden death in the animal models studied. For a good evaluation of the degree of dysrhythmicity, continuous Holter monitoring should be done, at least for several days after injection. No such study has been done in a model of myoblast transplantation.

Several potential disadvantageous side-effects need to be considered, and these must be resolved before moving the technique into clinical practice. For example, the transplantation procedure might affect organs other than the heart. Until now, no good study has been done on the biodistribution of myoblasts throughout the body after injection and the potential hazardous side-effects of engraftment in organs other than the heart.

Furthermore, the question remains to be answered of whether methods to recruit endogenous progenitor cells can give similar results to cell transplantation. More recently, endogenous circulating and bone marrow-derived cells have been found to contribute to regeneration of cardiomyocytes, as well as to endothelial and smooth muscle cells, by homing to the infarct area;[35,36] however, the amount of self-induced repair seems to be very low and incapable of meeting the functional demand post-infarct.

Carefully evaluating the benefits and side-effects provides an opportunity to define a new era in the treatment of cardiovascular disease. The current preclinical data raise the hope that myoblast transplantation will become a useful treatment for severe ischemic heart failure. Future research should be aimed at finding the best cell type, optimizing dose, timing and engraftment and designing injury-specific repair. In the clinic, designing a trial that evaluates the safety and efficacy of myoblast transplantation is crucial; doing it improperly could relegate the field to failure before its potential is realized.

References

1. Marelli D, Desrosiers C, El-Alfy M et al. Cell transplantation for myocardial repair: an experimental approach. Cell Transplant 1992; 1: 383–90.

2. Taylor DA, Atkins BZ, Hungspreugs P et al. Regenerating functional myocardium: improved performance after skeletal muscle myoblast transplantation. Nat Med 1998; 4: 929–33.

3. Ghostine S, Carrion C, Souza LC et al. Long-term efficacy of myoblast transplantation on regional structure and function after myocardial infarction. Circulation 2002; 106: I-131–6.

4. Murry CE, Wiseman RW, Schwartz SM, Hauschka SD. Skeletal myoblast transplantation for repair of myocardial necrosis. J Clin Invest 1996; 98: 2512–23.

5. Boheler KR, Czyz J, Tweedie D et al. Differentiation of pluripotent embryonic stem cells into cardiomyocytes. Circ Res 2002; 91: 189–201.

6. Reinecke H, Zhang M, Bartosek T, Murry CE. Survival, integration, and differentiation of cardiomyocyte grafts: a study in normal and injured rat hearts. Circulation 1999; 100: 193–202.

7. Strauer BE, Brehm M, Zeus T et al. Repair of infarcted myocardium by autologous intracoronary mononuclear bone marrow cell transplantation in humans. Circulation 2002; 106: 1913–18.

8. Mauro A. Satellite cells of skeletal muscle fibers. J Biophys Biochem Cytol 1961; 9: 493–7.

9. Zammit PS, Beauchamp JR. The skeletal muscle satellite cell: stem cell or son of stem cell? Differentiation 2001; 68: 193–204.

10. Grounds MA, White JD, Rosenthal N, Bogoyevitch MA. The role of stem cells in skeletal and cardiac muscle repair. J Histochem Cytochem 2002; 50: 589–610.

11. Howell JC, Yoder MC, Srour EF. Hematopoietic potential of murine skeletal muscle-derived CD45(-)Sca-1(+)c-kit(-) cells. Exp Hematol 2002; 30: 915–24.

12. Asakura A, Seale P, Girgis-Gabardo A, Rudnicki MA. Myogenic specification of side population cells in skeletal muscle. J Cell Biol 2002; 159: 123–34.

13. Csete M, Walikonis J, Slawny N et al. Oxygen-mediated regulation of skeletal muscle satellite cell proliferation and adipogenesis in culture. J Cell Physiol 2001; 189: 189–96.

14. Romero-Ramos M, Vourc'h P, Young HE et al. Neuronal differentiation of stem cells isolated from adult muscle. J Neurosci Res 2002; 69: 894–907.

15. Taylor DA, Silvestry SC, Bishop SP et al. Delivery of primary autologous skeletal myoblasts into the rabbit heart by coronary infusion: a potential approach to myocardial repair. Proc Assoc Am Physicians 1996; 109: 245–53.

16. Dib N, Diethrich EB, Campbell A et al. Endoventricular transplantation of allogenic skeletal myoblasts in a porcine model of myocardial infarction. J Endovasc Ther 2002; 9: 313–19.

17. Gussoni E, Blau HM, Kunkel LM. The fate of individual myoblasts after transplantation into muscles of DMD patients. Nat Med 1997; 3: 970–7.

18. Reinecke H, Poppa V, Murry CE. Skeletal muscle stem cells do not transdifferentiate into cardiomyocytes after cardiac grafting. J Mol Cell Cardiol 2002; 34: 241–9.

19. Balogh S, Naus CCG, Merrifield PA. Expression of gap junctions in cultured rat L6 cells during myogenesis. Dev Biol 1993; 155: 351–60.

20. Robinson SW, Cho PC, Levitsky HI et al. Arterial delivery of genetically labeled skeletal myoblasts to the murine heart: long-term survival and phenotypic modification of implanted myoblasts. Cell Transplant 1996; 5: 77–91.

21. Chiu RC, Zibaitis A, Kao RL. Cellular cardiomyoplasty: myocardial regeneration with satellite cell implantation. Ann Thorac Surg 1995; 60: 12–18.

22. Atkins BZ, Lewis CW, Kraus WE et al. Intracardiac transplantation of skeletal myoblasts yields two populations of striated cells in situ. Ann Thorac Surg 1999; 67: 124–9.

23. Terada N, Hamazaki T, Oka M et al. Bone marrow cells adopt the phenotype of other cells by spontaneous cell fusion. Nature 2002; 416: 485–7.

24. Pouzet B, Vilquin JT, Hagege AA et al. Factors affecting functional outcome after autologous skeletal myoblast transplantation. Ann Thorac Surg 2001; 71: 844–50.

25. Jain M, DerSimonian H, Brenner DA et al. Cell therapy attenuates deleterious ventricular remodeling and improves cardiac performance after myocardial infarction. Circulation 2001; 103: 1920–7.

26. Ellis MJ, Emani SM, Colgrove SL et al. Cell dosage is critical for improved contractility following cellular cardiomyoplasty. Circulation 2001; 104: II-336.

27. Reinecke H, MacDonald GH, Hauschka SD, Murry CE. Electromechanical coupling between skeletal and cardiac muscle, implications for infarct repair. J Cell Biol 2000; 149: 731–40.

28. Rajnoch C, Chachques JC, Berrebi A et al. Cellular therapy reverses myocardial dysfunction. J Thorac Cardiovasc Surg 2001; 121: 871–8.

29. Atkins BZ, Hueman MT, Meuchel JM et al. Myogenic cell transplantation improves in vivo regional performance in infarcted rabbit myocardium. J Heart Lung Transplant 1999; 18: 1173–80.

30. Hutcheson KA, Atkins BZ, Hueman MT et al. Comparison of benefits on myocardial performance of cellular cardiomyoplasty with skeletal myoblasts and fibroblasts. Cell Transplant 2000; 9: 359–68.

31. Suzuki K, Murtuza B, Heslop L et al. Single fibers of skeletal muscle as a novel graft for cell transplantation to the heart. J Thorac Cardiovasc Surg 2002; 123: 984–92.

32. Pouzet B, Vilquin JT, Hagege AA et al. Intramyocardial transplantation of autologous myoblasts: can tissue processing be optimized? Circulation 2000; 102: III-210–15.

33. Orlic D, Kajstura J, Chimenti S et al. Bone marrow cells regenerate infarcted myocardium. Nature 2001; 410: 701–5.

34. Jackson KA, Majka SM, Wang H et al. Regeneration of ischemic cardiac muscle and vascular endothelium by adult stem cells. J Clin Invest 2001; 107: 1395–402.

35. Quaini F, Urbanek K, Beltrami AP et al. Chimerism of the transplanted heart. N Engl J Med 2002; 346: 5–15.

36. Laflamme MA, Myerson D, Saffitz JE, Murry CE. Evidence for cardiomyocyte repopulation by extracardiac progenitors in transplanted human hearts. Circ Res 2002; 90: 634–40.

2. CELLULAR CARDIOMYOPLASTY: THE BIOLOGY AND CLINICAL IMPORTANCE OF MILIEU-DEPENDENT DIFFERENTIATION

Ray C-J Chiu and Jih-Shiuan Wang

Introduction

Cellular cardiomyoplasty

In a paper published in 1995 entitled 'Cellular cardiomyoplasty: myocardial regeneration with satellite cell implantation',[1] we suggested the term 'cellular cardiomyoplasty' to indicate a new therapeutic approach of using cells to repair damaged myocardium. Since then, in addition to the satellite cells derived from the skeletal muscle, many other stem cells and progenitor cells have been studied as donor cells to regenerate myocardial tissue. Notable among them are embryonic stem cells,[2] adult stem cells, particularly those derived from the bone marrow,[3] myoblasts[4] and pro-endothelial cells. In this chapter, we will focus on studies that have used the marrow stromal cells (MSCs) as the donor cells, for a number of reasons. First, autologous MSCs can be readily obtained from the patient, which avoids the need for immunosuppression and bypasses the ethical controversies encounted with the use of embryonic stem cells. Second, unlike the myoblasts and other progenitor cells, which undergo lineage-determined differentiation, the MSCs contain multipotent cells. They have been shown to differentiate into many phenotypes, including those of cardiomyocytes and endothelial cells, both of crucial importance in myocardial repair.

Milieu-dependent differentiation

One of the most intriguing questions in stem cell therapy is how pluripotent and multipotent cells determine which phenotype to express when they differentiate. Understanding the signaling mechanism for this is not only of profound biological interest but is also clinically relevant and important in determining how to prepare these cells and how to administer them to the patients. In general, the progenitor cells undergo lineage-dependent differentiation, so that, regardless of the environment, they will move along a predetermined pathway, such that a myoblast will become a myocyte, and a pro-endothelial cell will form an endothelial cell. The phenomenon of transdifferentiation occurs when an already differentiated mature cell transforms into a mature cell of another phenotype. Although the mechanism for such transformation is unknown, it is likely that environmental factors play important roles.

In this chapter, we will explore the hypothesis that the adult stem cells, such as those derived from the marrow stroma, will choose to express a specific phenotype as the result of a process known as milieu-dependent differentiation,[5] which has also been called in situ differentiation. This hypothesis posits that the differentiation is guided by the microenvironmental signal(s) such that the cells can express a specific phenotype depending on the anatomic topology that determines the nature of the microenvironment. At present, very little is known about the molecular signaling mechanisms for milieu-dependent differentiation. In the following discussion, we will examine two phenomenological observations which appear to offer some clue as to how such differentiation may take place. The first is an in vivo observation that we presented at the Annual Meeting of the American Heart Association in 2000,[6] but the full data have not been published to date. Thus the experiments in which our observations were made will be presented in some detail. The second is an in vitro study reported recently by Tomita et al at the 2002 Annual Meeting of the American Association for Thoracic Surgery,[7] and their paper is still in press at the time of writing. We hope that these complementary observations will generate hypotheses and will help in further exploring the underlying molecular mechanisms. Finally, we will discuss the clinical implications of these observations, which will deal with important considerations in bringing cellular cardiomyoplasty to the clinical arena.

In vivo observations

In this study, isogenic rat marrow stromal cells were isolated and expanded in vitro. After cell labeling, they were implanted into normal recipient hearts. We examined the hypothesis that different microenvironments of the implanted cells within a myocardium can have an impact on their differentiation and phenotype expression. Some of the findings from this study have been reported previously.[3]

Methods

Animals

Male inbred Lewis rats, 200–250 g, were obtained from Charles River Laboratories (Laprairie Co., Quebec, Canada). These isogenic rats were used as donors and recipients to simulate autologous implants clinically.

Isolation and culture of marrow stromal cells

Isolation and primary culture of MSCs were performed according to Caplan's method.[8] The MSCs were isolated from the femoral and tibial bones of donor rats. These cells, in 10 ml of complete medium, were then introduced into tissue culture dishes. Medium was replaced every 3 days and the non-adherent cells discarded. To prevent the MSCs from differentiating or slowing their rate of division, each primary culture was replated (first passaged) to three new plates when the cell density within colonies became 80–90% confluent, approximately 2 weeks after seeding. After the twice-passaged cells became nearly confluent, they were harvested and used for the implantation experiments described below after being labeled with 4',6-diamidino-2-phenylindole (DAPI).

Medium

The cells were cultured in complete medium consisting of Dulbecco's modified Eagle's medium (DMEM) containing selected lots of 10% fetal calf serum and antibiotics (100 U/ml penicillin G, 100 µg/ml streptomycin and 0.25 µg/ml amphotericin B) (Gibco Laboratories) at 37°C in a humidified atmosphere of 5% CO_2.

Marrow stromal cell labeling

Sterile DAPI[9] solution was added to the culture medium at a final concentration of 50 µg/ml on the day of implantation. The dye was allowed to remain in the culture dishes for 30 min. The cells were rinsed six times in Hanks' balanced salt solution (HBSS) to remove all excess, unbound DAPI. MSCs were collected (approximately 1 × 10⁶ cells for one implantation) and resuspended in a minimal volume of serum-free DMEM, ready for implantation into the myocardium.

Implantation of marrow stromal cells

Anesthesia was induced and maintained with isoflurane (MTC Pharmaceuticals). Animals were intubated with an 18-gauge catheter and connected to a Harvard rodent ventilator (Harvard Apparatus Co.) ventilated at 85 breaths/min. The heart was exposed via a 1.5-cm left thoracotomy incision. Under direct vision, the MSC suspension was injected into the left ventricular wall with a 28-gauge needle. The implantation site was marked with 8-0 polypropylene sutures. The wound was closed in layers.

Histology and immunohistochemistry
The rats were sacrificed at intervals 4 days to 12 weeks following the implantation. After the rats had been overdosed with pentobarbital, the hearts were exposed and injected with 100 ml saline (0.9%) through the posterior wall of the left ventricle, avoiding the transplant area, and then perfusion-fixed with 2% paraformaldehyde in phosphate-buffered saline (PBS). The lateral wall of the left ventricle was isolated from the remainder of the heart and cryoembedded after protection with 20% sucrose in PBS or embedded in paraffin. Frozen and paraffin sections 6 μm in thickness were collected across a set of glass slides to ensure that different stains could be carried out on successive sections of tissue cut through the implantation area. One of the sections was mounted without stain, to locate the DAPI-labeled donor cells under a fluorescence microscope. A consecutive section was stained with hematoxylin and eosin. Other sections were selected for immunostaining of sarcomeric myosin heavy chain molecules with MF20 (Courtesy of Donald A. Fischman, MD, Developmental Studies Hybridoma Bank, University of Iowa), connexin 43 with rabbit polyclonal antibody (Zymed) or smooth muscle α-actin (Sigma). Sections were incubated in primary antibodies overnight at 4°C. Detection was carried out with secondary antibodies conjugated to Texas Red for MF20 and fluorescein for anti-connexin 43 and anti-smooth muscle α-actin (Vector). Combined DAPI and Texas Red or DAPI and fluorescein images were made using a simultaneous excitation filter under a reflected light fluorescence microscope (BX-FLA, Olympus). Selected sections were stained in a saturated solution of Sudan Black (Sigma) in 70% ethanol for 15 min for detection of lipid. Digital images, transferred to a computer equipped with Image Pro software (Media Cybernetics, MA, USA), were obtained.

Results
Cultured MSCs were observed with a phase microscope to assess the level of expansion and to verify the morphology at each culture medium change. Most of the hematopoietic stem cells were not adherent to the culture plate and were removed with changes of medium. By the end of the second week, the colonies of adherent cells had expanded in size, with each colony containing several hundred to several thousand cells. Adherent MSCs had similar morphology, most being fibroblastic, with a few adipocytic, polygonal cells (Figure 2.1). This phenotype was retained throughout repeated passages under non-stimulating conditions.

We labeled twice-passaged MSCs with DAPI just before implantation

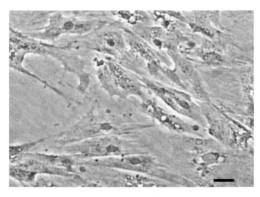

Figure 2.1 *Morphology of rat MSCs in culture. Phase contrast photomicrograph of twice-passaged culture of MSCs just before implantation. Most adherent MSCs are fibroblastic in appearance. Scale bar represents 60 μm.*

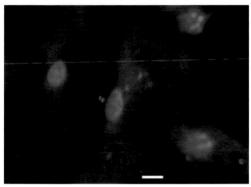

Figure 2.2 *In vitro labeling of MSCs before implantation into the recipient hearts. DAPI epifluorescence (blue fluorescence) of twice-passaged culture of MSCs. Note the intense nuclear and faint cytoplasmic blue fluorescence. Almost 100% of the cultured cells are labeled by DAPI. Scale bar: 15 μm.*

surgery. A DAPI-labeled MSC showed a clear nucleus and faint cytoplasmic blue fluorescence under an epifluorescence microscope (Figure 2.2). One hundred percent of the cultured cells were labeled by DAPI.

All rats with MSC implantation survived to the time scheduled for sacrifice. Gross examination of the specimen did not reveal any structural abnormalities except for several tiny fibrotic changes at needle puncture sites for implantation (marked by 8-0 suture).

Paraffin sections as well as frozen sections (for immunohistochemistry) of the implant sites of the hearts were made to evaluate the morphology and phenotypes of implanted MSCs. DAPI-labeled cells could be identified in specimens at all time points examined.

Four days after implantation, scattered blue fluorescent DAPI-labeled cells were found at the implantation site (Figure 2.3a). Hematoxylin and eosin (H & E) stain of the adjacent consecutive section showed concordance between dense hematoxylin staining and the presence of DAPI epifluorescence (Figure 2.3b). MSC-derived donor cells had an undifferentiated appearance with a large nucleus-to-cytoplasm ratio. Most cells were found within the needle puncture tract, but a few DAPI-labeled cells had infiltrated or migrated away

19

into the host myocardium surrounding the implantation site (Figure 2.3c,d). Four weeks after implantation, DAPI-labeled cells could be seen to remain at the implantation site (Figure 2.4a). The tract created by the trauma of earlier needle puncture for cell injection had undergone a healing process, with fibrous scar formation. H & E stain of the consecutive section (Figure 2.4b) demonstrated that MSC-derived donor cells had started to develop, with increased amounts of cytoplasm. However, they remained unorganized and were surrounded by the fibrous tissue of the needle tract scar. In contrast, adjacent to the implantation site, a few clearly DAPI-labeled cells could be seen to have been incorporated into myofibers with adjacent normal non-

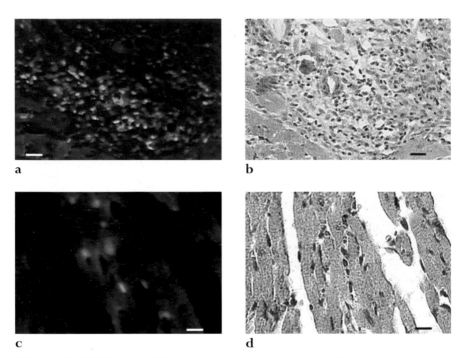

Figure 2.3 *MSCs engrafted into isogenic rat recipient hearts 4 days after implantation. (a,c) DAPI epifluorescence (blue fluorescence) photomicrographs. (b,d) H & E stain. (a) An implantation site of recipient heart. Note scattered DAPI-labeled cells present in this field. (b) Consecutive section to that shown in (a). Note the concordance between dense hematoxylin staining and the presence of DAPI epifluorescence. MSCs have an undifferentiated appearance with a large nucleus-to-cytoplasm ratio. (c) DAPI-labeled cells infiltrated within the host myocardium adjacent to the implantation site. (d) Consecutive section to that shown in (c). Scale bars: 30 μm in (a,b); 15 μm in (c,d).*

labeled host cardiomyocytes (CMs) (Figure 2.4c). The labeled cells had centrally located nuclei and mature morphology indistinguishable from that of the normal CMs, and had aligned themselves with non-labeled host CMs. H & E stain of consecutive sections confirmed that differentiated MSC-derived donor cells had acquired a morphology indistinguishable from that of the surrounding CMs (Figure 2.4d).

The phenotypes of implanted MSCs were further confirmed by immunohistochemistry. To view a section from the implantation site 6 weeks after MSC implantation, we used a simultaneous excitation filter to obtain combined DAPI (blue fluorescence) and Texas Red (red fluorescence) images in

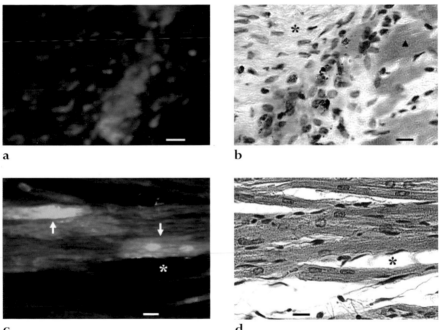

a   b

c   d

Figure 2.4 MSC grafts in isogenic rat recipient hearts 4 weeks after implantation. (a,c) DAPI epifluorescence (blue fluorescence) photomicrographs. (b,d) H & E stain. (a) An implantation site of recipient heart. DAPI-labeled cells gather in a cluster. (b) Consecutive section to that shown in (a). MSC-derived donor cells are unorganized, with increased amounts of cytoplasm. Arrowheads indicate host myocardium, and the asterisk indicates fibrous tissue at the implantation site. (c) Incorporation of DAPI-labeled cells into the host myocardiac fiber adjacent to the implantation site. Arrows indicate DAPI-labeled cells. (d) Consecutive section to that shown in (c). MSC-derived cells have the same structure as the surrounding cardiomyocytes. Asterisks in c & d indicate corresponding tissue clefts in this pair of images. Scale bars: 15 μm.

21

the same microscopic field. A few DAPI-labeled cells within the needle tract scar stained positive for sarcomeric myosin heavy chain molecules (using MF20 and Texas Red conjugated secondary antibody), although no cross-striation was noted. Most other DAPI-labeled cells within the needle scar were negative for this stain. The surrounding host myocardium, as expected, stained strongly positive (Figure 2.5a). However, adjacent to the implantation site, the sarcomeric myosin heavy chain-positive cells (red fluorescence) were seen all over the field (Figure 2.5b), including a few DAPI-labeled (i.e. MSC-derived) cells, all with clear striations, which indicated the presence of organized contractile sarcomeric proteins. Again, DAPI-labeled donor cells aligned in parallel with non-labeled host CMs and were incorporated into host myocardial fibers. To further confirm the integration of implanted MSCs with host CMs, other frozen sections were stained for connexin 43, a major gap junction protein in the intercalated disks, using fluorescein conjugated secondary antibody. Again, by using a simultaneous excitation filter, an image of

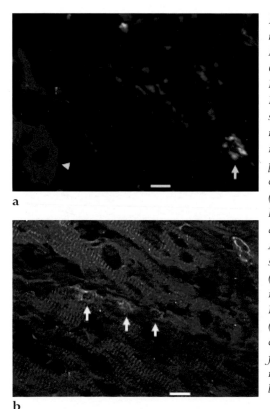

a

b

Figure 2.5 *Expression of sarcomeric myosin heavy chain molecules of MSC-derived donor cells in specimens 6 weeks after implantation. Combined DAPI (blue fluorescence) and Texas Red (red fluorescence) images in the same microscopic field. Anti-sarcomeric myosin heavy chain immunofluorescence using MF20 primary antibody and Texas Red conjugated secondary antibody.*
(a) An implantation site of recipient heart. Some of the DAPI-labeled cells are positively stained (arrow). Arrowhead indicates host myocardium surrounding implantation site.
(b) Myocardium away from implantation site. Arrows indicate DAPI-labeled cell nuclei. DAPI-labeled (MSC-derived) and non-labeled (host cardiomyocytes) cells are both positive for sarcomeric myosin heavy chain molecules with clear striations. Scale bars: 15 μm.

combined DAPI epifluorescence and fluorescein (green fluorescence) was
obtained from a section obtained 6 weeks after implantation (Figure 2.6). The
DAPI-labeled cells within the needle scar were negative for connexin 43.
However, outside of the scarred area, positive green fluorescence representing
connexin 43 was found at the interfaces between DAPI-labeled cells (MSC-
derived) and neighboring non-labeled cells (host CMs), as well as between non-
labeled cells.

We also used smooth muscle α-actin immunohistology to further evaluate
the phenotype expression of MSC-derived cells for their possible participation
in angiogenesis. At 6 weeks after implantation, some blood vessel formation
was found at the implantation site, along with smooth muscle α-actin positive
DAPI-labeled donor cells. This finding indicated the contribution of DAPI-
labeled donor cells to the structure of blood vessel walls (Figure 2.7).

Some MSC-derived donor cells at the implantation site contained many clear
yellow droplets in their cytoplasm which stained positive for Sudan Black,
indicating the presence of lipid. Thus, these cells were adipocytes (Figure 2.8).

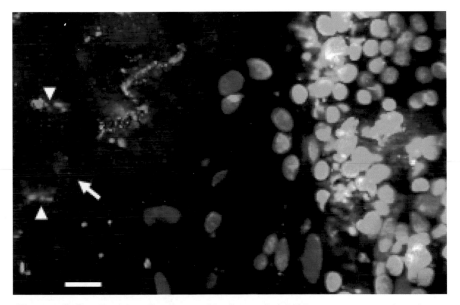

Figure 2.6 *Expression of connexin 43 of engrafted MSCs in a specimen 6 weeks
after implantation. Combined DAPI and fluorescein (green fluorescence) image. Anti-
connexin 43 immunofluorescence using fluorescein-conjugated secondary antibody. All
DAPI-labeled cells within the implantation site scar tissue are negative for connexin
43. Adjacent to the needle tract scar, positive connexin 43 staining (arrowheads) is
found at the interfaces between one DAPI-labeled cell (arrow) and neighboring non-
labeled cells (host cardiomyocytes) and between non-labeled cells. Scale bar: 15 μm.*

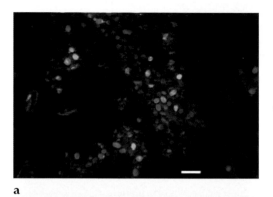

a

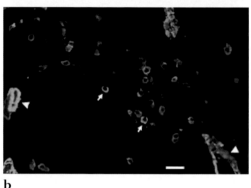

b

Figure 2.7 *Angiogenesis and expression of smooth muscle α-actin in MSC-derived donor cells 6 weeks after implantation. (a) DAPI epifluorescence (blue fluorescence) photomicrograph. (b) Fluorescein epifluorescence (green fluorescence) photomicrograph. (a) An implantation site of recipient heart. Note the scattered DAPI-labeled cells present in this field. (b) The same section as that in (a). Arrows indicate some DAPI-labeled donor cells stained positive for smooth muscle α-actin (green). Arrowheads indicate blood vessels. Scale bars: 15 μm.*

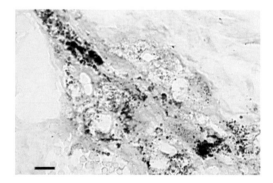

Figure 2.8 *MSC-derived donor cells express the phenotype of an adipocyte. Sudan Black stain of a section of heart 6 weeks after surgery. Clustered cells with black droplets indicate the presence of lipid. Scale bar: 15 μm.*

Discussion

In cellular cardiomyoplasty, one would like to see implanted donor cells perform specific physiologic roles to improve the function of a failing heart based on true regeneration of the myocardium. To achieve this goal, the phenotypes of the new cells and their spatial relationship to the host myocardial supracellular structure are critical for their efficacy. Under controlled in vitro conditions, MSCs have been guided to multiple mesenchymal lineages, including osteocytes, chondrocytes, adipocytes and myocytes.[10] In 1999, Makino et al[11] identified a clone of adherent fibroblast-like cells obtained from bone marrow that, when treated with 5-azacytidine, differentiated in vitro into cells with morphologic features of cardiac muscle cells and expression of a number of cardiac-specific genes. However, in our study described above, we did not pretreat the MSCs prior to their implantation in vivo. This is because we wanted to test our central hypothesis that MSCs can undergo cardiomyogenic differentiation spontaneously within the myocardial microenvironment, demonstrating that the microenvironment can have a major impact on their maturation and phenotype expression: namely, milieu-dependent differentiation. By using this model of needle injection of cells into a normal myocardium, we in effect created two different microenvironments for the implanted MSCs; those remaining within the implantation needle tract and thus surrounded by the fibrous scar tissue, and others which had infiltrated or migrated into the surrounding host myocardium, with close direct contact with native CMs. We were thus able to evaluate the in vivo differentiation of implanted MSCs in two different microenvironments. Our findings are consistent with the hypothesis that these cells obtained signal(s) from adjacent cells to express phenotypes similar to their in situ neighbors.

In contrast to this study, Tomita et al,[12] and more recently Bittira et al[13] from our laboratory, transplanted 5-azacytidine-pretreated MSCs into myocardial scars of rat hearts. Both studies found cardiomyogenic differentiation of these cells within the scar, with expression of cardiac-specific protein, troponin I-c. Thus such treatment in vitro prior to implantation may pre-program the gene expression such that the cells may undergo lineage rather than milieu-dependent differentiation, and no longer respond to microenvironmental signals.

In vitro observations and literature review

Co-culture studies

Recently, Tomita et al[7] used a co-culture system to determine the nature of signal(s) from the microenvironment which could guide the MSCs to differentiate into CMs. In group 1, MSCs derived from transgenic mice expressing green fluorescent protein (GFP) as a cell marker (GFP-BMs) were cultured alone. In group 2, GFP-BMs and CMs from neonatal rats were co-cultured, with the two cell populations being separated by a membrane filter which allowed exchange of macromolecules but not the cell populations. In group 3, GFP-BMs were mixed with CMs and cultured, allowing direct cell-to-cell contacts between these two cell populations. Over 7 days of observation, both group 1 and group 2 MSCs failed to show evidence of CM phenotypic expression. However, in group 3 during the first day of co-culture, myotube-like formations were noted, and on the second day some GFP-BMs started to contract synchronously with CMs, with a chronotropic response to isoproterenol of 80–100 contractions/min. Over the next several days, some of these GFP-positive cells progressively expressed myosin heavy chain, connexin 43 and ANP, as well as the cardiomyocyte-specific troponin I. However, overall, only about 2% of GFP cells appeared to express the cardiomyocytic phenotype after 7 days of co-culture, indicating that perhaps only a small fraction of MSCs are pluripotent. Purification of MSCs using cell surface markers such as CD34 etc. may increase the proportion of such cells. Nevertheless, the results of this interesting report are consistent with the hypothesis, derived from our in vivo observations described above, that cell-to-cell contact may play an important, and perhaps even essential, role in the milieu-dependent differentiation of MSCs, while soluble molecules, including growth factors per se, may not be sufficient to induce such an outcome.

The signaling mechanisms for milieu-dependent differentiation

Why and how the MSCs have different fates in different microenvironments are still not well understood at present. Previous studies had suggested that the MSCs may actually act as cycling stem cells and be involved in the mesengenic process of self-maintenance and repair of different mesenchymal tissues after birth.[14,15] Moreover, the progeny of MSCs express genes in a tissue-specific manner according to their destination.[16] This homing ability and the capacity to acquire the phenotypes of different target tissues suggest a significant role of the microenvironment in the differentiation of these cells. In embryonic stem cell biology, it is speculated that, for differentiation, certain specific molecules such as growth factors, as well as interactions among stem cells, host cells and extracellular matrix, are necessary for this process. Furthermore, these signals need to be presented to the stem cells in a coordinated temporal manner, in order to induce the expression of related developmental genes in sequence, driving them into specific phenotypes.[16,17] Our in vitro and in vivo findings cited above emphasize the important role of direct cellular contacts, at least for the adult stem cells.

Another issue that may affect the differentiation and maturation of implanted MSCs is the identity of MSCs used for such studies. Although some studies indicated that the MSCs isolated by this relatively simple procedure originally described by Caplan were multipotent and able to readily differentiate into osteoblasts, chondroblasts, adipocytes and myoblasts, others suggest that cultured MSCs contain different committed progenitor cells with limited potential for differentiation.[18] Using a 5-azacytidine-treated immortalized MSC model, Makino et al[11] found the percentages of cardiomyogenic differentiation to be distinct among the different subclones. In our study, not all the MSC-derived donor cells at the implantation site appeared to undergo myogenic differentiation, and some MSC-derived donor cells within normal myocardium did not show evidence of cardiomyogenic differentiation during the period of our observation. Furthermore, the differentiated myogenic MSCs at the implantation scar site and within normal myocardium often appeared in clusters, which could suggest that they were derived from a common precursor. Our results also showed that some MSC-derived donor cells changed into adipocytes, and they also appeared in clusters, which suggested again that they could have come from a common precursor. These observations indicate that implanted MSC-derived donor cells may contain subgroups of cells with various committed differentiation potentials. Such observations in vivo are also consistent with the in vitro co-culture study of Tomita et al,[7] which showed that only about 2% of MSCs co-cultured with new CMs expressed a cardiomyocytic phenotype. Nevertheless, the presence of some pluripotent mesenchymal stem cells in adult marrow has recently been confirmed convincingly by Verfaillie's group,[19] who termed such cells MAPCs (multipotent adult progenitor cells). Future advances in the classification and more precise definition of what we call 'stem cells', 'progenitor cells' etc. will be helpful in the further exploration of the signaling mechanisms for their differentiation, and such understanding will have important clinical implications, as discussed below.

Clinical implications

Progenitor and pre-programmed donor cells

Donor cells already committed to lineage-dependent differentiation, which may include progenitor cells and pre-programmed multipotent stem cells, may not be affected by the microenvironment in their ultimate phenotype expression. Thus skeletal myoblasts implanted within scar tissue have been shown to form striated muscle fibers, and MSCs pretreated with 5-azacytidine and implanted into a scar mature into cells expressing CM-specific markers such as troponin I-c. Although functional improvement has been attributed to such therapy, the challenge is to explain how such myofibers surrounded by scar tissue and not integrated into the native myocardial architecture can contribute to improved global cardiac function.[20] Although this approach is now undergoing early clinical trials, the pathophysiologic explanation for their efficacy, if any, remains to be confirmed.

Pluripotent and multipotent stem/progenitor cells

As discussed above, since these cells may undergo in situ, milieu-dependent differentiation, their phenotypic outcome would likely be determined by where and how they are implanted. Thus MSCs implanted into myocardial scar tissue may not readily express the cardiomyocytic phenotype, and instead may produce myofibroblasts and participate in the maturation of the myocardial scar tissue.[21] There is a preliminary observation that contact of MSCs with pre-existing blood vessels may enhance their participation in vasculogenesis (A. Al-Khaldi, personal communication). Thus one of the advantages of using such cells is their capacity to differentiate and replenish cell populations of various phenotypes to regenerate myocardium, which consists of many cell types. The feasibility of concomitant myogenesis and angiogenesis has been reported, and this seems therapeutically desirable.

Cell therapy strategy

Thus it is important not only to select the appropriate donor cells for cell therapy but also to match the cell administration strategy with the donor cells chosen and the therapeutic goals. Thus if the goal is to replace the scar tissue with muscle fibers, direct injection of myoblasts or pre-programmed adult stem cells seems reasonable. It would appear, in contrast, that injecting unaltered MSCs into the scar is undesirable, although maturing and strengthening the scar to prevent scar expansion or rupture may still be beneficial.

However, the strategy described above ignores a number of important capabilities of adult stem cells, including those derived from the marrow. It has been shown that these cells can be mobilized from the bone marrow, traffic through the bloodstream, migrate and home onto the injury site.[22] Thus MSCs injected intravenously following acute coronary artery ligation can appear at the infarct site (unpublished data), later expressing various phenotypes to participate in myogenesis and angiogenesis. The marrow-derived stem cells injected into peri-infarct myocardium have also been shown to migrate into the scar, and express the cardiomyocytic phenotype.[23] One may speculate that these cells received signals from the in vivo microenvironment to differentiate prior to their ultimate migration into the scar. Clearly, further studies are needed to explore such possibilities.

To date, there has been no quantitative study to compare various donor cells and the effect of routes of cell administration/implantation on their efficacy in improving impaired myocardial function. It seems both prudent and desirable to undertake such preclinical studies in order to optimize our strategy prior to large-scale clinical trials for cardiac cell therapy.

References

1.   Chiu RCJ, Zibaitis A, Kao RL. Cellular cardiomyoplasty: myocardial regeneration with satellite cell implantation. Ann Thorac Surg 1995; 60: 12–18.

2.   Leor J, Patterson M, Quinones MJ et al. Transplantation of fetal myocardial tissue into the infarcted myocardium of rat. A potential method for repair of infarcted myocardium? Circulation 1996; 94: II-332–6.

3.   Wang JS, Shum-Tim D, Galipeau J et al. Marrow stromal cells for cellular cardiomyoplasty: feasibility and clinical advantages. J Thorac Cardiovasc Surg 2000; 120: 999–1006.

4.   Taylor DA, Atkins BZ, Hungspreugs P et al. Regenerating functional myocardium: improved performance after skeletal myoblast transplantation. Nat Med 1998; 4: 929–33.

5.   Edelman GM. Topobiology: an introduction to molecular embryology. London: HarperCollins Basic Books, 1988: 18, 21.

6.   Wang J-S, Shum-Tim D, Chedrawy E et al. Marrow stromal cells for cellular cardiomyoplasty: the importance of microenvironment for milieu dependent differentiation. Presented at the 73rd Scientific Session of the American Heart Association in New Orleans, LA, 2000.

7.   Tomita S, Nakatani T, Fukuhara S et al. Bone marrow stromal cells can differentiate into cardiac lineage and contract synchronously with cardiomyocytes by direct cell-to-cell interaction in vitro. Presented at the 82nd Annual Meeting of the American Association for Thoracic Surgery, Washington, DC, 2002.

8.   Wakitani S, Saito T, Caplan AI. Myogenic cells derived from rat bone marrow mesenchymal stem cells exposed to 5-azacytidine. Muscle Nerve 1995; 18: 1417–26.

9.   Kapuscinski J. DAPI: a DNA-specific fluorescent probe. Biotechnic Histochem 1995; 70: 220–33.

10. Pittenger MF, Mackay AM, Beck SC et al. Multilineage potential of adult human mesenchymal stem cells. Science 1999; 284: 143–7.

11. Makino S, Fukuda K, Miyoshi S et al. Cardiomyocytes can be generated from marrow stromal cells in vitro. J Clin Invest 1999; 103: 697–705.

12. Tomita S, Li RK, Weisel RD et al. Autologous transplantation of bone marrow cells improves damaged heart function. Circulation 1999; 100: II-247–56.

13. Bittira B, Kuang JQ, Al-Khaldi A et al. In vitro preprogramming of marrow stromal cells for myocardial regeneration. Ann Thorac Surg (in press).

14. Caplan AI. The mesengenic process. Clin Plastic Surg 1994; 21: 429–35.

15. Pereira RF, Halford KW, O'Hara MD et al. Cultured adherent cells from marrow can serve as long-lasting precursor cells for bone, cartilage, and lung in irradiated mice. Proc Natl Acad Sci USA 1995; 92: 4857–61.

16. Fishman MC, Chien KR. Fashioning the vertebrate heart: earliest embryonic decisions. Development 1997; 124: 2099–117.

17. Smith AG, Henth JK, Donaldson DD et al. Inhibition of pluripotential embryonic stem cell differentiation by purified polypeptides. Nature 1988; 336: 688–90.

18. Conget PA, Minguell JJ. Phenotypical and functional properties of human bone marrow mesenchymal progenitor cells. J Cell Physiol 1999; 181: 67–73.

19. Jiang Y, Jahagirdar BN, Reinhardt RL et al. Pluripotency of mesenchymal stem cells derived from adult marrow. Nature advance online publication, 20 June 2002 (doi:10.1038/nature00870).

20. Chedrawy EG, Wang JS, Nguyen DM et al. Incorporation and integration of implanted myogenic and stem cells into native myocardial fibers: anatomical basis for functional improvement. J Thorac Cardiovasc Surg 2002; 124: 584–90.

21. Wang JS, Shum-Tim D, Chedrawy E, Chiu RCJ. The coronary delivery of marrow stromal cells for myocardial regeneration: pathophysiologic and therapeutic implications. J Thorac Cardiovasc Surg 2001; 122: 699–705.

22. Bittira B, Kuang JQ, Piquer S et al. The pathophysiological roles of bone marrow stromal cells (MSCs) in myocardial infarction. Circulation 2001; 104(suppl): II-523.

23. Orlic D, Kajstura J, Chimentl S et al. Bone marrow cells regenerate infarcted myocardium. Nature 2001; 410: 701–5.

3. Transplantation of Endothelial Progenitor Cells for Therapeutic Neovascularization

Atsuhiko Kawamoto, Douglas W Losordo and Takayuki Asahara

Therapeutic neovascularization by angiogenesis and vasculogenesis mechanisms

It has been well documented that the development of a collateral circulation can attenuate tissue ischemia in peripheral and coronary artery diseases. The classic mechanism of postnatal neovascularization had been considered to be limited to angiogenesis, i.e. proliferation and migration of pre-existing mature endothelial cells (ECs). Therefore, approaches by which one may augment collateral circulation in ischemic diseases in preclinical and clinical studies have been referred to as 'therapeutic angiogenesis'. Gene transfer of angiogenic growth factors, for example, has been reported to attenuate tissue ischemia through stimulation of angiogenesis at sites of neovascularization.[1–4]

Vasculogenesis, which indicates incorporation of circulating endothelial progenitor cells (EPCs) into foci of neovascularization and their proliferation, migration and differentiation into mature ECs, was believed to occur only during embryonic neovascularization, until postnatal vasculogenesis was first reported in 1997.[5] Our laboratory demonstrated that EPCs are mobilized from bone marrow into the circulation in response to tissue ischemia.[6] In addition to the mobilization of intrinsic EPCs in ischemic diseases, we have also reported that intravenous transplantation of exogenous EPCs, isolated as CD34+ cells from adult peripheral blood, results in the incorporation of the EPCs into foci of neovascularization of hindlimb ischemia.[5] These findings encouraged the therapeutic use of EPCs to augment collateral formation in ischemic diseases. On the other hand, administration of vascular endothelial growth factor (VEGF) was shown to increase the number of differentiated EPCs in vitro and to augment corneal neovascularization in vivo.[7] Recently, a pilot clinical study confirmed a similar beneficial effect of VEGF gene transfer in human patients. The number of circulating EPCs increased following VEGF gene transfer in patients with critical limb ischemia.[8] These findings suggest that vasculogenesis may be a key component in what was previously termed therapeutic angiogenesis. Thus, discerning the role of vasculogenesis in the pathophysiology and therapeutic neovascularization of ischemic diseases is now recognized as essential.

Isolation of endothelial progenitor cells for therapeutic neovascularization

Recently, EPCs were successfully freshly isolated from mononuclear cells (MNCs) of peripheral blood, bone marrow and cord blood using KDR, CD34 or AC133 antigen, which are shared by hematopoietic stem cells (HSCs). These cells differentiate into endothelial lineage cells in vitro, and incorporate into sites of neovascularization in vivo. Another method of obtaining EPCs is ex vivo expansion. Culture of the MNCs in EC basal medium allows these cells to proliferate and differentiate into endothelial lineage cells.[9]

The advantage of using cultured EPCs over freshly isolated cells lies in the fact that the number of EPCs obtained by ex vivo expansion (3.5×10^4 from 1 ml whole blood) exceeds the number of CD34$^+$ cells that can be freshly isolated (0.5×10^4/ml blood). The purity and quality of EPCs in a cultured population are also superior to those of freshly isolated CD34$^+$ cells, as HSCs may contaminate freshly isolated CD34$^+$ cells. The vast majority of these ex vivo expanded cells belong to the endothelial lineage, and contamination with other kinds of lineage cell is not significant. A theoretical advantage of the fresh isolation method is safety, which has already been established clinically for HSC transplantation. In contrast, the safety of ex vivo expansion has not yet been established for clinical use.

EPCs obtained by these methods have been utilized for experimental therapeutic neovascularization.

Intravenous transplantation of ex vivo expanded endothelial progenitor cells in hindlimb ischemia

The therapeutic application of EPCs was first attempted in a murine model of hindlimb ischemia.[9] One day following operative excision of one femoral artery, athymic nude mice, in which angiogenesis is characteristically impaired, received an intracardiac injection of 5×10^5 culture-expanded human EPCs (hEPCs). Two control groups were identically injected with either human microvascular ECs (HMVECs) or media from the culture plates employed for hEPC ex vivo expansion. Serial examination of hindlimb perfusion by laser doppler perfusion imaging (LDPI) performed at days 3, 7, 14, 21 and 28 disclosed profound differences in the limb perfusion within 28 days after induction of limb ischemia. At 3 days after the operation, limb perfusion was severely reduced in all three groups. By day 28, the ratio of ischemic/normal bloodflow in hEPC-transplanted mice had improved to 0.69 ± 0.08 versus 0.27 ± 0.08 and 0.34 ± 0.05 in mice receiving HMVECs and culture media respectively ($P < 0.003$). Histologic evaluation of skeletal muscle sections retrieved from the ischemic hindlimbs of mice sacrificed at days 7, 14 and 28 showed that capillary density, an index of neovascularization, was markedly increased in hEPC-transplanted mice.

Enhanced neovascularization in mice transplanted with hEPCs led to important biological consequences. Among mice in which induction of hindlimb ischemia was followed by administration of HMVECs, limb salvage was limited to 8% of animals, while the remainder developed extensive forefoot necrosis (42%), leading in 50% to spontaneous amputation. Likewise, a preserved limb was observed in only 7% of mice treated with culture media, while foot necrosis and/or autoamputation developed in 50% and 43% of mice respectively. In contrast, hEPC transplantation was associated with successful limb salvage in 59% of animals. Foot necrosis was limited to 29%, and only 12% of mice experienced spontaneous limb amputation. The difference in outcome between the hEPC-treated mice and both control groups was statistically significant (for hEPC versus HMVEC, $P = 0.006$; for hEPC versus control media, $P = 0.003$).

Murohara et al[10] reported similar findings, in which human cord blood-derived EPCs also augmented neovascularization in a hindlimb ischemic model of nude rats.

Intravenous transplantation of ex vivo expanded endothelial progenitor cells in myocardial ischemia

Similar outcomes have been demonstrated in rats with myocardial ischemia.[11] In this case, peripheral blood MNCs obtained from healthy human adults were cultured in EPC medium, and harvested 7 days later. Myocardial ischemia was induced by ligation of the left anterior descending coronary artery (LAD) in male Hsd:RH-rnu (athymic nude) rats. In two rats, 10^6 EPCs labeled with dialkylcarbocyanine (DiI) were injected intravenously 3 h after induction of myocardial ischemia. Seven days later, fluorescence-conjugated BS-1 lectin was administered intravenously and the rats were immediately sacrificed. Fluorescence microscopy revealed that transplanted

33

EPCs accumulated specifically in the ischemic area and incorporated into foci of myocardial neovascularization.

To determine the impact on left ventricular (LV) function, five rats (EPC group) were injected intravenously with 10^6 EPCs 3 h after induction of ischemia; five other rats (control group) received culture media. Echocardiography, performed just before and 28 days after induction of ischemia, showed ventricular dimensions that were significantly smaller and fractional shortening (FS) that was significantly greater in the EPC than in the control group by day 28. Regional wall motion was also better preserved in the EPC than in the control group. Following sacrifice on day 28, necropsy examination showed that capillary density was significantly greater in the EPC group than in controls. Moreover, the extent of LV scarring was significantly less in rats receiving EPCs than in controls. Immunohistochemistry revealed capillaries that were positive for human CD31 and UEA-1 lectin in the EPC-treated group. Thus, ex vivo expanded EPCs transplanted into ischemic myocardium incorporate into foci of myocardial neovascularization and have a favorable impact on preservation of LV function (Figure 3.1)

Transplantation of freshly isolated endothelial progenitor cells in small animal models of hindlimb and myocardial ischemia

Schatteman et al[12] performed local injection of freshly isolated human CD34+ MNCs (EPC-enriched fraction) into diabetic mice with hindlimb ischemia, and demonstrated an increase in the restoration of limb flow. Similarly, Kocher et al[13] have attempted intravenous transplantation of human CD34+ MNCs into nude rats with myocardial ischemia. Transplantation of the freshly isolated EPCs enhanced neovascularization in ischemic myocardium and preserved LV function associated with decreased cardiomyocyte apoptosis.

Preclinical studies of endothelial progenitor cell transplantation for therapeutic neovascularization of myocardial ischemia

Although these previous reports indicate a potential therapeutic role for EPCs in ischemic diseases, two major obstacles exist which must be overcome before considering actual clinical applications: dosage and immunologic

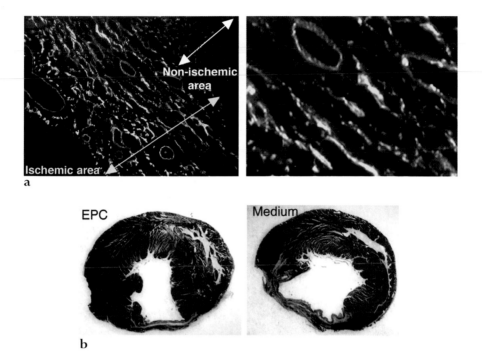

Figure 3.1 (a) Representative findings of fluorescent microscopy in the heart
sections of nude rats with myocardial ischemia. DiI-labeled human cultured EPCs
(red), which were intravenously transplanted 3h after ischemia, specifically homed to
the site of neovascularization and participated in new blood vessel formation with rat
intrinsic ECs which were positive for BS-1 lectin (green). (b) Representative findings of
elastic tissue trichrome staining of the heart samples obtained 4 weeks after ischemia.
The fibrosis area was significantly smaller in the EPC-treated rats than in controls.
Reprinted from Circulation 2001; 103: 634–7 with permission from American Heart
Association.

rejection. In the prior study by our laboratory,[17] 1×10^6 cultured EPCs were
used for each ~200-g rat. Kocher et al[13] have transplanted 1×10^6 freshly
isolated EPCs/100-g rat. On a weight-adjusted basis, this would translate into
$3–6 \times 10^8$ cells for an average-sized human, requiring 8.5–120 liters of
peripheral blood. Although there is a possibility of obtaining sufficient EPCs
from bone marrow in clinical situations, it is far from realistic to isolate
EPCs from peripheral blood using these previous methods. Moreover, these
prior studies employed an immunodeficient rat model to circumvent issues of
cell rejection.

Accordingly, we designed a series of in vivo investigations to address the
limitations of these prior approaches. First, we tested the hypothesis that local

transplantation of EPCs, rather than systemic infusion, would permit a significant reduction in the number of EPCs required. Second, we developed a strategy which relies on freshly isolated, autologous EPCs, thereby permitting evaluation of the therapeutic potential of autologous EPC transplantation. We therefore performed catheter-based transplantation of freshly isolated, autologous EPCs in a swine model of chronic myocardial ischemia.

Chronic myocardial ischemia was induced by ameroid constrictor placement around the left circumflex artery (LCX) of male Yorkshire swine. Four weeks after constrictor placement, 150 ml of peripheral blood was obtained from the ear vein of each pig. The MACS bead selection method for CD31 cell isolation was used to enrich the EPC fraction from peripheral blood MNCs (anti-swine CD34 antibody is not available). $CD31^+$ MNCs were cultured overnight in non-coated plastic plates. To remove macrophages, only non-adhesive $CD31^+$ (NA/$CD31^+$) MNCs were collected as the EPC-enriched fraction. $CD31^-$ MNCs were treated similarly, and non-adhesive $CD31^-$ MNCs (NA/$CD31^-$ MNCs) were obtained as a negative control. On the same day as the EPC isolation, NOGA non-fluoroscopic LV electromechanical mapping was performed to guide injections to foci of myocardial ischemia. The NOGA system (Biosense-Webster) of catheter-based mapping and navigation has been previously described in detail.[14–16] Immediately after the ischemic territory was identified by NOGA mapping, 10^7 NA/$CD31^+$ MNCs in 1 ml phosphate-buffered saline (PBS) ($n = 7$), 10^7 NA/$CD31^-$ MNCs in 1 ml PBS ($n = 8$) or 1 ml PBS without cells ($n = 9$) were injected into five sites within the ischemic myocardium (200 μl to each site) using the NOGA injection catheter (Biosense-Webster).

The ischemic area determined by NOGA mapping before transplantation was not significantly different between the NA/$CD31^+$, NA/$CD31^-$ and PBS groups. A decrease in the size of the ischemic area was observed only after NA/$CD31^+$ transplantation (before, 27.3 ±8.5%; after, 12.3 ±6.3%; $P = 0.0034$), whereas the zone of ischemia increased in size after NA/$CD31^-$ or PBS injection. Similarly, the percentage ischemic area after transplantation was significantly improved only in the $CD31^+$ group ($P = 0.0017$ versus NA/$CD31^-$ group and $P = 0.038$ versus PBS) (Figure 3.2). Selective left coronary angiography was performed to evaluate collateral development before and after transplantation in the swine study. The mean value of the Rentrop score of collateral development to the LCX territory at baseline was similar in all groups. Rentrop scoring was significantly improved only after NA/$CD31^+$ transplantation (0.6 ±0.4 versus 2.0 ±0.4, $P = 0.02$), and not after NA/$CD31^-$ or PBS injection. Similarly, the change in the Rentrop score was significantly greater in the NA/$CD31^+$ group than in either the NA/$CD31^-$ or PBS groups. Capillary density was significantly greater in the NA/$CD31^+$ group than in the

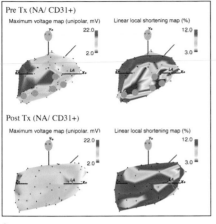

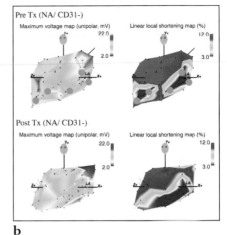

a

b

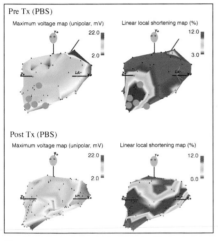

c

Figure 3.2 (a) Representative findings of NOGA electromechanical mapping before (top) and 4 weeks after (bottom) NA/CD31$^+$ MNC transplantation. The brown dots in the pretreatment map show the sites of cell transplantation. The red area on the pretreatment linear local shortening map (top right) indicates an area of decreased wall motion in the lateral wall of the left ventricle, consistent with ischemia in the territory of the LCX. Four weeks after local CD31$^+$ cell transplantation, this area of ischemia is no longer evident (bottom right panel). (b) Representative findings of NOGA electromechanical mapping before and 4 weeks after NA/CD31$^-$ MNC transplantation. The area of ischemia on the pretreatment map (top right) is unchanged/slightly increased 4 weeks following local transplantation of CD31$^-$ cells. (c) Representative findings of NOGA electromechanical mapping before and 4 weeks after PBS injection are similar to those for the CD31$^-$ transplant animals, with no improvement in the ischemic area. (d) Change in percent ischemic area 4 weeks after the treatment. NA/CD31$^+$, swine receiving NA/CD31$^+$ MNCs; NA/CD31$^-$, swine receiving NA/CD31$^-$ MNCs. *$P<0.05$; **$P<0.01$. Reprinted from Circulation 2003; 107: 461–8 with permission from American Heart Association.

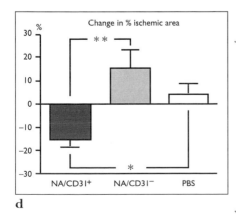

d

37

NA/CD31⁻ and PBS groups. Capillary density in the NA/CD31⁻ group was similar to that in the PBS group. LV ejection fraction measured by echocardiography in the NA/CD31+ group was similar to that in the NA/CD31⁻ and PBS groups 4 weeks after constrictor placement. However, LV ejection fraction significantly improved only after NA/CD31⁺ transplantation, and not after NA/CD31⁻ or PBS injection. LV ejection fraction 4 weeks after transplantation was significantly greater in the NA/CD31⁺ group than in the NA/CD31⁻ and PBS groups. Transplanted EPCs attenuated chronic myocardial ischemia and improved LV function through enhancement of histologic and angiographic myocardial neovascularization. Increased vascularity of the myocardium was observed only in animals in which EPCs were delivered. The notion of inflammation, induced either by needle injury or trauma resulting from injection of cells, is completely dispelled by these data. Thus, we demonstrated the therapeutic potential and technical feasibility of percutaneous, intramyocardial transplantation of autologous EPCs in the setting of chronic myocardial ischemia.[17]

The porcine model of chronic myocardial ischemia was chosen for the above preclinical studies to evaluate the strategy of local delivery using the NOGA injection catheter. Although CD34⁺ MNCs would be used in future clinical studies, anti-swine CD34 antibody is not available. Therefore, we performed cell selection with anti-swine CD31 antibody instead. To complement these studies and to verify that human CD34 selected cells could also yield similar clinical benefit, we transplanted freshly isolated human CD34⁺ cells into the myocardium in a nude rat model of myocardial ischemia achieved by LAD ligation. The locally transplanted CD34⁺ cells incorporated into foci of myocardial neovascularization, differentiated into mature ECs, enhanced vascularity in the ischemic myocardium, preserved LV systolic function and inhibited LV fibrosis.[17]

Taken together with the favorable outcomes in the swine study, percutaneous delivery of autologous, freshly isolated CD34⁺ MNCs targeted to sites of ischemia may represent a practical strategy for revascularization of patients with chronic myocardial ischemia.

Gene-modified EPC therapy

The observation that circulating EPCs home to foci of neovascularization suggests their potential utility as autologous vectors for gene therapy. For treatment of regional ischemia, neovascularization could be amplified by transfection of EPCs to achieve highly localized constitutive expression of angiogenic cytokines and/or provisional matrix proteins. For antineoplastic therapies, EPCs could be transfected with or coupled to antitumor drugs or angiogenesis inhibitors. Gene modification of EPCs has several advantages over conventional gene therapy. Ex vivo gene transfection of EPCs may avoid administration of vectors and vehicles into the recipient organism. Transcriptional or enzymatic gene modification may constitute effective means to maintain, enhance or inhibit the capacity of EPCs to proliferate or differentiate.

Our laboratory recently demonstrated that transplantation of VEGF gene-modified EPCs augments the therapeutic potential of EPCs for neovascularization. Human cultured EPCs were transfected with adenovirus encoding human VEGF165. VEGF-transfected EPCs were intravenously transplanted into nude mice with hindlimb ischemia. The gene-modified strategy resulted in enhancement of neovascularization determined by LDPI and histologic capillary density and in improvement in the frequency of limb salvage, compared to control groups. Notably, these favorable outcomes were achieved with VEGF-transfected EPCs in which the total cell number was less than the effective dosage of EPCs without gene modification.[18]

Conclusion

The discovery of EPCs in adults, increasing knowledge of the pathophysiologic role of EPCs in tissue ischemia and favorable outcomes of EPC transplantation in experimental peripheral and coronary artery diseases suggest a promising future for clinical applications of this cell-based regeneration strategy. However, there are still some issues to be addressed:

1. The optimal dose of EPCs to be transplanted has never been clarified. Dose–response studies should be considered.
2. Safety issues in both acute and chronic phases following EPC transplantation have not been fully explored.
3. Some of the risk factors of ischemic diseases, such as diabetes and hypercholesterolemia, were reported to impair EC function. In the case of autologous EPC transplantation, it is not clear whether EPCs obtained from atherosclerotic patients have significant therapeutic potential or not.
4. The most effective methods of EPC isolation, expansion and administration need to be established for optimal cell transplantation.

Considering these issues, clinical trials of EPC transplantation should be performed based on carefully examined preclinical research. Needless to say, discreet observation of adverse events following the cell transplantation is essential.

Acknowledgments

Atsuhiko Kawamoto is the recipient of a grant from the Japanese Ministry of Education. Takayuki Asahara is the recipient of Grant-in-Aid 0051121T from the American Heart Association.

References

1. Isner JM. Myocardial gene therapy. Nature 2002; 415: 234–9.

2. Losordo DW, Vale PR, Hendel RC et al. Phase 1/2 placebo-controlled, double-blind, dose-escalating trial of myocardial vascular endothelial growth factor 2 gene transfer by catheter delivery in patients with chronic myocardial ischemia. Circulation 2002; 105: 2012–18.

3. Morishita R, Nakamura S, Hayashi S et al. Therapeutic angiogenesis induced by human recombinant hepatocyte growth factor in rabbit hind limb ischemia model as cytokine supplement therapy. Hypertension 1999; 33: 1379–84.

4. Yanagisawa-Miwa A, Uchida Y, Nakamura F et al. Salvage of infarcted myocardium by angiogenic action of basic fibroblast growth factor. Science 1992; 257: 1401–3.

5. Asahara T, Murohara T, Sullivan A et al. Isolation of putative progenitor endothelial cells for angiogenesis. Science 1997; 275: 964–7.

6. Asahara T, Takahashi T, Chen D et al. Regulation of neovascularization with ischemia- or cytokine-induced mobilization of bone marrow-derived endothelial progenitor cells. Circulation 1998; 98: I-326.

7. Asahara T, Takahashi T, Masuda H et al. VEGF contributes to postnatal neovascularization by mobilizing bone marrow-derived endothelial progenitor cells. EMBO J 1999; 18: 3964–72.

8. Kalka C, Masuda H, Takahashi T et al. Vascular endothelial growth factor(165) gene transfer augments circulating endothelial progenitor cells in human subjects. Circ Res 2000; 86: 1198–202.

9. Kalka C, Masuda H, Takahashi T et al. Transplantation of ex vivo expanded endothelial progenitor cells for therapeutic neovascularization. Proc Natl Acad Sci USA 2000; 97: 3422–7.

10. Murohara T, Ikeda H, Duan J et al. Transplanted cord blood-derived endothelial precursor cells augment postnatal neovascularization. J Clin Invest 2000; 105: 1527–36.

11. Kawamoto A, Gwon HC, Iwaguro H et al. Therapeutic potential of ex vivo expanded endothelial progenitor cells for myocardial ischemia. Circulation 2001; 103: 634–7.

12. Schatteman GC, Hanlon HD, Jiao C et al. Blood-derived angioblasts accelerate blood-flow restoration in diabetic mice. J Clin Invest 2000; 106: 571–8.

13. Kocher AA, Schuster MD, Szabolcs MJ et al. Neovascularization of ischemic myocardium by human bone-marrow-derived angioblasts prevents cardiomyocyte apoptosis, reduces remodeling and improves cardiac function. Nat Med 2001; 7: 430–6.

14. Ben-Haim SA, Osadchy D, Schuster I et al. Nonfluoroscopic, in vivo navigation and mapping technology. Nat Med 1996; 2: 1393–5.

15. Botker HE, Lassen JF, Hermansen F et al. Electromechanical mapping for detection of myocardial viability in patients with ischemic cardiomyopathy. Circulation 2001; 103: 1631–7.

16. Vale PR, Losordo DW, Milliken CE et al. Left ventricular electromechanical mapping to assess efficacy of phVEGF(165) gene transfer for therapeutic angiogenesis in chronic myocardial ischemia. Circulation 2000; 102: 965–74.

17. Kawamoto A, Tkebuchava T, Yamaguchi JI et al. Intramyocardial transplantation of autologous endothelial progenitor cells for therapeutic neovascularization of myocardial ischemia. Circulation 2003; 107: 461–8.

18. Iwaguro H, Yamaguchi J, Kalka C et al. Endothelial progenitor cell vascular endothelial growth factor gene transfer for vascular regeneration. Circulation 2002; 105: 732–8

4. EMBRYONIC STEM CELL APPROACHES TO INDUCE MYOGENESIS: PRELIMINARY EXPERIMENTAL FINDINGS

Lior Yankelson, Izhak Kehat and Lior Gepstein

Introduction

The adult heart has limited regenerative capacity, and therefore any significant cell loss due to ischemic heart disease, viral infection or immunopathologic conditions is irreversible and may lead to progressive and irretrievable loss of ventricular function and finally to the development of heart failure. Bearing in mind that congestive heart failure is a growing epidemic that affects more than 5 million Americans[1] and is associated with significant morbidity and mortality, it is not surprising that much effort has been spent on the development of different therapeutic modalities. Yet, despite advances in pharmacologic, interventional and surgical therapeutic measures, the prognosis for these patients remains poor. Moreover, given the chronic lack of donors limiting the number of end-stage heart failure patients who could benefit from heart transplantation, the development of new therapeutic paradigms for these patients has become imperative.

Cell replacement therapy in general, and stem cell technology in particular, are promising and rapidly developing areas offering a possible novel method for the improvement of myocardial performance. This strategy is based on the assumption that an increase in the number and therefore mass of functioning cardiomyocytes within the damaged areas may improve the mechanical properties of these dysfunctional zones. Based on this assumption, several cell types have been suggested as potential sources for tissue grafting, including non-cardiomyocytes such as skeletal myoblasts,[2] fibroblasts and smooth muscle cells, fetal and neonatal cardiomyocytes[3] and embryonic[4] and adult stem cells.[5] Studies in animal models have demonstrated that cells originating from all of the above-mentioned sources may survive, differentiate and, in some cases, even improve cardiac function.

Why, if this is the case, use embryonic stem cells? Despite the fact that several cell sources have been examined in the aforementioned studies, the inherent electrophysiologic, structural and contractile properties of cardiomyocytes strongly suggest that they may be the ideal donor cell type. When fetal cardiomyocytes were transplanted into healthy mouse hearts in early studies, they were demonstrated to survive, align with host cells and form cell-to-cell contacts with host myocardium.[3] Later studies examined the feasibility of cardiomyocyte cell grafting into infarcted or cryoinjured hearts. These studies showed that cardiomyocyte transplantation was associated with smaller infarcts,[6] prevented ventricular dilatation and remodeling[7] and even improved the ventricular systolic function in some cases.[8] The mechanisms underlying these functional improvements are not clear and may include a direct contribution to contractility by the transplanted cells, attenuation of the remodeling process by changing the architectural and structural properties of the scar and improvement in the function of viable tissue within the border zone by induction of angiogenesis.

Despite the encouraging results obtained in animal studies with the use of fetal or neonatal cardiomyocyte transplantation, clinical application of this strategy may be hampered by the inability to obtain human cardiac cells in sufficient numbers. Apart from this, fetal and neonatal cardiomyocyte transplantation may also be restricted by their relatively limited proliferation aptitude in vitro, by their relative sensitivity to ischemic insult and by being prone to immune rejection.

The recent development of human embryonic stem (ES) cell lines[9,10] may potentially provide a solution to the above-mentioned cell-sourcing problem. This is because of the unique ability of these cells to be propagated in vitro in the undifferentiated state in large quantities and to be coaxed to differentiate to several cell lineages, including cardiomyocytes.[11,12] This chapter focuses on describing the unique properties of the human ES cell lines, the establishment of a reproducible cardiomyocyte differentiating system using these cells and the possible applications of this technology in the developing fields of cell therapy and tissue engineering.

What are embryonic stem cells?

All stem cells share two basic properties: prolonged self-renewal and the potential to differentiate into one or more specialized cell types. ES cells differ from other stem cell types (adult stem cells) in two important properties: (1) their ability to be propagated outside the body in the undifferentiated state for prolonged periods; and (2) their potential to differentiate into every cell type of the body, a property termed pluripotency. These unique cell lines were initially described in the mouse, some 20 years ago, by Evans and Kaufman,[13] and independently by Martin.[14]

These groups managed to isolate the pluripotent stem cells from early-stage mouse blastocysts. At this early developmental stage (Figure 4.1), some days after fertilization, an inner cluster of cells termed the inner cell mass (ICM) is formed by separation from the outer cell mass. The ICM cells will later give rise to the three germ layers and ultimately will create all tissues in the body. Interestingly, while the pluripotent ES cells possess unlimited multiplication ability in the culture dish, the ICM cells, from which they were derived, lose this property rather rapidly in vivo, as they disappear in favor of the emergence of specialized progenitor cell lines of the three germ layers.

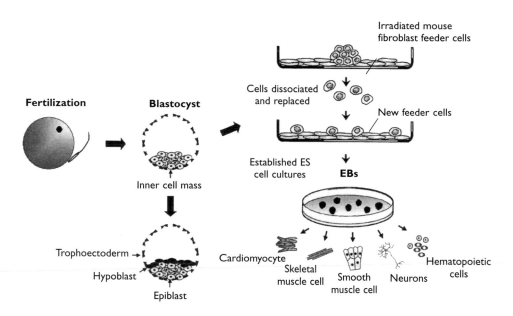

Figure 4.1 Early embryonic development, derivation of the human ES cell lines and in vitro differentiation. Human ES cells were generated from the early-stage embryo at the blastocyst stage. At this stage, the embryo is composed of the trophoectoderm and the inner cell mass (ICM), which eventually will give rise to all tissue types in the embryo. ICM cells isolated by immunosurgery and plated on the mouse embryonic fibroblast (MEF) feeder layer were used for the generation of the ES cell lines. The resulting colonies were propagated and expanded. Following establishment of the human ES cell lines, they can be propagated continuously in the undifferentiated state when grown on top of the MEF feeder layer. When removed from these conditions and grown in suspension, they form three-dimensional cell aggregates that are termed embryoid bodies (EBs). This in vitro differentiating system can be used to generate several tissue types, including cardiomyocytes.

Given the unique properties of the mouse ES cells and the large impact that they have had on modern biology, it is not surprising that much effort has been spent on the development of similar human pluripotent lines. This quest resulted in 1998 in the derivation of the first human ES cells.[15] The process of derivation of the human ES cell lines (Figure 4.1) consisted of selective removal by immunosurgery of the outer layer of the blastocyst's trophoectoderm produced by in vitro fertilization. The ICM cells were then isolated and plated on top of a mitotically inactivated mouse embryonic fibroblast (MEF) feeder layer. Cells were then selected from the periphery of the colonies formed, mechanically removed and plated again in the same manner until homologous colonies were formed, thus creating the ES cell lines.

By definition, there are three major properties that a cell line must possess in order to be considered as an ES cell line: (1) derivation from the preimplantation embryo; (2) the capability for longlasting undifferentiated proliferation, under the appropriate conditions in vitro; and (3) the ability to differentiate into derivatives of all three germ layers. The human ES cells, like their murine counterparts, were shown to fulfill all of the three conditions mentioned above. They were derived from human blastocytes and could be propagated in the undifferentiated state when cultivated on top of the MEF feeder layer.

The pluripotency of human ES cells was determined using two different approaches. In the first approach, human undifferentiated ES cells were injected into immunodeficient mice and were shown to generate benign teratomas containing highly advanced tissue types of all three germ layers.[9] The second approach established ES pluripotency during in vitro differentiation (Figure 4.1).[16] Both mouse and human ES cells, when removed from the MEF feeder layer and allowed to differentiate, could form three-dimensional cell aggregates, termed embryoid bodies (EBs). These structures were shown to contain tissue derivatives of endodermal, ectodermal and mesodermal origin.[16] Finally, in addition to the three basic properties described above, the human ES cells were also shown to maintain a stable diploid karyotype as well as high levels of telomerase activity when propagated in culture for prolonged periods.[9]

Creating cardiomyocytes – the next challenge

One of the most important aspects of ES cells in the context of the field of regenerative medicine is their incomparable ability to generate, ex vivo, diverse tissue types. Since the initial derivation of the human ES cells, several systems for in vitro differentiation to different tissue types, among them cardiac, neuronal, hematopoietic, endothelial and even beta islet cells, have been established.[17] For the murine ES cells, an even larger repertoire of cell types has been described.[18]

The most common method used to induce differentiation in the ES cell model is the EB system.[17,18] When ES cells are removed from the MEF feeder layer and cultivated in suspension, they tend to generate three-dimensional differentiating cell aggregates (EBs). The importance of these structures for differentiation is believed to result from the interactions and co-signaling between the cells within the EBs. Among other differentiating cell types, cardiomyocyte tissue can be detected within the EBs by the appearance of spontaneously contracting areas. Detailed studies in the murine model demonstrate that the development of cardiomyocytes in this in vitro model recapitulates many of the developmental processes observed in vivo.[18]

We have recently used slightly different methodologies from those reported in the mouse model to generate a similar cardiomyocyte-differentiating system in the human ES cell system.[11] Human ES cells were dissociated into small clumps of 3–20 cells and grown in suspension for 7–10 days, where they formed EBs. The EBs were then plated on gelatin-coated culture dishes and observed microscopically for the appearance of spontaneous contraction. Rhythmically contracting areas appeared at 4–22 days after plating in the EBs.

Several lines of evidence confirmed the cardiomyocyte phenotype of the contracting area within the EBs.[11] Cells from the contracting areas were demonstrated by RT-PCR to express cardiac-specific transcription factors such as GATA4 and Nkx2.5, as well as cardiac-specific genes such as cardiac troponin I and T, ANP, and atrial and ventricular myosin light chains (MLC). Other structural findings that support the cardiomyocyte phenotype include the positive immunostaining of dispersed cells isolated from the beating EBs with anti-myosin heavy chain α/β, cardiac troponin I (cTnI), desmin, α-actinin and ANP antibodies (Figure 4.2a) and the typical ultrastructural properties of the early-stage cardiac phenotype as determined by transmitting electron microscopy (Figure 4.2b). From the functional point of view, human ES displayed characteristics typical of early-stage human myocytes, with regard to the electrical activity (Figure 4.2c), calcium transients (Figure 4.2d) and response to adrenergic stimuli.

More recently, we have utilized a unique microelectrode array (MEA) mapping technique to study the network electrophysiologic properties of the ES-derived cardiomyocytes (Figure 4.2e,f). The MEA utilizes an array of 60 electrodes capable of describing the temporal spatial propagation of the electrical signal in a cell culture with extremely high resolution. Our results demonstrated that the human ES cell differentiating system is not limited to

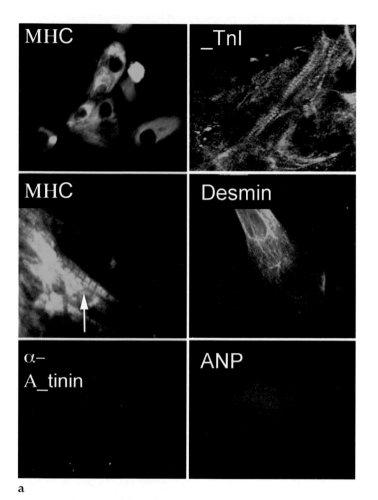

a

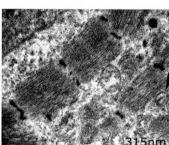

b

Figure 4.2 Structural and functional characterization of the human ES cell-derived cardiomyocytes. (a) Immunostaining for specific cardiac proteins. The presence of α/β myosin heavy chain, a-actinin, cTNi, desmin and ANP was noted in dispersed cells from the contracting areas. (b) Transmission electronmicrograph of human ES cell-derived cardiomyocytes. (c) Extracellular electrogram recording from the beating EB. (d) Calcium transients recorded from these cardiomyocytes. (e,f) Plating of the contracting EB on top of microelectrode array plates allowed the generation of a detailed activation map showing the generation of an excitable syncytium and pacemaking activity. (Reproduced with permission J Clin Invest 2001; 108: 407–14.)

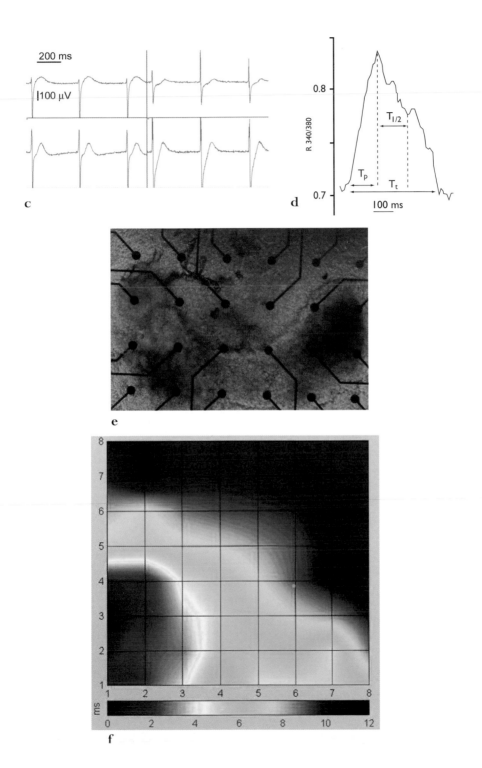

c

d

e

f

49

the generation of isolated cardiomyocytes, but rather that a functional syncytium can be generated with synchronous action potential propagation as well as spontaneous pacemaker activity.[19]

Human ES cell-derived cardiomyocytes for the regeneration of functional myocardium

The most attractive application of human ES cells and the one that captured the attention of the general public and the medical community is the promise that these cells hold in the field of regenerative medicine. This application may be of particular relevance to the cardiovascular field, since massive loss of terminally differentiated adult cardiomyocytes, as occurs, for example, during a large myocardial infarction, is mostly irreversible and may lead to permanent impairment in myocardial performance.

Although several cell preparations have been suggested as sources for tissue grafting, as discussed above, the use of human ES cell-derived cardiomyocytes has several potential advantages. First, as the ES cells possess an unlimited proliferation capacity as well as diverse differentiating capabilities, they currently represent the only cell source that can provide, ex vivo, large numbers of human cardiac cells for transplantation. Second, the ability of the ES cells to differentiate into a plurality of cell lineages may be utilized for transplantation of different cell types such as endothelial progenitor cells for induction of angiogenesis, and even specialized cardiomyocyte subtypes (pacemaking cells, atrial, ventricular, etc.) tailored for specific applications. Third, due to their clonal origin, the ES cell-derived cardiomyocytes could lend themselves to extensive characterization and genetic manipulation to promote desirable characteristics such as resistance to ischemia and apoptosis, improved contractile function, and specific electrophysiologic properties. Fourth, the ES cell-derived cells could also serve as a platform and a cellular vehicle for different gene therapy procedures aiming to manipulate the local myocardial environment by local secretion of growth-promoting factors, various drugs and angiogenic growth factors.

Last, the ability to generate potentially unlimited numbers of cardiomyocytes ex vivo from the human ES cells may also contribute to tissue-engineering approaches. This new discipline combines functional cells with three-dimensional polymeric scaffolds to create tissue substitutes.[20] The possible advantages of this approach versus direct cell transplantation may lie in the abilities to generate significantly thicker myocardial tissue grafts, to control graft shape and size, to provide adequate biomechanical support for

50

the cell graft, to manipulate the cell constitution and alignment and to promote vascularization of the graft. Recently, scaffolds that may allow mechanical contraction have also been described.[20]

Although the development of human ES cells holds great promise for the field of myocardial regeneration, several obstacles need to be overcome before this promising technology can be applied clinically. Among the targets that need to be addressed are the need to create an efficient strategy for directing ES cells into the cardiac phenotype, the development of selection and purification procedures for the generation of pure cardiomyocyte populations, upscaling the entire procedure to achieve clinically relevant numbers of cells, the development of strategies to combat immune rejection, and several issues related to the in vivo effects of cell transplantation.

Directing cardiomyocyte lineage differentiation, cell selection and mass production

Cardiomyocytes account for only a minority of the cells within the EBs, and spontaneously contracting areas are not observed in all EBs. Since the number of cardiomyocytes generated may have an important effect on the ultimate success of cell-grafting procedures, increasing the cardiomyocyte yield during ES differentiation may be of crucial importance. Possible strategies for increasing the cardiomyocyte yield during ES cell differentiation include the use of different ES cell lines or clones, modification of the protocols used during ES cell propagation and EB formation,[12] the use of different growth factors, transcription factors and feeder layers, and physical factors.

Both undifferentiated human ES cells and the more differentiated derivatives express receptors for various growth factors. Supplementation of the culture medium with appropriate growth factors may thus affect the differentiation pattern, although none of the growth factors tested directed differentiation exclusively to one cell type. Similarly, some in vitro and in vivo experimental evidence suggests a possible role for a number of soluble factors in promoting cardiomyocyte differentiation. These include members of the transforming growth factor family, retinoic acid, leukemia inhibitory factor and other factors when provided at the appropriate time and dosage. However, the extent to which these different factors may actually promote cardiogenesis is still unknown.

Although cardiomyocyte differentiation may be enhanced by one of the approaches described above, it is unlikely that the degree of purity achieved would be sufficient for clinical purposes. Consequently, obtaining relatively

51

pure cultures of cardiomyocytes would probably require some form of selection strategy. This selection strategy is required to increase the number of cardiomyocytes and to avoid the presence of other cell derivatives or remaining pluripotent stem cells within the graft.

In one approach,[4] a cardiomyocyte-specific promoter is used to drive a selection marker such as an antibiotic resistance gene (Neo[R]). Once a clone that stably expresses the vector is isolated, undifferentiated genetically modified ES cells can be propagated and expanded. The ES cells are then allowed to differentiate in vitro and are subjected to selection with the appropriate antibiotic (neomycin, G418). Klug et al,[4] using this approach, have shown that >99% pure cardiomyocyte cultures could be generated in the murine ES cell model. Using a different approach researchers have transfected murine ES cells with a construct encoding a cytomegalovirus (CMV) enhancer and a ventricular-specific (MLC-2V) promoter, driving the green fluorescent protein (GFP) product.[21] The use of Percoll gradient centrifugation and subsequent fluorescent-activated cell sorting (FACS) yielded 97% pure cardiomyocytic fractions. Approximately 80% of these cardiomyocytes displayed a typical ventricular action potential.

It is estimated that hundreds of millions of cardiomyocytes are typically lost in a large myocardial infarction that results in the development of heart failure. Moreover, transplantation of an even greater number of cells may be required to replace this cell loss because of the significant number of cardiomyocytes that die following cell grafting.[22] Therefore, a major barrier to the possible use of human ES cells in cell transplantation strategies is the generation of sufficient numbers of cardiomyocytes.

Strategies to increase the number of cardiomyocytes generated during ES cell differentiation may theoretically be employed at several levels: (1) by increasing the initial number of ES cells used for differentiation; (2) by increasing the percentage of ES cells differentiating to the cardiac lineage; (3) by increasing the ability of the cells to proliferate following cardiomyocyte differentiation; and (4) by upscaling the entire process using bioreactors and related technologies.

Issues related to in vivo transplantation

Cell death occurring after engraftment is believed to have a major negative impact on graft size.[22] Hence, cell survival after transplantation may depend on adequate vascularization of the graft, which may require additional revascularization procedures or induction of angiogenesis. In this respect, the ability to genetically manipulate the ES cell derivatives may be used to generate cell grafts that are more resistant to ischemia or apoptosis, that display larger proliferative capacity, that can secrete angiogenic growth factors, or that may be coupled with ES cell-derived endothelial progenitor cells.

Additional factors that remain to be determined in future studies include the ideal nature of the graft (individual cells, small cell clumps or combined with scaffolding biomaterials), the appropriate delivery method (epicardial, endocardial or via the coronary circulation) and the timing of cell delivery relative to the timing of the infarct.

Another barrier that has to be overcome is the prevention of immune rejection of the human ES cell-derived cardiomyocytic grafts.[23] An anti-rejection treatment will probably be needed for this type of allogeneic cell transplantation. However, the immunosuppressive regimens required may be relatively mild because of the expected small pool size of T cells alloreactive to pure stem cell-derived cardiomyocytes that are believed to express MHC class I, but not class II, at the time of transplantation. Strategies aimed at reduction of the mass of alloreactive T cells are being developed, and these and other novel therapies with particular relevance to the anticipated immune response mounted against ES cell-derived cell transplants will probably be employed.[23] These strategies may also include establishing 'banks' of MHC antigen-typed human ES cells, genetically altering ES cells to suppress the immune response such as by knocking out the MHCs, and possibly also nuclear transfer techniques (therapeutic cloning).

An important aspect related to the possible utilization of ES cell-derived cardiomyocytes for cell transplantation strategies relates to the safety of these procedures. A major safety concern is the possible development of ES cell-related tumors. As described above, injection of undifferentiated ES cells into immunodeficient mice has resulted in the generation of teratomas. Hence, as ES cells are coaxed to differentiate in vitro to terminally differentiated cardiomyocytes, efforts need to be made to ensure that the cell graft is depleted of any undifferentiated stem cells before transplantation.

A second major concern relates to the possible arrhythmogenic risk of cell transplantation. Besides the known increased risk for malignant ventricular arrhythmias in patients with reduced ventricular function, cell transplantation may modify the electrophysiologic properties of the scar and theoretically may change (increase or decrease) the propensity for development of arrhythmias. Possible mechanisms for generation of these arrhythmias are increased automaticity of the grafted cells, focal activity from injured host cells and generation of slow-conducting pathways within the scar that may form the basis for re-entrant arrhythmias.

Conclusion

The development of human ES cell lines and their ability to differentiate to cardiomyocyte tissue holds great promise for several research and clinical areas in the cardiovascular field, including developmental biology, gene and drug discovery, pharmacologic testing, cell therapy and tissue engineering. Nevertheless, as described in this chapter, several milestones have to be achieved and a number of hurdles need to be overcome before this approach can become a clinical reality.

References

1. Cohn JN, Bristow MR, Chien KR et al. Report of the National Heart, Lung, and Blood Institute Special Emphasis Panel on Heart Failure Research. Circulation 1997; 95: 766–70.

2. Taylor DA, Atkins BZ, Hungspreugs P et al. Regenerating functional myocardium: improved performance after skeletal myoblast transplantation. Nat Med 1998; 4: 929–33.

3. Soonpaa MH, Koh GY, Klug MG, Field LJ. Formation of nascent intercalated disks between grafted fetal cardiomyocytes and host myocardium. Science 1994; 264: 98–101.

4. Klug MG, Soonpaa MH, Koh GY, Field LJ. Genetically selected cardiomyocytes from differentiating embryonic stem cells form stable intracardiac grafts. J Clin Invest 1996; 98: 216–24.

5. Orlic D, Kajstura J, Chimenti S et al. Bone marrow cells regenerate infarcted myocardium. Nature 2001; 410: 701–5.

6. Li RK, Mickle DA, Weisel RD et al. Natural history of fetal rat cardiomyocytes transplanted into adult rat myocardial scar tissue. Circulation 1997; 96: II-179–86; discussion 186–7.

7. Etzion S, Battler A, Barbash IM et al. Influence of embryonic cardiomyocyte transplantation on the progression of heart failure in a rat model of extensive myocardial infarction. J Mol Cell Cardiol 2001; 33: 1321–30.

8. Scorsin M, Hagege AA, Marotte F et al. Does transplantation of cardiomyocytes improve function of infarcted myocardium? Circulation 1997; 96: II-188–93.

9. Thomson JA, Itskovitz-Eldor J, Shapiro SS et al. Embryonic stem cell lines derived from human blastocysts. Science 1998; 282: 1145–7.

10. Reubinoff BE, Pera MF, Fong CY et al. Embryonic stem cell lines from human blastocysts: somatic differentiation in vitro. Nat Biotechnol 2000; 18: 399–404.

11. Kehat I, Kenyagin-Karsenti D, Snir M et al. Human embryonic stem cells can differentiate into myocytes with structural and functional properties of cardiomyocytes. J Clin Invest 2001; 108: 407–14.

12. Xu C, Police S, Rao N, Carpenter MK. Characterization and enrichment of cardiomyocytes derived from human embryonic stem cells. Circ Res 2002; 91: 501–8.

13. Evans MJ, Kaufman MH. Establishment in culture of pluripotential cells from mouse embryos. Nature 1981; 292: 154–6.

14. Martin G. Isolation of a pluripotent cell line from early mouse embryos cultured in medium conditioned by teratocarcinoma stem cells. Proc Natl Acad Sci USA 1981; 78: 7635.

15. Thomson JA, Odorico JS. Human embryonic stem cell and embryonic germ cell lines. Trends Biotechnol 2000; 18: 53–7.

16. Itskovitz-Eldor J, Schuldiner M, Karsenti D et al. Differentiation of human embryonic stem cells into embryoid bodies compromising the three embryonic germ layers. Mol Med 2000; 6: 88–95.

17. Gepstein L. Derivation and potential applications of human embryonic stem cells. Circ Res 2002; 91: 866–76.

18. Boheler KR, Czyz J, Tweedie D et al. Differentiation of pluripotent embryonic stem cells into cardiomyocytes. Circ Res 2002; 91: 189–201.

19. Kehat I, Gepstein A, Spira A et al. High-resolution electrophysiological assessment of human embryonic stem cell-derived cardiomyocytes: a novel in-vitro model for the study of conduction. Circ Res 2002; 91: 659–61.

20. Zimmermann WH, Schneiderbanger K, Schubert P et al. Tissue engineering of a differentiated cardiac muscle construct. Circ Res 2002; 90: 223–30.

21. Muller M, Fleischmann BK, Selbert S et al. Selection of ventricular-like cardiomyocytes from ES cells in vitro. FASEB J 2000; 14: 2540–8.

22. Muller-Ehmsen J, Whittaker P, Kloner RA et al. Survival and development of neonatal rat cardiomyocytes transplanted into adult myocardium. J Mol Cell Cardiol 2002; 34: 107–16.

23. Strom TB, Field LJ, Ruediger M. Allogeneic stem cells, clinical transplantation, and the origins of regenerative medicine. Transplant Proc 2001; 33: 3044–9.

5. LONG-TERM EFFECTS OF FETAL AND NEONATAL CARDIAC MYOCYTE TRANSPLANTATION ON THE INFARCTED HEART

Robert A Kloner, Jochen Müller-Ehmsen, Mu Yao, Jonathan Leor, Thorsten Reffelmann, Sharon Etzion, Sharon Hale, Joan Dow, Boris Simkhovich, Kirk L Peterson and Larry Kedes

Following acute myocardial infarction, the necrotic myocardium gives way to non-contractile scar tissue over time. There may be small amounts of myocardial cell regeneration that occur in the border regions of infarcts, but certainly not enough to replace the lost muscle mass that infarcted. Numerous experimental studies have now shown that it is possible to replace or at least partially replace lost myocytes with immature cells, including fetal and neonatal cardiomyocytes, embryonic or mesenchymal stem cells, or skeletal muscle myoblasts.[1] The purpose of this chapter is to review our experience with transplantation of fetal and neonatal cardiomyocytes into an experimental myocardial infarct model, with emphasis on long-term effects on the heart. We will also review some early attempts to enhance the transplanted cells with fibroblast growth factor. The overall purpose of our studies was to determine whether immature cardiomyocytes could be injected into normal hearts or hearts with myocardial infarction, survive in a hostile milieu, differentiate, contribute to left ventricular (LV) mass by way of thickening the infarct wall, reduce LV dilatation and remodeling, and ultimately contribute to improved LV ejection fraction.

The basic infarct model

The basic model used in all of these studies was the anesthetized open chest rat model. In early studies we utilized Sprague Dawley rats, which required immunosuppression with cyclosporin A. Later, we switched to Fischer 344 rats, which are syngeneic and did not require immunosuppression. Rats were anesthetized, usually with ketamine and xylazine, intubated and then ventilated. A left thoracotomy was performed, the pericardium was incised and a suture was placed under the proximal left coronary artery. The left coronary artery was isolated just under the left atrial appendage in the interventricular groove. The suture was tied in order to ligate the coronary artery and induce an acute myocardial infarction. Using this model, it is possible to infarct 30–50% of the left ventricle – primarily the anterior free wall of the left ventricle. These infarcts are large in the rat, in part due to a general lack of coronary collateral flow, a large risk area and a high metabolic demand of the heart. The infarcted wall gradually thins as the necrotic tissue is reabsorbed. In large infarcts, the necrotic tissue not only thins but stretches, resulting in LV dilatation. The early phase of infarct thinning and stretching is termed myocardial infarct expansion. Patients who demonstrate this phenomenon, which can be observed non-invasively with such techniques as echocardiography, typically have a worse prognosis and may be prone to congestive heart failure.

Following coronary artery ligation, the chest is closed under sterile conditions and the rats are allowed to survive for varying periods of time, depending upon the protocol. Some rats die, usually related to the infarct itself, with arrhythmias or pump failure. In some rats, no infarct develops if the coronary artery was missed. Usually, at 1 week, the rats are reanesthetized, the chests are opened and the infarct is examined. In most cases, the infarct is readily visible as a pale gray non-beating or dyskinetic area of the free wall of the anteroapical portion of the left ventricle. If the coronary artery ligation was unsuccessful, this will usually be obvious by a lack of a visible infarction. Isolated fetal or neonatal myocytes are then injected directly into the infarct. We usually use cells that have been isolated and cultured for several days. In some studies, preplating has been used to purify the cells and remove fibroblasts. The cells are injected using a tuberculin syringe through a 26- or 27-gauge needle. We place a 30–45° bend at the end of the needle, which allows us to better visualize the tip of the needle once we penetrate the LV wall. Successful injection of the cells is associated with the immediate appearance of a pale bleb that blanches the myocardium. A lack of this bleb usually means that the operator has pushed the needle into the LV cavity. Also, if the needle is pushed through the wall of the left ventricle, bleeding will occur. The chest is then closed and the rats are allowed to survive.

Feasibility of cell transplant

Leor in our group[2] determined the feasibility of fetal cardiomyocyte transplantation into the rat model of myocardial infarction. In these initial studies, the coronary artery was occluded for 60 min; this was followed by reperfusion, and fragments of fetal ventricular tissue were injected into the infarcts. Tissue had been cultured for 7–10 days, and viable, contracting fragments were selected for injection. Transplantation took place 7–24 days after myocardial infarction; at 7, 14, 32 and 65 days after tissue transplantation, rats were euthanized for histology, electronmicroscopy and immunohistochemistry. Clumps of transplanted cells were readily visible within the scar by staining with smooth muscle α-actin (which stains embryonic cardiac cells but not adult cardiac cells) as well as by identifying the fetal phenotypes within the scar (myocytes with large nuclei, large nucleoli and myofilaments located primarily at the periphery of the cell). In one protocol, cells were implanted 1–3 weeks after occlusion; 11 hearts were examined 7 days after transplantation and four hearts were examined 14 days after transplantation. Engrafted fetal cardiomyocytes were detected in 55% of rats after 7 days and in 100% after 14 days. In another protocol, 11 rats received fetal tissue at 9, 13 and 17 days after infarction. Engrafted fetal cardiac tissue was observed at 8 (1 of 2), 14 (1 of 2), 32 (1 of 1) and 65 (2 of 2) days after transplantation. Four hearts were excluded due to a lack of myocardial infarction. Overall graft survival rate in this experiment was 71%. Control animals injected with saline did not demonstrate areas of engrafted fetal cells by immunocytochemistry, routine histology or ultrastructural analysis. While this study demonstrated the feasibility of implanting fetal cells, the finding that these cells often appeared in rounded clumps and relatively undifferentiated raised the issue of whether differentiation and a meaningful contribution to cardiac function would be feasible.

Etzion et al[3] isolated and cultured fetal rat cardiomyocytes from 14- to 15-day-old embryos. The cells were incubated with 5-bromo-2'-deoxyuridine (BrdU) overnight; other cells were transfected with adenovirus carrying the nuclear LacZ reporter gene. Experimental myocardial infarction was created in Sprague Dawley rats as described above. Seven days after myocardial infarction, cultured cells (1.5×10^6) or culture medium alone was injected directly into the infarct scar. The chest was closed and rats were allowed to survive for 8 weeks. Transthoracic echocardiography was done 5–7 days after induction of myocardial infarction, but prior to cell therapy and 8 weeks after cell therapy. A 7.5-MHz phased-array transducer was utilized. The following echocardiographic measures were obtained: maximal LV end-diastolic dimension, minimal LV end-systolic dimension, fractional shortening and change in LV area. Pulmonary artery Doppler flow and diameter were utilized to calculate cardiac output and stroke volume. The survival rate was 11 out of 11 in the cell transplant group versus 12 out of 16 for the medium-treated rats ($P = 0.12$).

Grafted cells could be identified at 8 weeks within the infarcted myocardium by smooth muscle α-actin positive staining. The cells appeared relatively round with large nuclei. Some of these cells appeared more elongated, with cross-striations typical of sarcomeres. In other studies, rats euthanized after transplantation were studied for the presence of ß-galactosidase and BrdU staining. In specimens where prelabeled cells were implanted, microscopic examination confirmed that scar tissue contained clusters of embryonic cells that stained positive for ß-galactosidase and BrdU. Cells within the scar that appeared to have early sarcomeres stained positive for myosin heavy chain. Connexin 43 staining within the graft appeared punctate and scattered but did not show connections between the transplanted cells and the host myocardium. There was a trend towards greater capillary and arteriolar density in the areas of cell transplantation, suggesting that the transplants stimulated an angiogenic response.

In the control (medium) group, LV diastolic diameter increased from 0.710 cm to 0.839 cm from the baseline to the final echocardiogram ($P=0.024$). There was less dilatation in the cell-treated group (0.710 cm to 0.760 cm; $P=0.25$). LV systolic internal diameter increased from 0.402 cm to 0.562 cm ($P=0.019$) in control animals over the course of the study, and less so for treated animals (0.410 cm to 0.506 cm; $P=0.06$). Fractional shortening deteriorated over the course of the study in control animals (43% to 31%; $P=0.04$) and less so for cell transplant animals (42% to 36%; $P=0.21$). Stroke volume did not change in the control group (0.25 ml to 0.25 ml; $P=0.92$) but improved in cell-treated rats (0.21 ml to 0.27 ml; $P=0.15$). There were non-significant changes in cardiac output, with a trend towards a fall in the control group (71 to 59 ml/min; $P=0.17$) and a trend towards an increase in the cell-treated group (61 to 77 ml/min; $P=0.19$). While the anterior wall thinned according to echocardiography in the control group (0.10 cm to 0.085 cm; $P=0.05$), it did not thin in the cell-treated group (0.096 cm to 0.097 cm; $P=0.92$). These results suggested that, when studied over a period of 2 months, transplanted fetal cardiomyocytes survived in an infarct scar, attenuated LV dilatation and infarct thinning, and improved some parameters of global LV function. However, by histology, many cells appeared immature and appeared to be isolated by scar from the host tissue. This study was also one of the first to suggest that fetal cell transplantation might stimulate angiogenesis. A newer study with neonatal cardiac myocytes has confirmed an increase in capillary density and regional myocardial bloodflow at the site of transplantation.[4]

Yao et al[5] have recently extended these findings and have observed that, as late as 10 months after fetal cell transplantation, these cells survived, differentiated further, thickened the infarct wall, reduced the degree of LV

dilatation and improved ejection fraction. However, regional wall motion
analysis suggested that much of this benefit was due to passive thickening of
the infarct wall rather than active systolic contraction of the cells.

Neonatal rat cardiomyocytes

A second series of studies was performed using neonatal rat cardiomyocytes
rather than fetal heart cells. An advantage of neonatal cells may be that they
are more mature than fetal cells. A disadvantage is that they will not divide
appreciably. Müller-Ehmsen et al[6] transplanted male donor neonatal
cardiomyocytes (isolated 1–2 days after birth) from Fischer 344 rats into
adult female Fischer 344 rats. In an initial series of studies, they injected
these cells into adult hearts to observe the time course of their differentiation
and then used qualitative (Figure 5.1) or quantitative TaqMan PCR to
establish their survival. This later technique measures quantitatively the Sry
gene of the Y chromosome of the male neonatal cells within the milieu of
the female heart. Within 24 h of transplantation into the left ventricle of non-

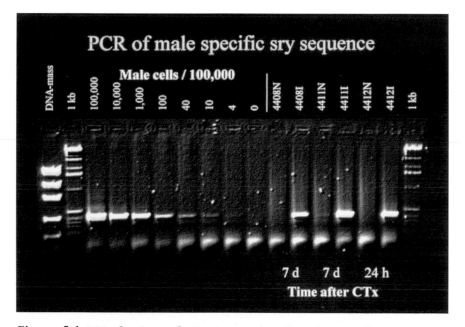

Figure 5.1 PCR of male specific Sry sequence that allows detection of the Y
chromosome. About four male cells per 100 000 cells can be identified in vitro. The
positive Sry gene signal for male neonatal cardiomyocytes was observed within the infarct
(I) versus non-infarcted tissue (N) at 7 h and 24 h after cell transplantation (CTX).

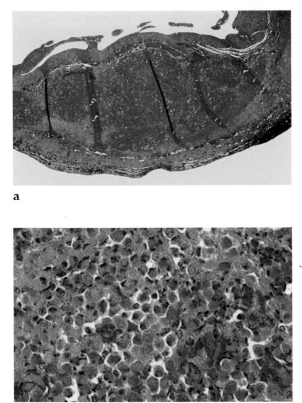

a

b

Figure 5.2

(a) Appearance of neonatal cell implant (hematoxylin and eosin, ×4 objective) within 24 h of injection into an infarcted rat that died. The plane of the myocardial infarct scar is disrupted, and the cells occupy the central portion of the scar, resulting in what appears to be a thickened LV wall. The endocardium is towards the top and the epicardium is towards the bottom of the figure. (b) Higher-power view of cells within the first 24 h after transplantation shows a round, immature appearance and large nuclei (original magnification ×40). (Reprinted from Müller-Ehmsen et al.[7] Used with permission of the American Heart Association.)

infarcted or infarcted hearts, the cells appeared rounded (Figure 5.2). Within 1–2 weeks, the neonatal cells became elongated and showed early cross-striations (sarcomeres; Figure 5.3). By 4–6 weeks, the sarcomeres became well developed. The nuclei of the transplanted cells initially demonstrated a rounded appearance but became elongated with time. However, even later, the transplanted cardiomyocytes remained thinner than host cells, and the nuclei appeared rounder than host cells. It is somewhat sobering that, immediately after injection and at 1 h after injection into normal (non-infarcted) hearts, 57% and 58% of cells survived as assessed by quantitative TaqMan analysis. This suggests that there is some initial failure due to retention of cells in the syringe's dead space, cell washout through the vasculature or lymph, or injection of some cells into the LV cavity or some cell disruption at the time of injection. At 24 h, cell survival was 24%; it remained at this level for 4 weeks and was then further reduced to 15% at 12 weeks. Pretreatment of the isolated neonatal cells with an anti-apoptotic caspase inhibitor did not improve survival in this study. We do not believe

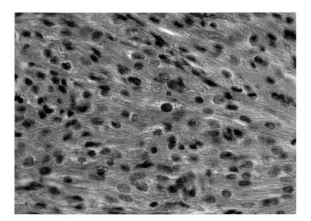

Figure 5.3 *Implanted neonatal cardiomyocytes at day 7 after implantation into non-infarcted tissue. Instead of a rounded morphology, the cells have taken on a cylindrical shape, and early cross-striations are visible (right-hand side of figure). (Reprinted from Müller-Ehmsen et al,[6] with permission.)*

that graft rejection played a role, since syngeneic animals were used and there was no sign of inflammation over the course of the study. As will be discussed below, we now believe that significant washout of cells may have occurred when they were injected into high-flow non-ischemic tissue, whereas when injected into an infarct the cells were more likely to be retained there.

Müller-Ehmsen et al[7] recently assessed the long-term effects of neonatal cardiac cell transplantation on ventricular function in an infarct model. Male Fischer rat neonatal cardiomyocytes were isolated 1–2 days after birth, and purified by preplating. Female syngeneic Fischer 344 rats underwent proximal left coronary artery ligation and at 1 week were randomized to receive intracardiac injection of either neonatal cardiomyocytes ($3–5 \times 10^6$ in 50 μl medium) or medium (50 μl) alone. At 6 months, the rats underwent hemodynamic and LV angiographic measures with a XiScan 1000 C-arm X-ray system (XiTech, Inc.) and nonionic contrast injected into the jugular vein. This technique allows evaluation of an LV angiogram in the rodent without having to advance a catheter into the left ventricle (Figure 5.4). LV ejection fraction was determined and regional wall motion was calculated using the Sheehan centerline method.[8] Post-mortem LV volumes, infarct size and wall thickness were measured. The percentages of the LV circumference occupied by infarcted and non-infarcted tissue were determined from histologic images of transverse LV sections. In some hearts, real-time fluorescence TaqMan PCR was used to determine cell survival.

The post-mortem LV volume, which used fluid to measure the cavity, was 0.42 ml in transplanted rats and 0.45 ml in control rats ($P = NS$).

Histologic analysis, including staining with hematoxylin and eosin as well as picrosirius red (enhances ability to see collagen), showed, in control rats, thin-walled collagenous scars that, in general, were transmural. Hearts injected with cells demonstrated well-delineated clumps of cells within the scar (Figure 5.5).

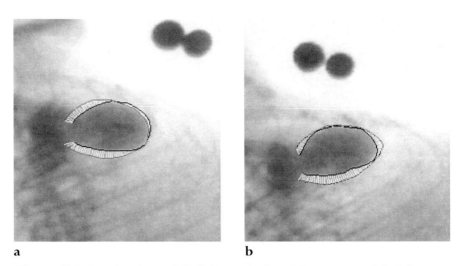

a   b

Figure 5.4 *Centerline Regional Wall Motion Analysis. LV angiograms of the left ventricle of a medium-treated heart and neonatal cell-treated heart, showing inward motion of the apex of the cell-treated heart. (a) Media-treated animal. (b) Neonatal cell-treated animal. Red, end-diastole; black, end-systole.*

Figure 5.5 *Low-power view of transmural slices of left ventricles stained with hematoxylin and eosin (left column) or picrosirius red (right column). The muscle appears pink in hematoxylin and eosin-stained slides. The muscle appears yellow and the collagen red in picrosirius red-stained slides. (a) and (b) are from a control heart that received medium injection. Note the thin free wall of the left ventricle, composed primarily of collagen. (c) and (d) are from a cell transplant heart. Note two discrete lumps of myocardial cells (c) within the scar that increase wall thickness at the site of cells. (e) and (f) are from a control heart that received medium. Again, note that the free LV wall is thin and composed of collagen. (g) and (h) are from a heart that received cell injections into the scar. Note discrete lumps of cells (c) within the scar. Note improved wall thickness. (Reprinted from Müller-Ehmsen et al,[7] with permission of the American Heart Association.)*

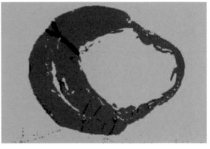

a

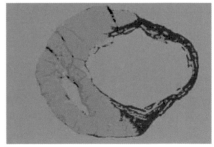

b

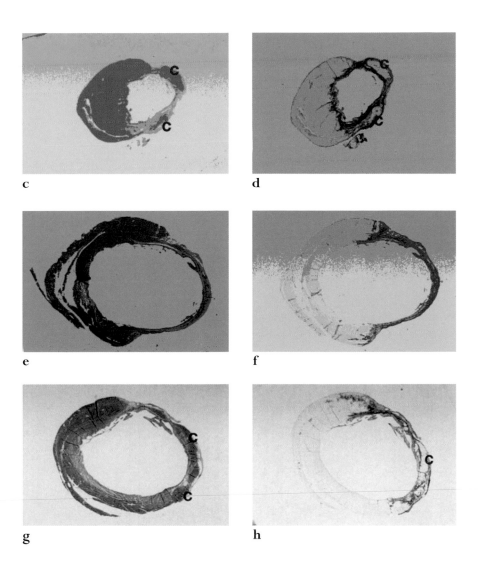

These clumps appeared to thicken the wall of the infarct and appeared to have dissected the plane of collagen of the scar, so that they were sandwiched between an endocardial and epicardial layer of infarct collagen.

The infarct scar at its thickest portion measured 619 μm in the medium-treated hearts but was 909 μm in cell-treated hearts ($P < 0.02$), and the mid lateral portion of the scar was increased from 324 μm to 531 μm ($P < 0.02$) in cell-treated hearts. There was no difference in scar circumference between groups. The transplanted myocytes appeared lengthened, with typical striations. However, their diameter appeared smaller and their nuclei rounder than in adult myocardial cells. Connexin 43 staining was positive for junctions between grafted cells but not between grafted cells and host myocardium. At 6 months, the survival rate of injected cells was estimated at 62%, based on TaqMan PCR. (Hence survival rate was actually greater in this study, to our surprise, than when cells were injected into normal hearts. Again, we postulate that when cells are injected into normal myocardium, cell washout through the vasculature and lymphatics may be a serious issue. When they are injected into a low-flow or no-flow tissue such as scar, they are trapped there.)

Ejection fraction by area length measurement was 0.25 in the medium-treated animals and 0.36 in the cell-transplanted animals ($P = 0.009$). Stroke volume was 71 μl in the medium-treated rats and 97 μl in cell-transplanted animals ($P = 0.09$). dP/dt was unchanged. Cell-treated animals showed a small but significant increase in average chordal shortening of the infarct-related area (Figure 5.6). There was a significant decrease in paradoxical systolic bulging of the anterior wall and apex of the left ventricle. Dyskinesis in the lateral wall as a fraction of the perimeter of the left ventricle was 0.244 in the media group versus 0.111 in the cell-transplant group ($P = 0.018$).

This study showed that the long-term effects of neonatal cardiomyocytes transplanted into an infarct scar were improvements in global and regional in vivo cardiac function and thickening of the wall of the infarct scar.

Efforts to enhance transplanted cells

While cell transplantation is feasible, it is clear from our results that it is not yet optimal. Cell survival remains an issue and in our hands was not amenable to antiapoptotic therapy. Another approach would be to manipulate the cells prior to transplantation with various growth hormones. In this regard, we have studied the effect of fibroblast growth factor (bFGF) on cultured fetal heart cells and cultured fetal ventricular tissue samples.

Isolated cardiomyocytes from rat fetuses (16–18 days) were either cultured with bFGF at 300 ng/ml or not treated for 3 days. To examine cell proliferation in the culture, BrdU at 10 μg/ml was added to the culture 20 h prior to collection. The cells were harvested and immunostained for myosin heavy chain (MHC) and BrdU (Figures 5.7 and 5.8). Phenotypic myocytes were defined as MHC positive; proliferating cells were defined as BrdU positive (Figures 5.7 and 5.8). Proliferating myocytes were identified as both BrdU- and MHC-positive cells (Figure 5.9). Treatment with bFGF increased

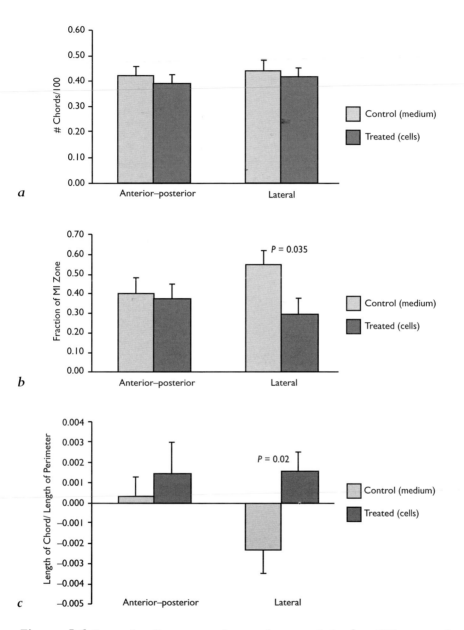

Figure 5.6 *Regional wall motion analysis in the myocardial infarct (MI) zone at 6 months after media injection or cardiomyocyte transplantation. (a) MI zone as a fraction of total perimeter of the left ventricle (P = NS between groups). (b) Fraction of the MI zone that was found to demonstrate paradoxic systolic bulging (dyskinesis). P = 0.035 on lateral projection, where anteroapical wall motion is best seen in profile. (c) Average chordal shortening in MI zone. P = 0.02 on lateral projection. (Reprinted from Müller-Ehmsen et al,[7] with permission of American Heart Association.)*

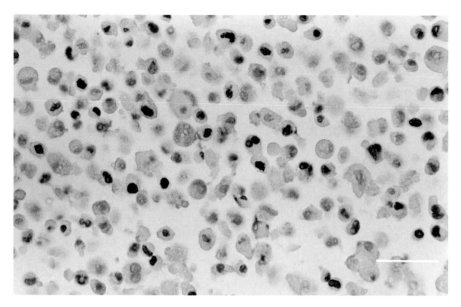

Figure 5.7 *An illustration of myocytes that are positive for myosin heavy chain (MHC). The myocytes are indicated by the red color in the cytoplasm. The non-muscle cells appear blue by counterstaining. Bar = 50µm.*

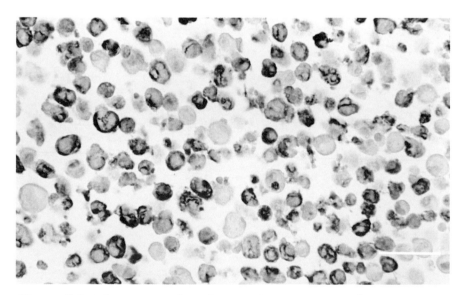

Figure 5.8 *A demonstration of proliferating cells that are positive for BrdU labeling. The positively stained cells have reddish nuclei, an indication of BrdU being incorporated into newly synthesized DNA. The nuclei of non-proliferating cells have no incorporated BrdU and they appear blue with hemotoxylin counterstaining. Bar = 50 µm.*

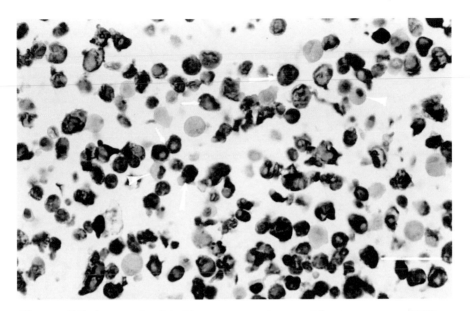

Figure 5.9 *An example of double staining to detect proliferating myocytes. MHC appears red in the cytoplasm and BrdU brownish in the nuclei. While the proliferating non-muscle cells are only stained for BrdU in their nuclei, the proliferating myocytes are shown by the colocalization of both MHC and BrdU staining. The examples of proliferating myocytes and proliferating non-muscle cells are indicated by large arrows and arrowheads respectively. In the non-proliferating myocytes (small arrows), the cytoplasm is positive for MHC but the nuclei are negative for BrdU labeling. Bar = 50 μm.*

the percentage of cardiomyocytes (MHC-positive cells) from $45.7 \pm 9.4\%$ to $56.4 \pm 9.6\%$ ($P < 0.01$). bFGF also enhanced the percentage of proliferating myocytes (both MHC and BrdU positive) from $10.0 \pm 3.5\%$ to $13.6 \pm 4.3\%$ ($P < 0.05$). Thus bFGF therapy may be a useful means of promoting the formation of new myocardium from fetal heart cells destined for transplantation.

In a separate study,[9] ventricular fragments from fetal rats (approximately 1 mm³) were cultured in bFGF or were not supplemented. Five days of incubation in bFGF increased graft size from 2.0 mm to 4.1 mm in diameter ($P < 0.001$) and increased BrdU incorporation from 0.6% in controls to 5.7% in bFGF-treated tissue. Ultrastructural analysis showed an increase in myofilaments and early sarcomeres. Treated tissue also demonstrated an increased expression of myocyte-related antigens.

Conclusion

In conclusion, our studies suggest that transplantation of fetal or neonatal cardiomyocytes into the hostile environment of a myocardial infarction is feasible. These cells will survive long-term, thicken the wall of the infarct and improve global LV function. Neonatal cells improved regional wall motion, while a recent study by our group suggests that fetal heart cells are less likely to do this. Fetal cells did have a more prominent effect on reducing LV dilatation. Both types of cells appear to stimulate their own blood supply. bFGF may enhance the growth of these grafts, and future studies should concentrate on how to optimize cell transplantation.

There is now a host of literature on the cell transplant into infarct or heart concept using fetal, neonatal, stem, bone marrow and skeletal muscle cells.[1] There are several recent excellent reviews that cover the findings from numerous laboratories and that describe some ongoing clinical trials as well.[1,10,11] What we have tried to accomplish in this chapter is to review the experience of this technique in one laboratory. Our studies have continued and we are currently assessing mesenchymal stem cells as a potential source of cells for rebuilding the damaged heart.

Acknowledgment

This work was funded in part by grant NHLBI HL61488.

References

1. Etzion S, Kedes LH, Kloner RA, Leor J. Myocardial regeneration. Present and future trends. Am J Cardiovasc Drugs 2001; 1(4): 233–44.

2. Leor J, Patterson M, Quinones MJ et al. Transplantation of fetal myocardial tissue into the infarcted myocardium of rat. A potential method for repair of infarcted myocardium? Circulation 1996; 94(suppl II): II-332–6.

3. Etzion S, Battler A, Barbash IM et al. Influence of embryonic cardiomyocyte transplantation on the progression of heart failure in a rat model of extensive myocardial infarction. J Mol Cell Cardiol 2001; 33: 1321–30.

4. Reffelmann T, Dow JS, Dai W et al. Transplantation of neonatal cardiomyocytes after permanent coronary artery occlusion increases regional blood flow of infarcted myocardium. J Mol Cell Cardiol 2003; 35: 607–13.

5. Yao M, Dieterle T, Hale SL et al. Long-term outcome of fetal cell transplantation on postinfarction ventricular remodeling and function. J Mol Cell Cardiol 2003; 35: 661–70.

6. Müller-Ehmsen J, Whittaker P, Kloner RA et al. Survival and development of neonatal rat cardiomyocytes transplanted into adult myocardium. J Mol Cell Cardiol 2002; 34: 107–16.

7. Müller-Ehmsen J, Peterson KL, Kedes L et al. Rebuilding a damaged heart: long-term survival of transplanted neonatal rat cardiomyocytes after myocardial infarction and effect on cardiac function. Circulation 2002; 105: 1720–6.

8. Sheehan FH, Bolson EL, Dodge HT et al. Advantages and applications of the centerline method for characterizing regional ventricular function. Circulation 1986; 74: 293–305.

9. Patterson MJ, Kloner RA. Basic fibroblast growth factor and differentiation of fetal cardiac myocytes: a potential improvement for fetal cell transplant therapy. Cardiac Vasc Regeneration 2000; 1: 170–7.

10. Reffelmann T, Kloner RA. Cellular cardiomyoplasty–cardiomyocytes, skeletal myoblasts or stem cells for regenerating myocardium and treatment of heart failure? Cardiovasc Res 2003; 58: 358–68.

11. Müller-Ehmsen J, Kedes L, Schwinger RHG, Kloner RA. Cellular cardiomyoplasty – a novel approach to heart disease. Congest Heart Failure 2002; 8: 220–7.

71

6. THE ROLE OF CARDIAC FIBROBLASTS IN CARDIAC REGENERATION

Mahboubeh Eghbali-Webb

The diversity of cell types in the myocardium offers a complex context for the intricate and highly coordinated cell–cell and cell–environment interactions that are necessary for regenerative processes. The population of cells in the myocardium includes cardiac myocytes, endothelial cells, smooth muscle cells and cardiac fibroblasts. Cardiac fibroblasts play a central and multifaceted role in cardiac regeneration that is characterized by their trophic and protective effects on the one hand and their phenotypic plasticity on the other. The environmental factors necessary for muscle and vascular regeneration include extracellular matrix and an array of soluble factors consisting of matrix metalloproteases, cytokines and diverse growth factors necessary for cell growth and differentiation. Because cardiac fibroblasts constitute the majority of non-myocyte cells in the heart[1,2] they are the principal source of the extracellular matrix and soluble factors[1–7] (Figure 6.1). Most importantly, the demonstrated resilience of cardiac fibroblasts under environmental stress, including hypoxia and hypothermia, enhances their potential to influence muscle and vascular regeneration in response to pathophysiologic stimuli during development, normal growth, aging, ventricular hypertrophy and heart failure after myocardial infarction. As the result of their proven phenotypic plasticity and their predisposition to transform into cells with features characteristic of myocytes, cardiac fibroblasts can directly enter into myogenic pathways and contribute to the regeneration of cardiac muscle. This chapter is aimed at providing insights into the mechanisms by which cardiac fibroblasts may regulate various aspects of muscle and vascular regeneration in the heart. Specifically, the role of the extracellular matrix and soluble factors and the effects brought about as the result of the phenotypic plasticity of cardiac fibroblasts will be discussed (Figure 6.2).

The extracellular matrix and its regulation

In most tissues, the interaction of cells with the surrounding extracellular matrix, mainly via integrin-mediated pathways, is a critical bi-directional

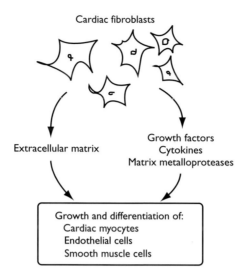

Figure 6.1 Biological properties of cardiac fibroblasts. Cardiac fibroblasts, by producing soluble factors and the extracellular matrix, may regulate proliferation, growth and differentiation in cardiac myocytes and vascular endothelial cells thereby actively participate in the process of muscle and vascular regeneration.

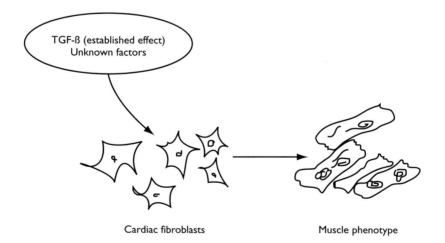

Figure 6.2 Phenotypic plasticity of cardiac fibroblasts. Cardiac fibroblasts are predisposed to transform into cells with phenotypic properties characteristic of cardiac myocytes. TGF-β has been established as an inducer of phenotypic change in cardiac fibroblasts (see text for reference).

exchange vital for cell growth and differentiation. In the heart, the ability of cardiac fibroblasts to deposit an intricate and highly organized extracellular matrix is perhaps the best evidence of their central role in cardiac regeneration. This matrix serves multiple functions. On the one hand, as shown by electron microscopy,[8] it forms a highly specialized structure that interconnects cardiac myocytes to one another and to their capillaries. This structure also provides support for cardiac myocytes and maintains their alignment during a cardiac cycle. On the other hand, the interaction between the extracellular matrix and cardiac cells provides an essential component necessary for cell growth, proliferation, differentiation, motility and apoptosis. The integrin-mediated interaction between cardiac myocytes and the extracellular matrix may also serve as a link between the contractile elements of adjacent cardiac myocytes and as a conduit of information necessary for cell function.

Hormonal regulation of collagen matrix

The production of the extracellular matrix by cardiac fibroblasts is subject to regulation by hormonal and hemodynamic factors. Fibrillar collagen type I is the most abundant protein of the extracellular matrix in the heart. Of a large number of growth factors and hormones that alter production of collagen type I by cardiac fibroblasts, transforming growth factor-beta (TGF-β_1), thyroid hormones and angiotensin II are the most extensively studied. Cardiac fibroblasts are both the source and target for TGF-β_1.[4,9–11] TGF-β_1 stimulates collagen type I gene expression in cardiac fibroblasts, and this effect is dependent on de novo synthesis of proteins.[10] Thyroid hormones, on the other hand, have an inhibitory effect on collagen gene expression. This effect is consistent with the findings that, of all known forms of pathologic ventricular hypertrophy, thyroid hormone-induced hypertrophy is distinct by the lack of fibrosis.[12] In vitro studies from our laboratory showed decreased levels of collagen type I mRNA with moderate changes in mRNA stability and a significant decrease in the activity of collagen type I promoter in thyroid hormone-treated cardiac fibroblasts.[12] Analysis of 5′-flanking regions and the intronic segments of pro-α_1(l) collagen gene showed that proximal (−15/+115) sequences of pro-α_1(l) collagen promoter which bind to thyroid hormone receptor type ß and an AP-1 (activator protein-1) response element located at +92/+97 are necessary for the T_3-induced inhibition of promoter activity.[13] These findings provide insights into the mechanisms responsible for in vivo downregulation of collagen biosynthesis by circulating thyroid hormones, as shown in rats with hyperthyroidism,[12] in thyroidectomized rats[14] and in tight skin mouse, a genetic model of cardiac fibrosis.[15]

Angiotensin II is an important regulator of matrix production by cardiac fibroblasts. In human heart with interstitial fibrosis, the expression of AT2 receptor is associated with the extent of interstitial fibrosis.[16] The association of AT2 receptors with collagen production is also shown in failing hamster heart, where AT2 receptor activation caused a decrease in the progression of interstitial fibrosis during cardiac remodeling.[17] Captopril, an angiotensin-converting enzyme (ACE) inhibitor, causes a significant decrease in collagen synthesis in cardiac fibroblasts of cardiomyopathic hamsters, which have a significantly higher level of collagen than cells from normal hamsters.[18] Angiotensin II-induced release of prostacyclin from cardiac fibroblasts causes a decrease in the expression of collagen type I and III. This suggests a role for eicosanoids in modulating collagen synthesis.[19] Angiotensin II also promotes collagen gel contraction by adult rat cardiac fibroblasts via induction of osteopontin and β_3 integrin expression.[20]

Effect of mechanical stress

It is suggested that in cardiac fibroblasts integrins act as mechanotransducers, converting mechanical stimuli into biochemical signals. This notion is based on data demonstrating stretch-induced activation of integrin-dependent ERK1/2 and c-Jun NH2 terminal kinases in rat cardiac fibroblasts.[21] It is shown that equibiaxial strain and the rate at which the strain is applied stimulate early activation of G proteins in cardiac fibroblasts. Thus it is suggested that G proteins may be the mediators that transform mechanical stretch into biochemical response.[22] Together, these results suggest that in cardiac fibroblasts mechanical stimuli could be coupled to biological responses including collagen matrix production (see ref. 23 for review). The ratio of collagen type III/I mRNA increases significantly in mechanically stretched cardiac fibroblasts.[24] Stretch also affects the expression and activity of neutral transmembrane matrix metalloproteases and tissue plasminogen activator in cardiac fibroblasts.[25]

Effect of hypoxia

Hypoxia, a condition of myocardial ischemia, is a powerful regulator of gene expression, at transcriptional and post-transcriptional levels. It is now established that hypoxia regulates both basal and factor-induced collagen production in cardiac fibroblasts.[26] In our laboratory, we determined the effect of hypoxia (2% oxygen) on collagen type I production in human cardiac fibroblasts, under basal conditions of cell culture and in response to growth factors.[26] Hypoxia caused an increase in the basal level of pro-α_1(l) collagen mRNA and protein. However, the TGF-β_1-induced increase in the level of pro-α_1(l) collagen mRNA that was achieved under normoxia was absent under hypoxia. Furthermore, the inhibitory effect of thyroid hormones on pro-α_1(l) collagen mRNA was reversed under hypoxia. Under normoxia, TGF-β_1 and thyroid hormones diminished the levels of collagen type I protein. This effect of both factors was reversed under hypoxia.[26] These findings suggest that, in human cardiac fibroblasts, hypoxia, by increasing the basal level of collagen type I gene expression on the one hand and by reversing the TGF-β_1- and T_3- induced inhibition of collagen type I gene expression on the other, may cause an overall increase in collagen type I production. Other studies have shown that atrial natriuretic factor (ANF) inhibits hypoxia-induced enhanced expression of collagen type I and type III in cardiac fibroblasts.[27] It is suggested that paracrine effects of ANF produced by cardiac myocytes may play a role in the prevention of cardiac fibrosis in ischemic heart diseases.[27]

Soluble factors released by cardiac fibroblasts

In a growing list of soluble factors involved in the development of heart muscle, those with known effects on the growth and differentiation of cardiac myocytes and endothelial cells include vascular endothelial growth factor (VEGF), fibroblast growth factor (aFGF, bFGF), TGF-β_1, platelet-derived growth factor (PDGF), angiopoietin-1 and thrombospondin-1/2. Studies from our laboratory have shown that a significant number of these factors are released by human cardiac fibroblasts in culture.[28] Using western analysis of human cardiac fibroblast-conditioned medium (CF-CM), we showed that cardiac fibroblasts release VEGF, bFGF, PDGF, TGF-β_1, fibronectin and thrombospondin-1.[28] Cardiac fibroblasts are also the source of matrix metalloproteases (MMPs).[5,6,25] This property points to the role of cardiac fibroblasts in proteolytic mechanisms that are essential in regenerative processes such as endothelial cell migration. Fibronectin is a matrix component with an established role in chemotaxis in several cell–cell interaction systems. Fibronectin fragments released from phorbol ester-stimulated pulmonary endothelial cells promote neutrophil chemotaxis.[29] Cardiac fibroblasts are the cellular source of fibronectin[30] that may provide chemotactic stimuli necessary for endothelial cell migration in the myocardium. Cardiac fibroblasts are also the source of endothelin-1, a trophic factor. Studies utilizing cyclic mechanical stretch have indicated that the stretch-induced hypertrophic effect on cardiac myocytes is mediated by increasing endothelin-1 production by cardiac fibroblasts.[31]

The role of cardiac fibroblasts in vascular regeneration

In most tissues, vascular regeneration is accompanied by malignancies. In the heart, however, vascular regeneration is most desirable. The formation of new

77

collaterals in the infarct zone after myocardial infarction could improve vascular supply and protect the myocardium from ischemic injury. New collaterals can sprout from pre-existing microvasculature by the process of 'angiogenesis' or they can evolve from existing coronary anastomoses.[32] Angiogenesis necessitates a sequence of complex and precisely programmed events that regulate biological responses of endothelial cells. These events include the release of MMPs by endothelial cells, degradation of basement membrane, proliferation and migration of endothelial cells into the surrounding tissue and, finally, reconstruction of matrix and assembly of endothelial cells into capillary tubes.[32,33] Until recently, the effects of cardiac fibroblasts with direct impact on endothelial cell biology and on the process of angiogenesis remained, for the most part, unexplored. Although studies in three-dimensional gels had shown that cardiac fibroblasts regulate the in vitro sprouting of vascular endothelial cells,[34] the mechanisms by which cardiac fibroblasts may regulate specific steps of angiogenesis were not determined. The results of a recent study from our laboratory (described below) clearly demonstrated that human cardiac fibroblasts, via their soluble factors and the extracellular matrix, could indeed regulate distinct stages of angiogenesis, including proliferation, migration and differentiation of human endothelial cells.[28]

The effect of soluble factors on the proliferation capacity of human endothelial cells

Human umbilical vein endothelial cells (HUVECs), when incubated with cardiac fibroblast-conditioned medium (CF-CM), showed a significant increase in DNA synthesis as determined by [^{3}H-]thymidine incorporation.[28] This effect was dependent on de novo protein synthesis and activation of MAP kinases. Consistently, CF-CM induced the expression and activation of MAP kinase ERK2 in HUVEC. The stimulatory effect of CF-CM from which heparin-binding proteins were removed was significantly enhanced compared to that of 'whole CF-CM'. The individual immunodepletion of VEGF, bFGF, aFGF, PDGF, fibronectin and TGF-β_1 from 'whole CF-CM' showed that all factors were necessary for full activity. Our results also showed that an important role of soluble factors released by cardiac fibroblasts appears to be the protection of endothelial cells against hypoxia. This notion was supported by data demonstrating that, in addition to stimulation of DNA synthesis under normal conditions of cell culture, CF-CM caused a significant reversal of hypoxia-induced inhibition of DNA synthesis in HUVEC.[28] Furthermore, CF-CM caused an enhancement in the expression of survival-associated protein, Bcl$_2$, in HUVECs. In summary, these data established that cardiac fibroblasts release an ensemble of factors, the net effect of which is an enhancement of DNA synthesis in endothelial cells. Furthermore, soluble factors released by cardiac fibroblasts may play a role in protecting human endothelial cells under hypoxia. Together, these results suggest that cardiac fibroblasts, by releasing an array of growth factors and soluble forms of matrix proteins, may regulate the proliferation capacity of endothelial cells, an important stage of angiogenesis.

Effect of soluble factors and the cardiac fibroblast monolayer on the migration of endothelial cells

In vivo, the migration of endothelial cells within the surrounding tissue depends on complex processes including proteolysis, and a series of path-finding events led by adhesion molecules and chemotactic factors. The activation of MMPs produced locally or by endothelial cells is an essential step in the process of angiogenesis. Since cardiac fibroblasts produce MMPs, we tested the influence of CF-CM and that of the cardiac fibroblast monolayer on the migratory properties of HUVECs in a modified Boyden migration assay. The results showed a significant increase in the number of migratory endothelial cells in the presence of both CF-CM and cardiac fibroblast monolayer compared to the number in the presence of fetal bovine serum (Lei Zhao and Mahboubeh Eghbali-Webb, unpublished data).

Effect of matrix, deposited by cardiac fibroblasts (CF-matrix), on DNA synthesis in HUVECs

In our studies aimed at understanding the effect of cardiac fibroblast matrix (CF-matrix) on the proliferation capacity of endothelial cells, HUVECs were seeded and grown in 'CF-matrix'-coated culture dishes and their DNA synthesis was compared to that in HUVECs seeded on uncoated dishes. The results showed that, unlike soluble factors, the matrix deposited by cardiac fibroblasts decreased the level of DNA synthesis in HUVECs significantly (45%, $P < 0.0001$) (Lei Zhao and Mahboubeh Eghbali-Webb, unpublished data). The presence of a synthetic peptide containing the RGD sequence did not reverse this inhibitory effect but enhanced it (Figure 6.3), suggesting that the matrix interactions with endothelial cells are not via RGD-sensitive α5ß1, αvß3 and α3ß1 integrins.[35] Together, these results demonstrate that the extracellular matrix deposited by cardiac fibroblasts may play an important role in reducing the proliferation capacity of endothelial cells as part of their preparation for subsequent differentiation and tube formation.

Formation of tube-like structures by endothelial cells grown on matrix deposited by cardiac fibroblasts

Because cell proliferation and differentiation are mutually exclusive events, we tested the possibility that the observed inhibition of DNA synthesis by 'CF-matrix' in HUVECs may eventually lead to their differentiation. Cells

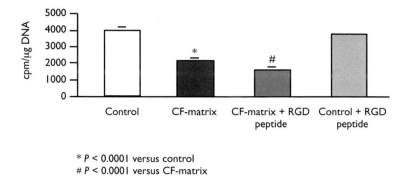

* $P < 0.0001$ versus control
# $P < 0.0001$ versus CF-matrix

Figure 6.3 *Effect of matrix deposited by human cardiac fibroblasts (CF-matrix) on proliferation of human endothelial cells. Human vascular endothelial cells (HUVECs) were seeded and grown in 'CF-matrix'-coated culture dishes and their DNA synthesis, as determined by [³H-]thymidine incorporation, was compared to that in HUVECs seeded on uncoated dishes.*

were seeded on 'CF-matrix' and monitored over a period of 7–10 days in culture. HUVECs grown on 'CF-matrix' demonstrated an elongated arrangement that in most instances resembled tube-like structures (Figure 6.4) (Lei Zhao and Mahboubeh Eghbali-Webb, unpublished data). The endothelial nature of cells in these structures was confirmed by staining the cells with a monoclonal anti-Von Willebrand factor antibody and immunofluorescent light microscopy. All cells in the tube-like structures stained positively with the antibody (Figure 6.4). The tube-like structures were not observed in HUVECs grown in the absence of 'CF-matrix' for a comparable length of time (Figure 6.4).

The role of cardiac fibroblasts in muscle regeneration

Similar to their role in vascular regeneration, cardiac fibroblasts, using their soluble factors and the extracellular matrix, and via a combination of trophic and protective mechanisms, provide permissive conditions of growth and differentiation for cardiac myocytes, and hence regeneration of cardiac muscle. Their most important impact, however, is brought about by their phenotypic plasticity, which allows them to directly enter the myogenic pathways.

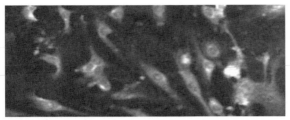

HUVECs grown in the absence of 'CF-matrix'

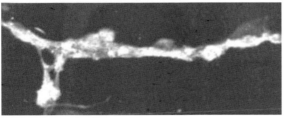

HUVECs grown on 'CF-matrix'

Figure 6.4 *Formation of tube-like structures by endothelial cells grown on matrix deposited by cardiac fibroblasts (CF-matrix). Endothelial cells were visualized by immunofluorescent light microscopy using anti-factor VIII antibody.*

Effects of the extracellular matrix

Based on in vitro findings, there is now significant evidence suggesting the influence of cardiac fibroblasts on growth capacity and survival of cardiac myocytes. Studies in which cardiac myocytes were cultured on a continuous collagen matrix showed that the expression of the tissue-like pattern of organization in cardiac myocytes was dependent on the tertiary structure of the matrix and the extracellular domains of α and ß integrins.[36] These data suggest that phenotypic information is stored within the tertiary structure of the extracellular matrix and is transduced to the myocytes via integrin molecules. In vivo findings demonstrating a coordinated regulation of the expression of integrin molecules and the extracellular matrix during heart development provide additional support for this notion.[37] Recent studies have shown that the effect of extracellular matrix as an inducer of cardiac myocyte growth and differentiation may be exploited in in vitro engineering of heart muscle.[38,39]

Effect of soluble factors

Several studies using co-culture of cardiac fibroblasts and cardiac myocytes, along with those using developing animal heart, have produced compelling evidence in support of the notion that soluble factors released by cardiac fibroblasts exert trophic effects on cardiac myocytes. In one study, co-culture of neonatal cardiac myocytes with cardiac fibroblasts led to enhanced surface area and suppressed beating rate in cardiac myocytes.[40] Both features are associated with the growth and differentiation of cardiac myocytes during development. These data also point to the role that cardiac fibroblasts may play in modulation of cardiac myocyte growth in developing heart.[40] Whether soluble factors of cardiac fibroblasts act directly and/or via mediators is not fully understood. There is, however, significant evidence supporting the role of angiotensin II as an important mediator of trophic effects of cardiac fibroblasts. Such a role was established by co-culture studies in which angiotensin II enhanced the stimulatory effect of cardiac fibroblasts on protein synthesis in cardiac myocytes. Angiotensin II alone, however, did not have the same trophic effect on cardiac myocytes.[41] Later studies showed that angiotensin II induces the release of endothelin-I and TGF-ß$_1$ from cardiac fibroblasts and that endothelin-1 acts in a paracrine fashion as a hypertrophic factor for cardiac myocytes.[42–44] Cardiac fibroblasts express angiotensin II receptors, and it has been shown that, in the embryonic heart, blocking the angiotensin II receptors results in reduced ventricular development.[45] While these findings clearly point to the role of angiotensin II in the early embryonic development of the heart, they also provide strong evidence in support of the role that cardiac fibroblasts, via their angiotensin II system, may play in early cardiac development. The communication between cardiac myocytes and cardiac fibroblasts, via angiotensin II, has been clearly demonstrated by in vivo studies using chimeric mice that have both the homozygous intact and null mutants of the angiotensin A1 receptor.[46] In those studies it was shown that cardiac fibroblasts proliferate in response to local and systemic actions of angiotensin II and that this effect is determined by the angiotensin II receptors located on the neighboring cardiac myocytes. The results also indicated that a communication between cardiac fibroblasts and cardiac myocytes via angiotensin II can play an important role during angiotensin II-dependent ventricular remodeling.[46]

Protective effect of cardiac fibroblasts on cardiac myocytes

In addition to their trophic function, cardiac fibroblasts may also protect cardiac myocytes from injury under stressful conditions. There is mounting evidence demonstrating the resilience of cardiac fibroblasts under environmental stress. For example, although mechanisms of apoptosis in cardiac fibroblasts are not fully understood, it is evident that the extracellular inducers and intracellular mechanisms of apoptosis in cardiac fibroblasts are not similar to those in postmitotic cardiac myocytes. Indeed, concurrent apoptosis of cardiac myocytes and enhanced proliferation of cardiac fibroblasts in failing heart is a clear demonstration of differential responses of both cell types under identical environmental stimuli. This effect is best shown by studies demonstrating that, while superoxide induces apoptosis in cardiac myocytes, it causes proliferation and expression of TGF-ß in cardiac fibroblasts.[47] Another example is the response of cardiac fibroblasts to hypoxia, a known inducer of apoptosis in cardiac myocytes.[48] We showed that although hypoxia diminishes both protein synthesis and proliferation in human cardiac fibroblasts, it fails to induce DNA fragmentation and morphologic criteria of apoptosis in those cells.[26] Others have also reported the lack of hypoxia-induced expression of apoptosis-associated transcription factor, p53, in cardiac fibroblasts.[48] Our separate studies, however, have shown that hypoxia indeed induces p53 in cardiac fibroblasts but in a gender-specific manner.[49] Similar to hypoxia, a specific inhibitor of vacuolar proton ATPase that induces apoptosis in cardiac myocytes failed to induce apoptosis in cardiac fibroblasts.[50] Oxidative stress also causes greater injury and cell death in cardiac myocytes than in cardiac fibroblasts. It is suggested that the signaling differences via mitogen-activated protein kinases may partly mediate the observed differences in vulnerability.[51] Together, these findings demonstrate the resilience of cardiac fibroblasts under environmental stress and suggest that they have the potential to protect the fragile cardiac myocytes via, perhaps, stimulation of compensatory mechanisms. In support of this notion, studies in our laboratory showed that, while the beating rate of cardiac myocytes decreases under hypoxia, the presence of cardiac fibroblast-conditioned medium prevents the hypoxia-induced inhibition of beating rate (A. Agocha and M. Eghbali-Webb, unpublished data). Similarly, neonatal cardiac fibroblasts have been shown to restore the hypothermia-induced decreased beating rate in cardiac myocytes.[52] In addition, the release of creatine phosphokinase and lactate dehydrogenase from cardiac myocytes in response to hypothermia was significantly lower in the presence of cardiac fibroblasts.[52] These data, in turn, suggest a role for cardiac fibroblasts in protection of cardiac myocytes during hypothermic conditions of pre-transplant preservation of cardiac tissue.

Phenotypic plasticity of cardiac fibroblasts

The mechanisms governing the growth of cardiac muscle in postnatal periods remain vastly unclear. Although the precise pathways through which terminal differentiation of cardiac fibroblasts into cardiac myocytes is possible are yet to be identified, mounting evidence demonstrating their transformation into cells with characteristic features of myocytes provides strong support for the notion that cardiac fibroblasts, as a result of their phenotypic plasticity, have the potential to enter into the myogenic pathways. Earlier studies from our laboratory showed that cardiac fibroblasts, when exposed to TGF-ß$_1$, display

83

phenotypic features characteristic of cardiac myocytes.[11] The determination that such phenotypic modulation occurs was based on: appearance of morphologic features characteristic of cardiac myocytes in TGF-ß$_1$-treated cells; induction of sarcomeric actin mRNA and sarcomeric actin filaments in TGF-ß$_1$-treated cells; disappearance of intermediate filament vimentin following treatment with TGF-ß$_1$; and continued expression of muscle-specific morphologic features and sarcomeric actin filaments in the second generation of cells stemmed from TGF-ß$_1$-treated cells, even in the absence of TGF-ß$_1$. While expression of sarcomeric actin mRNA and appearance of sarcomeric actin filaments in cardiac fibroblasts could be attributed to the regulatory effects of TGF-ß$_1$ on actin gene expression, the loss of vimentin filaments in TGF-ß$_1$-treated cells combined with their altered morphology is an indication of phenotypic modulation. This effect of TGF-ß$_1$ on cardiac fibroblasts is cardiac-specific, because it was not induced in skin fibroblasts and NIH 3T3 cells. Furthermore, other factors to which cardiac fibroblasts are naturally exposed did not produce the same effect.[11] More recent studies by other investigators have confirmed phenotypic transformation of cardiac fibroblasts and also shown that, during their transformation, TGF-ß$_1$ induces angiotensin-converting enzyme synthesis in cardiac fibroblasts.[53] Furthermore, the transformation of cardiac fibroblasts is also characterized by stimulation of collagen production.[54] Whether these in vitro findings are translated into in vivo effects depends on the effects of TGF-ß$_1$ in the context of antagonistic and/or cooperative effects of other growth factors and hormones in vivo. In addition to factor-induced transformation, phenotypic plasticity in cardiac fibroblasts is also shown to be associated with developmental stage and their regional distribution in the heart. Differences in proliferation and collagen synthesis in cardiac fibroblasts obtained from epicardium versus atrioventricular valves in developing chick myocardium have been reported.[55] It is suggested that these differences were caused by the impact of the microenvironment.[55] Also, two subsets of cardiac fibroblasts, isolated from ventricular tissue, differed in their growth rate, angiotensin II receptor and angiotensin II responsiveness. These differences were also attributed to differences in phenotype.[56] Another example of phenotypic plasticity in cardiac fibroblasts is the reduced proliferation of neonatal cardiac fibroblasts in the postnatal period that is also associated with the expression of insulin-like growth factor receptors.[57]

Summary and future directions

Cardiac fibroblasts are multifunctional and resilient cells that provide an ensemble of environmental factors, including extracellular matrix, growth factors, MMPs and cytokines that are necessary for cell growth, proliferation and differentiation in the myocardium. Their trophic effects on cardiac myocytes via extracellular matrix and the soluble factors have been established. Most importantly, their established phenotypic plasticity and predisposition to transform into cells with features characteristic of cardiac myocytes point to the possibility of their direct participation in myogenic pathways. In addition to their role in myogenesis, their effects on several stages of angiogenesis, including proliferation, migration and tube formation by endothelial cells, have been established. These effects strongly support the notion that cardiac fibroblasts are actively involved in regeneration of vasculature. The diversity of factors produced by cardiac fibroblasts and the wide spectrum of their effects point to their unique potential in providing a balanced microenvironment that could not be otherwise maintained by any single biological factor. Future studies must now determine whether cardiac fibroblasts can be used as stem cells in cell therapy and if their transplantation into an infarct zone may provide a microenvironment conducive to the growth of cardiac myocytes and outgrowth of new microvasculature from pre-existing vessels. The use of cardiac fibroblasts in cell therapy aimed at alleviation of myocardial diseases may prove to be a preferred strategy compared with the use of other cells. We have shown that human cardiac fibroblasts can be obtained and grown from biopsy specimens.[58] Therefore, patients at risk for myocardial infarction can provide samples in advance for subsequent propagation of their own cardiac fibroblasts. Those cells can then be preserved under liquid nitrogen for future autograft when needed. This process eliminates the risk of immunologic complications associated with the use of foreign tissues or proteins.

References

1. Eghbali M, Czaja MJ, Zeydel M et al. Collagen mRNAs in isolated adult heart cell. J Mol Cell Cardiol 1988; 20: 267–76.

2. Eghbali M, Blumenfeld OO, Seifter S et al. Localization of types I, III and IV collagen mRNAs in rat heart cells by in situ hybridization. J Mol Cell Cardiol 1989; 21: 103–13.

3. Long CS, Henrich CJ, Simpson PC. A growth factor for cardiac myocytes is produced by cardiac non-myocytes. Cell Regul 1991; 2: 1081–95.

4. Eghbali M. Cellular origin and distribution of transforming growth factor β_1 in the normal rat myocardium. Cell Tiss Res 1991; 265: 553–8.

5.   Tomek RJ, Rimar S, Eghbali-Webb M. Nicotine regulates collagen gene expression, collagenase activity, and DNA synthesis in cultured cardiac fibroblasts. Mol Cell Biochem 1994; 136: 97–103.

6.   Chua CC, Chua BH, Zhao ZY et al. Effect of growth factors on collagen metabolism in cultured human heart fibroblasts. Connective Tiss Res 1991; 26: 271–81.

7.   Tsuruda T, Kato J, Kitamura K et al. An autocrine or a paracrine role of adrenomeduline in modulating cardiac fibroblast growth. Cardiovasc Res 1999; 43: 958–67.

8.   Robinson TF, Cohen-Gould L, Factor SM et al. Structure and function of connective tissue in cardiac muscle: collagen type III in endomysial struts and pericellular fibers. Scanning Microsc 1988; 2: 1005–15.

9.   Sigel VA, Centrella M, Eghbali-Webb M. Regulation of proliferative response of cardiac fibroblasts by transforming growth factor-β_1. J Mol Cell Cardiol 1996; 28: 1921–9.

10. Eghbali M, Tomek R, Sukhatme VP et al. Differential effects of transforming growth factor-β_1 and phorbol myristate acetate on cardiac fibroblasts: regulation of fibrillar collagen mRNAs and expression of early transcription factors. Circ Res 1991; 69: 483–90.

11. Eghbali M, Tomek R, Woods C, Bhambi B. Cardiac fibroblasts are predisposed to convert into myocyte phenotype: specific effects of transforming growth factor-beta. Proc Natl Acad Sci USA 1991; 88: 795–9.

12. Yao J, Eghbali M. Decreased collagen gene expression and absence of fibrosis in thyroid hormone-induced myocardial hypertrophy: response of cardiac fibroblasts to thyroid hormone in vitro. Circ Res 1992; 71: 831–9.

13. Lee H-W, Klein LE, Raser J, Eghbali-Webb M. An activator protein-1 (AP-1) response element on pro α_1(l) collagen gene is necessary for thyroid hormone-induced inhibition of promoter activity in cardiac fibroblasts. J Mol Cell Cardiol 1998; 30: 2495–506.

14. Klein LE, Sigel VA, Douglas JA, Eghbali-Webb M. Up-regulation of collagen type I gene expression in the ventricular myocardium of thyroidectomized rats of both genders. J Mol Cell Cardiol 1996; 28: 33–42.

15. Yao J, Eghbali M. Decreased collagen mRNA and regression of cardiac fibrosis in the ventricular myocardium of the tight skin mouse following thyroid hormone treatment. Cardiovasc Res 1992; 26: 603–7.

16. Tsutsumi Y, Matsubara H, Ohkubo N et al. Angiotensin II type 2 receptor is upregulated in human heart with interstitial fibrosis, and cardiac fibroblasts are the major cell type for its expression. Circ Res 1998; 83: 1035–46.

17. Ohkubo N, Matsubara H, Nozawa Y et al. Angiotensin type 2 receptors are reexpressed by cardiac fibroblasts from failing myopathic hamster hearts and inhibit cell growth and fibrillar collagen metabolism. Circulation 1997; 96: 3954–62.

18. Shinohara T, Shimizu M, Yoshio H et al. Collagen synthesis by cultured cardiac fibroblasts obtained from cardiomyopathic hamsters. Jpn Heart J 1998; 39: 97–108.

19. Yu H, Gallagher AM, Garfin PM, Printz MP. Prostacyclin release by rat cardiac fibroblasts: inhibition of collagen expression. Hypertension 1997; 30: 1047–53.

20. Nunohiro T, Ashizawa N, Graf K et al. Angiotensin II promotes integrin-mediated collagen gel contraction by adult rat cardiac fibroblasts. Jpn Heart J 1999; 40: 461–9.

21. MacKenna DA, Dolfi F, Vuori K, Ruoslahti E. Extracellular signal-regulated kinase and c-jun NH2-terminal kinase activation by mechanical stretch is integrin-dependent and matrix-specific in rat cardiac fibroblasts. J Clin Invest 1998; 101: 301–10.

22. Gudi SR, Lee AA, Clark CB, Frangos JA. Equibiaxial strain and strain rate stimulate early activation of G proteins in cardiac fibroblasts. Am J Physiol 1998; 274: C1424–8.

23. MacKenna D, Summerour SR, Villarreal FJ. Role of mechanical factors in modulating cardiac fibroblast function and extracellular matrix synthesis. Cardiovasc Res 2000; 46: 257–63.

24. Carver W, Nagpal ML, Nachtigal M et al. Collagen expression in mechanically stimulated cardiac fibroblasts. Circ Res 1991; 69: 116–22.

25. Tyagi SC, Lewis K, Pikes D et al. Stretch-induced membrane type matrix metalloproteinase and tissue plasminogen activator in cardiac fibroblast cells. J Cell Physiol 1998; 176: 374–82.

26. Agocha A, Eghbali-Webb M. Hypoxia regulates DNA synthesis and collagen type I production in human cardiac fibroblasts: effects of transforming growth factor-beta$_1$, thyroid hormone, angiotensin II and basic fibroblast growth factor. J Mol Cell Cardiol 1997; 29: 2233–44.

27. Tamamori M, Ito H, Hiroe M et al. Stimulation of collagen synthesis in rat cardiac fibroblasts by exposure to hypoxic culture conditions and suppression of the effect of natriuretic peptides. Cell Biol Int 1997; 21: 175–80.

28. Zhao L, Eghbali-Webb M. Release of pro- and anti-angiogenic factors by human cardiac fibroblasts: effects on DNA synthesis in human endothelial cells. Biochim Biophys Acta 2001; 1538: 273–82.

29. Odekon LE, Frewin MB, Del Vechio P et al. Fibronectin fragments released from phorbol ester-stimulated pulmonary artery endothelial cell monolayers promote neutrophil chemotaxis. Immunology 1991; 74: 114–20.

30. Zeydel M, Puglia K, Eghbali M et al. Heart fibroblasts of adult rats: properties and relation to deposition of collagen. Cell Tissue Res 1991; 265: 353–9.

31. Harada M, Saito Y, Nakagawa O et al. Role of cardiac nonmyocytes in cyclic mechanical stretch-induced myocyte hypertrophy. Heart Vessels Suppl 1998; 12: 198–200.

32. Risau W. Mechanisms of angiogenesis. Nature 1997; 386: 671–4.

33. Stetler-Stevenson WG. Matrix metalloproteases in angiogenesis: a moving target for therapeutic intervention. J Clin Invest 1999; 103: 1237–41.

34. Nehls V, Herrmann R, Huhnken M, Palmetshofer A. Contact-dependent inhibition of angiogenesis by cardiac fibroblasts in three-dimensional fibrin gels in vitro: implications for microvascular network remodeling and coronary collateral formation. Cell Tissue Res 1998; 293: 479–88.

35. Romanov VI, Goligorsky MS. RGD-recognizing integrins mediate interactions of human prostate carcinoma cells with endothelial cells in vitro. Prostate 1999; 39: 108–18.

36. Simpson DG, Terracio L, Terracio M et al. Modulation of cardiac myocyte phenotype in vitro by the composition and orientation of the extracellular matrix. J Cell Physiol 1994; 161: 89–105.

37. Carver W, Price RL, Raso DS et al. Distribution of beta-1 integrin in the developing rat heart. J Histochem Cytochem 1994; 42: 167–75.

38. Zimmermann WH, Schneiderbanger K, Schubert P et al. Tissue engineering of a differentiated cardiac muscle construct. Circ Res 2002; 90: 223–30.

39. Kofidis T, Akhyari P, Boublik J et al. In vitro engineering of heart muscle: artificial myocardial tissue. J Thorac Cardiovasc Surg 2002; 124: 63–9.

40. Orita H, Fukasawa M, Hirooka S et al. Modulation of cardiac myocyte beating rate and hypertrophy by cardiac fibroblasts isolated from neonatal rat ventricle. Jap Circ J, English Ed 1993; 57: 912–20.

41. Kim NN, Villarreal FJ, Printz MP et al. Trophic effects of angiotensin II on neonatal rat cardiac myocytes are mediated by cardiac fibroblasts. Am J Physiol 1995; 269: E426–37.

42. Lee AA, Dillmann WH, McCulloch AD, Villarreal FJ. Angiotensin II stimulates the autocrine production of transforming growth factor-beta 1 in adult rat cardiac fibroblasts. J Mol Cell Cardiol 1995; 27: 2347–57.

43. Gray MO, Long CS, Kalinyak JE et al. Angiotensin II stimulates cardiac myocyte hypertrophy via paracrine release of TGF-beta 1 and endothelin-1 from fibroblasts. Cardiovasc Res 1998; 40: 352–63.

44. Harada M, Itoh H, Nakagawa O et al. Significance of ventricular myocytes and nonmyocytes interaction during cardiocyte hypertrophy: evidence for endothelin-1 as a paracrine hypertrophic factor from cardiac nonmyocytes. Circulation 1997; 96: 3737–44.

45. Price RL, Carver W, Simpson DG et al. The effects of angiotensin II and specific angiotensin receptor blockers on embryonic cardiac development and looping patterns. Dev Biol 1997; 192: 527–84.

46. Matsusaka T, Katori H, Inagami T et al. Communication between myocytes and fibroblasts in cardiac remodeling in angiotensin chimeric mice. J Clin Invest 1999; 103: 1451–8.

47. Li PF, Dietz R, von Harsdorf R. Superoxide induces apoptosis in cardiomyocytes, but proliferation and expression of transforming growth factor-beta1 in cardiac fibroblasts. FEBS Lett 1999; 448: 206–10.

48. Long X, Boluyt MO, Hipolito ML et al. p53 and the hypoxia-induced apoptosis of cultured neonatal rat cardiac myocytes. J Clin Invest 1997; 99: 2635–43.

49. Zhao X, Eghbali-Webb M. Gender-related differences in basal and hypoxia-induced activation of signal transduction pathways controlling cell cycle progression and apoptosis in cardiac fibroblasts. Endocrine 2002; 18: 137–45.

50. Long X, Crow MT, Sollott SJ et al. Enhanced expression of p53 and apoptosis induced by blockade of the vacuolar proton ATPase in cardiomyocytes. J Clin Invest 1998; 101: 1453–61.

51. Zhang X, Azhar G, Nagano K, Wei JY. Differential vulnerability to oxidative stress in rat cardiac myocytes versus fibroblasts. J Am Coll Cardiol 2001; 38: 2055–62.

52. Orita H, Fukasawa M, Hirooka S et al. Protection of cardiac myocytes from hypothermic injury by cardiac fibroblasts isolated from neonatal rat ventricle. J Surg Res 1993; 5: 654–8.

53. Petrov VV, Fagard RH, Lijnen PJ. Transforming growth factor-beta(1) induces angiotensin-converting enzyme synthesis in rat cardiac fibroblasts during their differentiation to myofibroblasts. J Renin Angiotensin Aldosterone Syst 2000; 1: 342–52.

54. Lijnen P, Petrov V. Transforming growth factor-beta 1-induced collagen production in culture of cardiac fibroblasts is the result of appearance of myofibroblasts. Methods Find Exp Clin Pharmacol 2002; 24: 333–44.

55. Choy M, Oltjen S, Ratcliff D, Armstrong P. Fibroblast behavior in the embryonic chick heart. Develop Dynam 1993; 198: 97–107.

56. Klett CP, Palmer AA, Dirig DM et al. Evidence for differences in cultured left ventricular fibroblast populations isolated from spontaneously hypertensive and Wistar-Kyoto rats. J Hypertens 1995; 13: 1421–31.

57. Reiss K, Cheng W, Kajstura J et al. Fibroblast proliferation during myocardial development in rats is regulated by IGF-1 receptors. Am J Physiol 1995; 269: H943–51.

58. Agocah E, Eghbali-Webb M. A simple method for preparation of cultured cardiac fibroblasts from adult human ventricular tissue. Mol Cell Biochem 1997; 172: 195–8.

7. Transplantation of Satellite Cells for Myocardial Regeneration

Race L Kao

Despite the precipitous drop in death rates from heart attacks and strokes during the past decades, cardiovascular disease still exceeds all other causes of death in the USA. It is estimated that 12.6 million Americans alive today have coronary heart disease and more than one million people will suffer a heart attack every year. Restoring bloodflow, improving perfusion, reducing clinical symptoms and augmenting ventricular function are the common treatments after acute myocardial infarction. With longer life-expectancy for the US population, a further increase is anticipated for cardiovascular disease. Other than replacing the whole heart (cardiac transplantation), no standard clinical procedure is available to restore or regenerate the damaged myocardium following a heart attack.

Adult mammalian ventricular myocytes lack regenerative capability, so an injured heart is normally repaired by scar formation, hypertrophy of surviving myocytes and hyperplasia of non-muscle cells. Recently, the possible existence of stem cells or progenitor cells for myocardium has been suggested; however, it is clear that functionally significant myocardial regeneration has not been documented in diseased or injured heart. The contribution of other cells to the formation of ventricular myocytes appears to be negligible, as evidenced by the consistent formation of scar after myocardial infarction. Satellite cells are adult stem cells responsible for growth, repair and maintenance of homeostasis of skeletal muscle. We have been using autologous satellite cells for myocardial regeneration since 1989 in dogs and we applied this procedure to patients in 2001.

Satellite cells

Since the identification of satellite cells in skeletal muscle in 1961,[1] satellite cells have been confirmed as myogenic precursor cells responsible for growth, repair and adaptation to the physiologic demands of skeletal muscle.[2,3] Satellite cells of normal adult skeletal muscle are mitotically quiescent and located under the basal lamina but outside the sarcolemma of individual muscle fibers

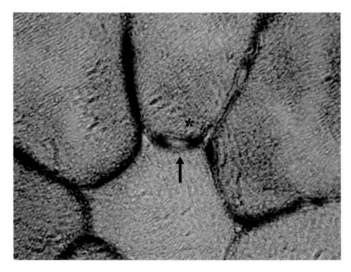

Figure 7.1
Satellite cell (➤)
associated with a
muscle fiber (*)
located under the
basal lamina but
outside the
sarcolemma in
canine skeletal
muscle. Original
magnification
×800.

(Figure 7.1). Satellite cells are found in skeletal muscle samples obtained from all ages and species of normal mammals. The spindle-shaped satellite cell is about $25 \times 5\,\mu m$, and contains a heterochromatic nucleus and scanty cytoplasm with few organelles. The cytoplasm is dominated by large quantities of free ribosomes with small amounts of rough endoplasmic reticulum. After activation, satellite cells produce myogenic progenitor cells which undergo several rounds of cell division before fusing with existing muscle fibers or forming new muscle fibers before complete terminal differentiation.

Shortly after birth, the number of muscle cells in growing skeletal muscle ceases to increase and the number of muscle fibers remains relatively constant during one's lifetime. Normal muscle growth takes place through increases in the length and diameter of the existing muscle fibers. Accompanying this increase in muscle mass is a 2–4-fold increase in the number of muscle nuclei. Because true muscle nuclei are postmitotic, these additional nuclei are derived from the multiplication and differentiation of satellite cells. Radioautographic studies reveal that the dividing satellite cells are able to fuse with the existing muscle fibers and provide new myonuclei during growth. Satellite cells regenerate injured skeletal muscle by repairing surviving fibers and/or by forming new fibers.[2,3]

Muscle stem cells are cells that do not express markers of muscle differentiation (myogenic regulatory factors, desmin, etc.) but are able to produce both new muscle stem cells (i.e. self-renewal) and progeny destined to become myoblasts and myofibers. The muscle satellite cell appears to fulfill many of the criteria demanded of a stem cell, such as clonogenicity, self-renewal and production of differentiated progeny.[4–6] Although satellite cells have been considered as monopotential stem cells, recent in vivo and in vitro studies clearly indicate that satellite cells from adult mammalian skeletal muscle are multipotential stem cells. Satellite cells isolated from adult mice possess multipotential mesenchymal stem cell activity and are capable of forming osteocytes, adipocytes and myocytes.[7] The plasticity of adult stem cells has been well summarized in review papers.[8,9]

Recent studies have identified a subpopulation of multipotential stem cells called side-population (SP) cells, obtained from adult skeletal muscle preparations using methods to isolate and culture satellite cells. The muscle-derived SP cells are isolated from satellite cells by fluorescence-activated cell sorting (FACS) based on Hoechst dye exclusion. The SP cells derived from muscle exhibit the capacity of hematopoietic stem cells and myogenic stem cells.[10] These putative stem cells may be identical to muscle satellite cells and lack the hematopoietic marker CD45. Satellite cell preparations contain heterogeneous cells; whether a subpopulation of cells or certain stem cells are responsible for the success of myocardial regeneration is under current investigation.

Labeling of cultured satellite cells

To identify the muscle cells formed from transplanted satellite cells at the site of injured myocardium, it is necessary to have long-term stable labeling of cells with high intensity and specificity. Satellite cells that have been enriched by and have proliferated in culture (Figure 7.2a) can be labeled with 0.49-μm fluorescent microspheres (Polyscience Inc., Warrington, PA, USA) or [³H]thymidine, as reported in our earlier studies.[11–16] Cultured satellite cells can form multinucleated myotubes (Figure 7.2b) under differentiation conditions, which clearly indicates the myogenic potential of the cells. The thymidine analogue 5-bromo-2'-deoxyuridine (BrdU) has been used to label the dividing cells in several recent investigations.[17] The advantage of BrdU is the immediate revealing of its incorporation after antibody application (without the need for radioautography). A fluorescent stain, 4', 6-diamidino-2-phenylindole (DAPI), has been used to visualize DNA in living and fixed cells. After exposure to DAPI (1 μg/ml) for 24h, the labeling efficiency for satellite cells is outstanding (Figure 7.2c) without detectable damage after 6 weeks in culture.[18,19] The advantages of DAPI are the high efficiency of labeling and the ability to detect the viable labeled cells under the fluorescent microscope. Dialkylcarbocyanine (DiI) and other membrane markers (Molecular Probes, Inc., Eugene, OR, USA) have also been used to label the cells with success. The disadvantage of all these labeling procedures is the

93

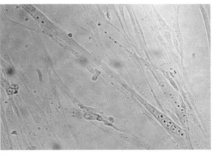
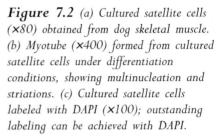

a   b

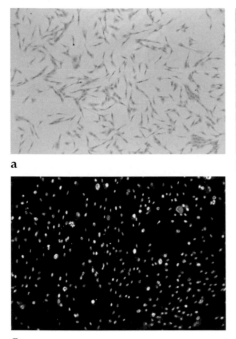

Figure 7.2 (a) Cultured satellite cells (×80) obtained from dog skeletal muscle. (b) Myotube (×400) formed from cultured satellite cells under differentiation conditions, showing multinucleation and striations. (c) Cultured satellite cells labeled with DAPI (×100); outstanding labeling can be achieved with DAPI.

c

loss of labeling intensity as the cell divides (assuming equal division into daughter cells, 50% lower intensity for each cell cycle). Therefore, better labeling methods have been established in our laboratory.

The *lacZ* gene, which encodes ß-galactosidase in *Escherichia coli* is a commonly used reporter gene in molecular biology. The mammalian reporter vector pCMVß can be purchased from Clontech Laboratory Inc. (Palo Alto, CA, USA) and the lipofectamine reagent can be obtained from Gibco BRL (Gaithersburg, MD, USA). Very good labeling of cultured cells has been achieved by this procedure, and satellite cell proliferation or differentiation has not been affected by *lacZ* transfection.[11,18,19] Myocardial infarction alone can also produce ß-galactosidase staining, and *lacZ* labeling lacks specificity. However, the endogenous ß-galactosidase activity of eukaryotic cells is not detectable at higher pH (≥ 7.0), while the prokaryotic (*E. coli*) enzyme can be measured.[20] Therefore, if *lacZ* is used to label the cells, an X-gal reaction should be performed at pH ≥ 7.0 with a reaction time of 3–4 h to prevent false-positive results. Green fluorescent protein (GFP) is a 238 amino acid, 28-kDa protein with remarkable resistance to physicochemical denaturing conditions. The fluorescence properties of GFP have been extensively studied, and GFP has been demonstrated to be an efficient biological marker.

LacZ, nuclear targeted *lacZ*, nuclear targeted GFP, AdenoLacZ, and

AdenoGFP have been used for labeling satellite cells to compare their labeling efficiency and to follow them for 8 weeks[19] (normally, 6 weeks are needed for satellite cells to form myocytes in the injured heart). Although nuclear targeted *lacZ* and GFP have higher specificities of labeling, the low efficiency of labeling prohibited their selection. AdenoLacZ and AdenoGFP both have excellent labeling efficiency and retain the label for 8 weeks in cultured cells. However, the existence of endogenous ß-galactosidase in eukaryotic cells and the need to fix the cells before the X-gal reaction are limitations to the use of AdenoLacZ.

Satellite cells labeled with AdenoGFP can be observed in living cells and do not interfere with their proliferation or differentiation capabilities. However, AdenoGFP cannot be used for long-term in vivo studies, due to the strong inflammatory reactions and expression of viral proteins. The helper-free adeno-associated virus containing humanized Renilla GFP (AAV-hrGFP), purchased from Stratagene (La Jolla, CA, USA) has all the advantages of AdenoGFP plus the non-toxicity of hrGFP and long-term stable in vivo expression. AAV-hrGFP was selected for our study, with excellent outcomes (Figure 7.3). In addition, retrovirus and lentivirus can be used to label the cells. The Y chromosome is an endogenous cell marker with high specificity; however, inbred or syngeneic animals must be used to avoid rejection. All of the labeling procedures are compared in Table 7.1.

Table 7.1 Comparison of labeling procedures

Compound	Dividing cells	Non-dividing cells	Efficiency of labeling	Long-term labeling
Microsphere	+	+	±	−
[³H]Thymidine	+	−	−	−
BrdU	+	−	−	−
DAPI	+	+	+	−
DiI	+	+	±	−
Liposome	+	+	−	−
Adenovirus	+	+	+	−
AAV	+	+	+	+
Retrovirus	+	−	±	±
Lentivirus	+	+	+	+
Y chromosome	+	+	+	+

BrdU, 5-bromo-2′-deoxyuridine; DAPI, 4′,6-diamidino-2-phenylindole; DiI, dialkylcarbocyanine; AAV, adeno-associated virus.
+, yes or high; ±, medium; −, no or low.

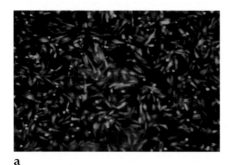

a

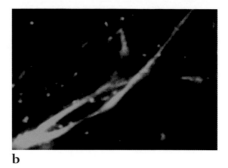

b

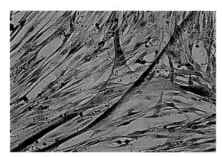

c

Figure 7.3 *AAV-hrGFP-labeled satellite cells (a) (×100) and formation of multinucleated myotubes under differentiation conditions viewed under the fluorescent (b) (×200) and light (c) (×200) microscope.*

Injury of the heart and satellite cell implantation

It is necessary to have a reproducible animal model of cardiac injury that simulates clinical conditions for the study of myocardial regeneration. Cardiac cryolesions that were described many years ago healed into a fibrous scar with little disruption of the surrounding tissue. This method produced an injury of well-controlled size and location with a sharp visual demarcation between damaged and normal tissue. Cryoinjury to the heart was selected for the initial satellite cell implantation study,[11–16] because of the advantage of total destruction of muscle cells in the injured myocardium. Since cryoinjury did not entirely mimic a clinical infarct, an ischemic model was developed to better simulate the heart attack condition.

Owing to the rich collateral bloodflow in dog myocardium, obstruction of both arterial and venous flow was necessary to develop a consistent and reliable myocardial infarction. The left anterior descending coronary artery (LAD) and vein were occluded for 4h before reperfusion. The site of occlusion was just below the first branch of the LAD at a distance about two-thirds from the apex of the heart. The lack of myocardial perfusion after coronary occlusion was further documented by using isolated heart perfused with buffer containing Evans blue under Langendorff preparation.[18] The site of coronary occlusion and the location of the flow probe, ultrasound crystals and

96

Millar pressure transducers (Millar Instruments, Inc., Houston, TX, USA) are shown in Figure 7.4. The computerized Crystal Biotech VF-1 hemodynamic system (Data Science Int., St Paul, MN, USA) was used to integrate the pressure, bloodflow, contractility and systolic wall thickening fraction of each cardiac cycle. A flow probe placed below the ligation site of the LAD confirmed the drastic reduction in coronary flow (normal flow 53 ± 2.6 ml/min; during occlusion 1.4 ± 0.3 ml/min) after coronary occlusion. The ischemic myocardium was easily identified by its cyanosis and hypokinesis.

The ischemic area was visually divided into 30–40 0.25-cm^2 areas before 0.1 ml (containing approximately one million cells) of the labeled autologous satellite cells were injected at the center of each area. In total, 30 million to 40 million satellite cells were grafted into the myocardial infarction through a 25-gauge hypodermic needle (a needle smaller than 25-gauge can cause significant damage to the isolated satellite cells). Serum-free culture medium was injected into the control heart by the same procedure. Electrocardiograms (Figure 7.5) were recorded using the PageWriter Cardiograph and showed typical ST elevation or depression during ischemia. For the control dogs, ST depression was observed at 6 weeks after the

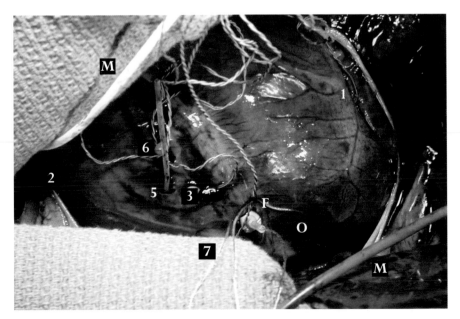

Figure 7.4 Instrumentation in the canine heart for hemodynamic measurement, showing Millar pressure transducers (M), flow probe (F), site of occlusion (O) and ultrasound crystals (1–7). The ultrasound crystal 4 is located under the heart directly opposite to crystal 3.

97

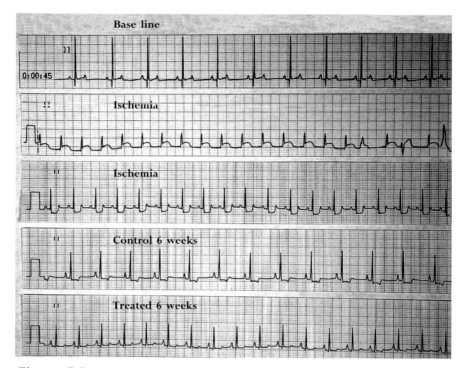

Figure 7.5 Electrocardiograms obtained before coronary occlusion (Baseline), during coronary occlusion (Ischemia) and at 6 weeks after the procedure for animals treated with culture medium (Control) or satellite cells (Treated). Clear ST elevation or depression was observed during Ischemia, and only Treated animals had normal electrocardiograms.

procedure, while a normal electrocardiogram was restored in the cell-implanted dogs. Echocardiographs before and after coronary occlusion also showed significant depression of contractility (Figure 7.6) and further supported the validity of our animal model. Ejection fraction, percentage thickening fraction and fractional shortening were all significantly decreased during ischemia, but returned to normal levels only in satellite cell-implanted animals during termination. Left ventricular end diastolic diameter was significantly increased during ischemia and returned to baseline value in treated animals but not in the control dogs.

Myocardial regeneration

At 1 day to 14 weeks after myocardial injury and satellite cell implantation, dogs were sacrificed under general anesthesia. Each heart was perfused

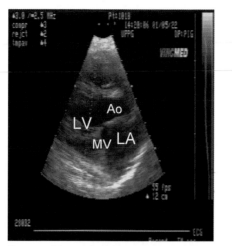

Parasternal long-axis view

Parasternal short-axis view

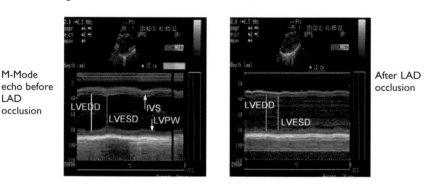

M-Mode echo before LAD occlusion

After LAD occlusion

Figure 7.6 *Echocardiographs of dog heart before and after coronary occlusion. Ejection fraction, percentage thickening fraction, fractional shorting and left ventricular end systolic and diastolic dimensions were obtained from echocardiographs.*

through the aortic root with 4°C cardioplegic solution at a pressure of 150 mmHg before being cut into slices, and samples were obtained for frozen sections, paraffin sections and ultrathin sections. Labeled cells were identified at the sites of injections and gradually filled the needle tracts and diffused out of the initial injection sites in the myocardium after cell implantation. Multiple areas of necrotic myocardium were surrounded and infiltrated by labeled tissue at a later date. By 6 weeks, neomyocardium with clear labeling mixed with some fibrous tissue (scar) was observed for the cell-implanted dogs[18] while dense scars were found for the control animals (Figure 7.7). The maintenance of normal morphology, with labeled cells replacing the scar tissue, was found for the treated animals. Thinning of the ventricular wall with massive dense scar tissue was observed for the control dogs. Immunohistologic, histologic and ultrastructural evaluations indicated the presence of viable muscle cells with clear labeling and aligned parallel with the host cardiac myocytes from cell-implanted animals.[18] The labeled muscle cells showed intercalated disks and gap junctions between the muscle cells and cardiac myocytes.

During ischemic insult, the systolic thickening fraction was significantly impaired. At 6 weeks after ischemic injury and satellite cell implantation, the

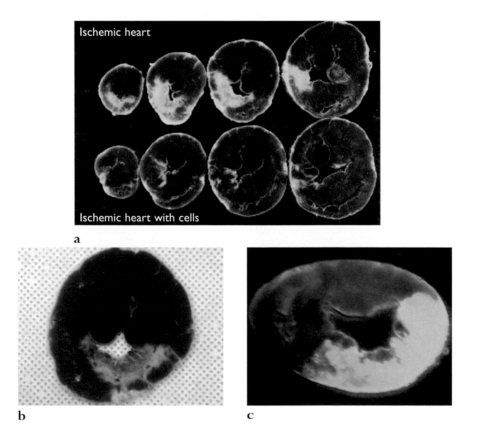

Figure 7.7 *Ventricular slices of canine myocardium at 6 weeks after ischemic injury with or without satellite cell implantation (a). Thinning of the ventricular wall with massive dense scarring was seen for the ischemic heart (b), while maintenance of normal morphology with cell therapy (c) was achieved. Transplantation of autologous satellite cells labeled with GFP into injured heart resulted in the formation of neomyocardium that also expressed GFP (c).*

regional wall systolic thickening was not different from that in the normal heart. In dogs without satellite cell implantation, the systolic thickening fraction was markedly lower than the initial value.[18] A digital sonomicrometer (Sonometrics Co., London, Canada) was used for real-time segment length or volume measurements. The pressure–volume and pressure–length loops (Figure 7.8) clearly showed the recovery of contractile function after autologous satellite cell implantation into the injured heart. A significant improvement in contractile function was observed only in the animals with successful cell transplantation.[11,13,14,18,21] The delivery of autologous skeletal myoblasts (satellite cells) into rabbit heart as a potential approach for myocardial repair has been confirmed by other investigators.[22] The contractile functions were significantly improved only in the animals with successful engraftment.[22] In general, satellite cell transplantation into injured heart significantly reduced scar area and markedly improved contractile function by new muscle formation.[21]

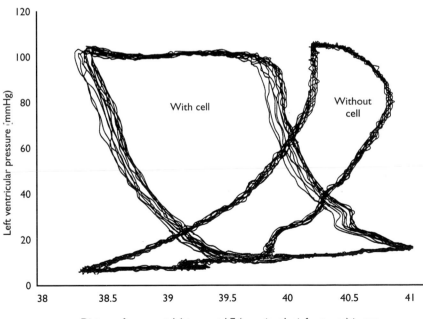

Distance from crystal 6 to crystal 7 (covering the infarct area) in mm

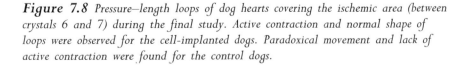

Figure 7.8 Pressure–length loops of dog hearts covering the ischemic area (between crystals 6 and 7) during the final study. Active contraction and normal shape of loops were observed for the cell-implanted dogs. Paradoxical movement and lack of active contraction were found for the control dogs.

Clinical observations

Menasche et al[23] performed the world's first clinical case of cellular cardiomyoplasty on 15 June 2000; they completed more than 10 cases, with highly encouraging outcomes. A skeletal muscle biopsy was obtained from the vastus lateralis to isolate satellite cells and produce large numbers of myoblasts (800×10^6 of most CD56$^+$ cells). During coronary artery bypass grafting, the cell suspension was injected at 33 sites into and around the white spots of necrotic or fibrotic myocardium. After recovery and during follow-up examination, it was found that the patients' clinical status improved, there were no substantial arrhythmias, ejection fraction increased, segmental contractility improved, and metabolic activity ([^{18}F]deoxyglucose) and perfusion were markedly enhanced. When additional patients were given the same treatment, a 13% increase in ejection fraction (range: 5–24%), systolic thickening of the akinetic scars and increased metabolic activity were observed.

We have successfully performed five cases since 2001. Autologous satellite cells were implanted into myocardium during coronary artery bypass grafting while the heart was still under hypothermic cardioplegia. This offered the advantages of eliminating arrhythmia during cell injection and significantly improving cell retention. All patients survived the procedure and had an uneventful recovery before being discharged from the hospital. During follow-up examinations, significant increases in ejection fraction (by two-dimensional echo), improvements in perfusion (^{99m}TC-MIBI) and metabolic activity ([^{18}F]/deoxyglucose) and reductions in left ventricular end diastolic diameter were observed.[24] If the favorable outcomes could be confirmed by rigorous clinical trials, autologous satellite cells for myocardial regeneration might be a generally applicable procedure for patients suffering heart attacks or heart failure.

Discussion

By replacing, repairing or enhancing the biological function of damaged tissue or organs, cell therapy has emerged as a strategy for the treatment of many human diseases. Satellite cells have been shown to regenerate skeletal muscle in all ages and species of mammals that have been investigated. Cellular cardiomyoplasty using autologous satellite cells offers several advantages: (1) they are autologous cells, and immunorejection is not a concern; (2) they are not transformed cells, and tumorigenesis may not occur; (3) they form gap junctions with the cardiac myocytes, and arrhythmia has not been a complication; (4) they are not fetal tissue and will not raise ethical issues; (5) they are readily available from all patients, and donor availability is not a limitation for autologous cells; and (6) they are highly resistant to ischemic and anoxic conditions and their survival after transplantation is much better than that of other types of cell.

It has been well documented from recent observations that only a small fraction of transplanted satellite cells survive at the recipient tissue.[25] This minority of cells are slowly dividing in culture, but rapidly proliferate after grafting and cover the entire injured tissue to form differentiated cells. Whether a subpopulation of satellite cells or true adult stem cells can be isolated from the satellite cell preparation and improve the outcomes awaits future study. In addition, transfection of the cells with angiogenic factors or growth factors (i.e. cell therapy + gene therapy) and pretreatment of the cells with factors that regulate their proliferation, differentiation, survival or function may also improve the outcomes of cellular cardiomyoplasty. However, the factors for activation, mobilization, homing, differentiation and integration of satellite cells at injured myocardium have not yet been identified.

We have been using the autologous satellite cells from skeletal muscle for myocardial regeneration in dogs since 1989.[12] Satellite cells have been successfully isolated, labeled and implanted into injured heart, with neomyocardial formation and functional improvement.[11,13,14,18,21] Viable muscle cells with clear labeling were found in the infarct area after cell implantation. The labeled muscle cells showed intercalated disks at cellular junctions. Significant improvement in contractile function was observed only in the animals receiving cell transplantation.[18] The delivery of autologous skeletal myoblasts (satellite cells) into rabbit heart as a potential approach for myocardial repair has been confirmed by other investigators.[22] The contractile functions were significantly improved only in the animals with successful engraftment.[22] Early clinical applications have offered highly encouraging results;[23,24] however, additional studies are needed before satellite cell implantation can be considered a standard clinical procedure.

Acknowledgment

Our studies were supported by NIH grant HL54286, HL72138, American Heart Association grant 0051458B, 0255009B and a VA Merit Review Grant.

References

1.   Mauro A. Satellite cell of skeletal muscle fibers. J Biophys Biochem Cytol 1961; 9: 493–8.

2. Bischoff R. The satellite cell and muscle regeneration. In: Engel AG, Frazini-Armstrong C, eds. Myology. New York: McGraw-Hill, 1994: 97–118.

3. Hawke TJ, Garry DJ. Myogenic satellite cells: physiology to molecular biology. J Appl Physiol 2001; 9: 534–51.

4. Zammit P, Beauchamp J. The skeletal muscle satellite cell: stem cell or son of stem cell? Differentiation 2001; 68: 193–204.

5. Asakura A, Komaki M, Rudnicki MA. Muscle satellite cells are multipotential stem cells that exhibit myogenic, osteogenic, and adipogenic differentiation. Differentiation 2001; 68: 245–53.

6. Jankowski RJ, Deasy BM, Huard J. Muscle-derived stem cells. Gene Ther 2002; 9: 642–7.

7. Qu-Petersen Z, Deasy B, Jankowski R et al. Identification of a novel population of muscle stem cells in mice: potential for muscle regeneration. J Cell Biol 2002; 157: 851–64.

8. Blau HM, Brazelton TR, Weimann JM. The evolving concept of a stem cell: entity or function? Cell 2001; 105: 829–41.

9. Goodell MA, Jackson KA, Majka SM et al. Stem cell plasticity in muscle and bone marrow. Ann NY Acad Sci 2001; 938: 208–18.

10. Gussoni E, Soneoka Y, Strickland CD et al. Dystrophin expression in the mdx mouse restored by stem cell transplantation. Nature 1999; 401: 390–4.

11. Kao RL, Chiu RC-J, eds. Cellular cardiomyoplasty: myocardial repair with cell implantation. Austin, TX: Landes, 1997; 109–28.

12. Kao RL, Rizzo C, Magovern GJ. Satellite cells for myocardial regeneration. Physiologist 1989; 32: 220.

13. Chiu RC, Zibaitis A, Kao RL. Cellular cardiomyoplasty: myocardial regeneration with satellite cell implantation. Ann Thorac Surg 1995; 60: 12–18.

14. Yoon PD, Kao RL, Magovern GJ. Myocardial regeneration. Transplanting satellite cells into damaged myocardium. Texas Heart Inst J 1995; 22: 119–25.

15. Marelli D, Desrosier C, El-Alfy M et al. Cell transplantation for myocardial repair: an experimental approach. Cell Transplant 1992; 1: 383–90.

16. Zibaitis A, Chiu RC-J, Kao RL. Cellular and molecular cardiomyoplasty: new approaches to regenerate lost cardiac muscle. In: Carpentier A, Chachques C, Grandjean PA, eds. Cardiac bioassist. New York, NY: Futura Publishers, 1997: 591–610.

17. Reinecke H, Murry CE. Transmural replacement of myocardium after skeletal myoblast grafting into the heart. Too much of a good thing? Cardiovasc Pathol 2000; 9: 337–44.

18. Kao RL, Chin TK, Ganote CE et al. Satellite cell transplantation to repair injured myocardium. Cardiac Vasc Regen 2000; 1: 31–42.

19. Zhao R, Kao RL. Comparison of labeling procedures for myogenic cells. Cardiac Vasc Regen 2000; 1: 85–95.

20. Al-Khaldi A, Lachapelle K, Galipeau J. Endogenous B-galactosidase enzyme activity in normal tissue and ischemic myocardium. Cardiac Vasc Regen 2000; 1: 283–90.

21. Kao RL. Autologous satellite cells for myocardial regeneration. J Reg Med 2001; 2: 1–8.

22. Taylor DA, Atkins BZ, Hungspreugs P et al. Regenerating functional myocardium: improved performance after skeletal myoblast transplantation. Nat Med 1998; 4: 929–33.

23. Menasche P, Hagege AA, Scorsin M et al. Myoblast transplantation for heart failure. Lancet 2001; 357: 279–80.

24. Zhang F, Yang Z, Chen Y et al. Clinical cellular cardiomyoplasty: technical considerations. J Cardiac Surg 2003; 18: 268–73.

25. Beauchamp JR, Morgan JE, Pagel CN, Partridge TA. Dynamics of myoblasts transplantation reveal a discrete minority of precursors with stem cell-like properties as the myogenic source. J Cell Biol 1999; 144: 1113–22.

8. Myogenic Cardiac Fibroblasts for Myocardial Infarction

Race L Kao, John J Laffan, Thomas K Chin,
D Glenn Pennington and Charles E Ganote

The heart functions as a muscular pump that generates flow and maintains the pressure of blood in the circulatory system. Its function is dependent upon the rapid and continuous energy supply to the myocardium and efficient oxidative phosphorylation in cardiomyocytes supported by adequate coronary flow. Coronary heart disease can severely reduce or completely stop blood perfusion to the myocardium, resulting in myocardial infarction. Coronary heart disease is the single leading cause of death in the USA and heart attacks result in more than 500,000 deaths each year.[1] After an acute myocardial infarction, the healing process can be divided into four phases: (1) cardiomyocyte death; (2) acute inflammation; (3) tissue granulation; and (4) remodeling/repair.[2,3] Since adult mammalian ventricular myocytes lack regenerative capability, injured myocardium consistently forms scar tissue after a heart attack. The scar is living tissue consisting of metabolically active myofibroblasts nourished by the neovasculature and innervated by postganglionic nerve fibers.[3]

After myocardial infarction, the death of cardiomyocytes occurs by both cell necrosis and cell apoptosis, with the release of cellular proteins into the blood. The majority of the apoptotic cells after infarction cannot be completely phagocytosed by neighboring cells, and secondary cell necrosis occurs by acute inflammation. Subsequently, new extracellular matrix proteins are deposited along with the myofibroblasts and neovascularization during granulation tissue formation. The last phase of wound healing can continue for a long time, with the remaining myofibroblasts and cross-linked collagen fibers forming the mature scar. Ventricular remodeling after a heart attack involves expansion of the infarction, dilatation of the ventricle and thinning of the ventricular wall, all of which contribute to the development of heart failure. Turning the scar (cardiac fibroblasts or myofibroblasts) into viable myocardium is an innovative idea to reverse scar formation, prevent ventricular remodeling and eliminate heart failure.

Cardiac fibroblasts

Cardiac fibroblasts constitute more than 90% of non-muscle cells in the myocardium. They are responsible for the synthesis of extracellular matrix, growth factors, matrix metalloproteases, chemokines and cytokines in the heart.[4,5] Cardiac fibroblasts produce collagen types I, III and IV as well as laminin and fibronectin, which organize the intricate interstitial matrix to interconnect cardiac myocytes to one another and to their neighboring capillaries, thus preventing cardiac myocyte slippage and maintaining their alignment during the cardiac cycle. Gene expression and proliferation of cardiac fibroblasts are regulated by physical (mechanical stretch, hypoxia) and humoral (transforming growth factor-beta$_1$ (TGF-ß$_1$), basic fibroblast growth factor (bFGF), platelet-derived growth factor (PDGF), angiotensin II, thyroxin, estrogen, etc.) factors.[5]

Myofibroblasts are mesenchymal cells with properties of both smooth muscle cells and non-muscle cells (fibroblasts). They play an important role in organogenesis, oncogenesis, inflammation, repair and fibrosis in most organs and tissues. Myofibroblasts are highly plastic and diverse in their phenotypes, depending on their tissue of origin and the condition of the tissue (normal or pathologic). Numerous cell types have been characterized as myofibroblasts, including stromal cells, pericytes, stellate cells, interstitial cells, mesangial cells and granulation tissue fibroblasts. Myofibroblasts have abundant rough endoplasmic reticulum, have modestly developed peripheral myofilaments with focal densities (stress fibers), and are connected to each other by adherens and gap junctions. It is unclear whether myofibroblasts originate from progenitor stem cells or transdifferentiate from other cells; Figure 8.1 shows the possible origin of myofibroblasts.

Myogenic transdifferentiation of fibroblasts

The formation of functional striated muscle cells from mouse embryo fibroblasts C3H 10T1/2 Clone 8 (10T1/2) after 5-azacytidine treatment was initially reported in 1977.[6] In addition to 10T1/2 cells, Swiss 3T3 cells, adult mouse cell line and keratinocytes could also form contractile striated muscle cells after 5-azacytidine or 5-aza-2'-deoxycytidine treatment.[7–9] Myogenic cells derived from rat bone marrow mesenchymal stem cells and cardiomyocytes generated from marrow stromal cells after 5-azacytidine treatment were also reported recently.[10] Most cells in the body have identical genotypes; gene expression and development determine the special phenotypes of individual cells. It is possible for undifferentiated cells to

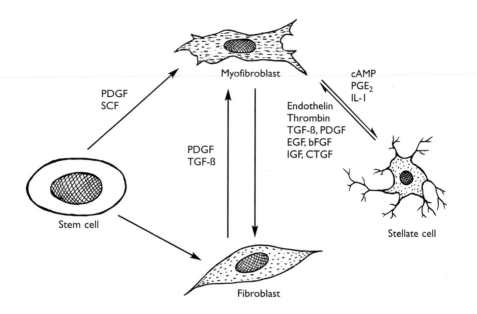

Figure 8.1 Schematic drawing showing the origin, transdifferentiation and transformation of fibroblasts. PDGF, platelet-derived growth factor; TGF-β, transforming growth factor-beta; SCF, stem cell factor; EGF, epidermal growth factor; bFGF, basic fibroblast growth factor; IGF, insulin-like growth factor; CTGF, connective tissue growth factor; PGE_2, prostaglandin E_2; IL-1, interleukin-1.

differentiate into other types of cells (plasticity). The plasticity of adult stem cells has been well summarized by several review papers.[11,12] The phenotypic plasticity of cardiac fibroblasts has demonstrated the feasibility of using them for cardiac muscle regeneration.[4,13]

Vertebrate DNAs contain 5-methylcytosine in 5′-CpG-3′ dinucleotide, and the complementary 3′-GpC-5′ that makes the base pairs is also methylated symmetrically. The methyl groups have a three-dimensional structure projecting into the major groove of the DNA. Approximately 60–90% of all CpG sequences in the vertebrate genome are methylated, while non-methylated CpGs are mainly clustered in the dense regions of CpGs, known as CpG islands. About 60% of genes have promoters and transcription start sites included within the CpG islands. Gene expression is completely repressed when this region becomes hypermethylated. Furthermore, the methylation pattern present in the parental strand is semiconservatively copied after replication and passed into the daughter cells. It is well recognized that DNA methylation is one of the key mechanisms regulating gene transcription.[14]

Cytidine analogs that can inhibit DNA methylation will induce myogenic

109

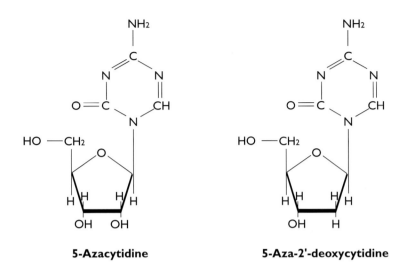

Figure 8.2 *Chemical structures of 5-azacytidine and 5-aza-2′-deoxycytidine.*

transdifferentiation of non-muscle cells.[15,16] After 5-azacytidine (Figure 8.2) converts to its deoxynucleotide (5-aza-2′-deocycytidine), it can be incorporated into DNA and block methylation by non-competitive inhibition of DNA methyltransferase.[15-17] This explains why 5-aza-2′-deoxycytidine is 10 times more potent than 5-azacytidine at inducing myogenic transdifferentiation. The methylation of cytosine involves the covalent binding of the DNA methyltransferase through a nucleophilic attachment of a cysteine thiolate at the C-6 position of the cytosine ring. The covalent binding of the enzyme at C-6 allows the attachment and transfer of a methyl group from the donor S-adenosylmethionine and subsequent release of the enzyme. When 5-aza-2′-deoxycytidine is incorporated into the DNA, the nitrogen atom at position 5 cannot be methylated and the enzyme remains covalently bound under physiologic conditions that result in lost enzyme activity and DNA hypomethylation. The hypomethylation of DNA is thought to induce gene activation and expression that, in turn, regulates cell differentiation.[14]

MyoD was identified after the treatment of 10T1/2 fibroblasts with 5-azacytidine. Transfection of 10T1/2 cells with DNA from 5-azacytidine-induced myoblasts or from C2C12 myoblasts resulted in myogenic conversion of 10T1/2 cells. When one of the cDNAs was transfected into 10T1/2 fibroblasts, it was sufficient to convert the fibroblasts into stable myoblasts, and the transfected gene was termed *MyoD*.[18] *MyoD* is normally expressed only in skeletal muscle in vivo and in myogenic cells in vitro transfection of

MyoD cDNA into a variety of cell lines induced myogenesis. When human and murine fibroblasts from skin, muscle or bone marrow were transfected with an adenoviral vector containing *MyoD* cDNA, a high efficiency of myogenic conversion was achieved.[19]

MyoD was known for years to be the master gene of skeletal muscle differentiation, and could convert cardiac fibroblasts or granulation tissue (myofibroblasts) to functional skeletal myocytes.[20] We selected 5-aza-2'-deoxycytidine for myocardial regeneration, based on its activation of other genes in addition to *MyoD*, for possible development of cardiac myocytes from cardiac fibroblasts. The phenotypic plasticity of cardiac fibroblasts demonstrated the possibility of using them for cardiac muscle regeneration.[4,13] This point was further supported by the observation of muscle formation from dermal fibroblasts[21] and myogenic conversion of cardiac fibroblasts after *MyoD* transfection. [22]

Experimental animals

Mongrel dogs weighing 25–30 kg were purchased for the project. Humane care and proper treatment were applied to all experimental animals. The 'Principles of Laboratory Animal Care', formulated by the National Society for Medical Research, and the 'Guide for the Care and Use of Laboratory Animals' prepared by the National Research Council in 1996 were followed. The proposed study was approved by the Animal Care and Use Committee of East Tennessee State University. After overnight fasting and preoperative antibiotic treatment, each dog was anesthetized with sodium pentobarbital (15 mg/kg) through a catheter inserted percutaneously into the leg vein. Following intubation with a cuffed endotracheal tube, crystalloid infusate was given through the venous catheter. The electrocardiogram was monitored using the PageWriter cardiograph, the body temperature was recorded with a rectal probe (Yellow Springs Co., Yellow Springs, OH, USA), and anesthesia was maintained with 1% isoflurane on a ventilator (Narkovet 2, North American Drager, Telford, PA, USA). Following preparation of the surgical area with povidone-iodine (Betadine), arterial and central venous pressures were monitored using Millar pressure transducers.

Isolation and culture of cardiac fibroblasts

Dogs were anesthetized and prepared for a sterile surgical procedure to obtain myocardial biopsy samples through a partial sternotomy. A sample

($\sim$1 g) was removed from the apex of the hearts without injury to the major vessels for control and experimental animals. The cell isolation procedures were carried out inside a laminar flow hood. The muscle was rinsed three times in Hanks' balanced salt solution without Ca^{2+} and Mg^{2+} but containing 1% of penicillin–streptomycin. The tissue was minced ($\sim$1 mm^3) before being incubated with 10 ml of enzyme solution in a sterile 15-ml plastic centrifuge tube. The enzyme solution was composed of buffered medium 199 containing 1% collagenase and 0.2% hyaluronidase that had been filtered through a 0.2-μm filter and equilibrated with 95% O_2/5% CO_2. After 15 min of incubation at 37°C in a shaking water bath, the cardiac cells were harvested by pouring the solution through layers of sterile gauze into a sterile container and pelleted by centrifugation.

The remaining tissue was incubated for another 15 min to complete the enzymatic release of heart cells from the muscle. The cardiac fibroblasts were isolated by differential centrifugation (to remove muscle cells) before being washed with medium 199 containing serum (10% fetal bovine serum) and 1% antibiotic antimycotic solution (Sigma Chemical Co., St Louis, MO, USA) three times by centrifugation and resuspension. The viability of isolated cells was checked by trypan blue exclusion, and the cell number was determined with a hemocytometer. After proper dilution, 1×10^6 cells were cultured with 8 ml of medium in a 25-cm^2 culture flask and subcultured every 3–4 days to maintain them at low density.

Myogenic conversion of cardiac fibroblasts in vitro

Culture medium containing cytidine, 5-azacytidine or 5-aza-2'-deoxycytidine was used to induce myogenic conversion of the cultured cardiac fibroblasts. Cytidine did not induce myogenic transdifferentiation, and 5-aza-2'-deoxycytidine was much more effective than 5-azacytidine. Owing to the highly labile nature of 5-azacytidine and 5-aza-2'-deoxycytidine at physiologic pH, it was necessary to make a stock solution of them in Ringer's lactate solution and store at low temperature (–80°C). Just before use, the stock solution was diluted with Ringer's lactate solution and added to the culture flasks. Cultured primary cardiac fibroblasts (Figure 8.3a) obtained from dogs were treated with medium containing the optimal concentration of 5-aza-2'-deoxycytidine (0.3 μmol/l) for myogenic conversion. At 2 weeks after treatment, formation of multinucleated myotubes (Figure 8.3b) from cultured cardiac fibroblasts was clearly seen. At higher magnification, multinucleation and striations of the myotubes were quite evident (Figure 8.3c).

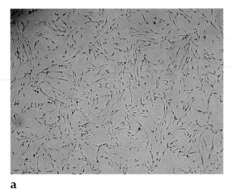

a

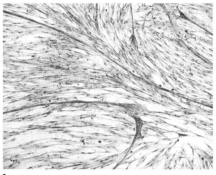

b

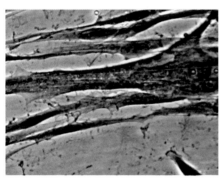

c

Figure 8.3 Cultured canine cardiac fibroblasts (a) transdifferentiated into myotubes (b) after treatment with 5-aza-2'-deoxycytidine, showing multinucleation and striations at higher magnification (c).

Labeling the cultured cardiac fibroblasts with AAV-hrGFP

The helper-free adeno-associated virus containing humanized green fluorescent protein (GFP) (AAV-hrGFP) was purchased from Stratagene (La Jolla, CA, USA) for the labeling procedure (detailed in Chapter 7). Two to three days before the cardiac fibroblasts were harvested for transplantation, culture medium containing AAV-hrGFP was used to replace the regular medium. After another 24–48 h, the GFP was easily observed in the labeled cells (Figure 8.4a) using a fluorescent microscope with a fluorescein isothiocyanate (FITC) filter set. When cardiac fibroblasts were labeled with GFP and treated with 5-aza-2'-deoxycytidine, myotubes with GFP were also found in culture (Figures 8.4b,c), indicating that the GFP labeling did not interfere with the myogenic conversion of cultured cardiac fibroblasts.

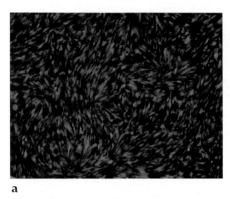

a

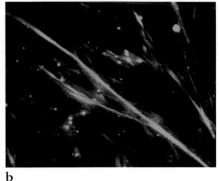

b

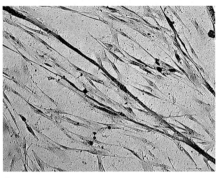

c

Figure 8.4 *Cardiac fibroblasts labeled with AAV-hrGFP (a), and the formation of multinucleated myotubes after myogenic transdifferentiation in the same area observed under a fluorescent microscope (b) and a light microscope (c). Labeling the cells with AAV-hrGFP did not interfere with the myogenic conversion of the cells.*

Implantation of myogenic cardiac fibroblasts

Under full anesthesia and sterile surgical conditions, the heart was exposed through a median sternotomy. The pericardium was opened and the edges attached to the chest wall to allow good exposure of the left ventricle. After administration of heparin (100 U/kg) and lidocaine (2 mg/kg), the left anterior descending coronary artery (LAD) and vein were temporarily occluded for 4 h before reperfusion.[23] It has been reported that the dog has significant collateral bloodflow in the myocardium, and the generation of a reproducible ischemic or infarct zone is problematic. Occlusion of both the LAD and left anterior descending coronary vein was necessary to develop a relatively consistent infarct zone. The site of occlusion was just below the first branch of the LAD that was about two-thirds of the distance from the apex of the heart. From our previous experience, this created a reproducible myocardial infarction with low mortality (< 5%) in dogs. The ischemic myocardium was easily identified by its cyanosis and hypokinesis. The ischemic area was marked with 5-0 polypropylene epicardial sutures for future identification.

After release of the occluded coronary vessels, cardiac function was stabilized before cell implantation. The infarct zone was visually divided into 30–40 areas of ~0.25 cm² before 0.1 ml (approximately one million cells suspended in serum-free medium) of the labeled (AAV-hrGFP) and treated (5-aza-2′-deoxycytidine) autologous cardiac fibroblasts was injected (five dogs) into the center of each area through a 25-gauge hypodermic needle. The control animals (five dogs) were subjected to the same treatment, but serum-free culture medium was used.

Assessment of hemodynamic function

The left ventricular volume, segmental length, wall thickness and regional shortening before and after myocardial ischemia, as well as during and after recovery, were measured with the digital ultrasonic measurement system (Sonometrics Co., London, ON, Canada). The major advantages of this system were that there is no need to perfectly align the crystals and three-dimensional reconstruction is possible. A pair of 2-mm implantable sonomicrometer crystals (transducers) was placed at the base and the apex for continuous measurement of the external left ventricular (LV) long axis. A 1-mm crystal was inserted tangentially (~45°) through the myocardium into the subendocardium and another one was sutured to the epicardial surface directly above the inner crystal (ultrasonic transit time shortest between the two crystals). The fifth crystal was placed on the LV posterior wall opposite to the epicardial crystal for the external LV short axis. A pair of crystals was positioned at the border of the ischemic area to determine the changes in segmental length of the ischemic zone. Another pair of crystals was placed for transmyocardial measurement of percentage thickening fraction and regional contractile function of a normal area.

With the computerized Crystal Biotech VF-1 hemodynamic system (Data Science Int., St Paul, MN, USA) integrated with the Sonometrics system, it was possible to measure the regional contractile functions in real time. Millar microtip pressure transducers (Millar Instruments, Inc., Houston, TX, USA) were used for pressure measurements. It was possible to measure the beat-to-beat changes in bloodflow, ejection fraction, wall thickness, regional shortening, ventricular pressure, dP/dt, pressure–volume loops and pressure–length loops.[23,24] The pressure–volume loops from the normal heart, from the heart at 6 weeks after transplantation with myogenic cardiac fibroblasts and from the heart without cell implantation (injected with culture medium) clearly indicated the restoration of LV function by the cell therapy (Figure 8.5).

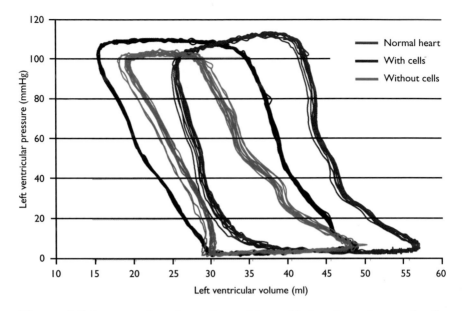

Figure 8.5 *Pressure–volume loops of normal heart (blue), ischemic heart with cell implantation (red) and ischemic heart without cell therapy (green) at 6 weeks after the treatment. Significant decreases in stroke work and stroke volume were found for the heart without cell implantation. Transplantation of autologous myogenic cardiac fibroblasts restored left ventricular function. The left ventricular volume was derived by the formula for a general ellipsoid and subtracting the wall volume determined by water displacement of the isolated heart.*

Histologic evaluations

After hemodynamic evaluations and administration of heparin (100 U/kg), hearts were flushed and arrested with cold (2°C) cardioplegic solution by retrograde perfusion through the aorta. The hearts were sliced into 0.25-cm-thick sections in a plane parallel to the atrioventricular groove, using a commercial meat slicer. Images of each slice (both sides) were scanned into a computer for determining the fractions of normal, GFP-positive (observed under UV light), scar and necrotic tissues. The individual quantity and volume as well as chamber size or wall thickness were derived using the computer after three-dimensional reconstruction of the scanned data (Figure 8.6). Autologous cardiac fibroblasts after 5-aza-2′-deoxycytidine treatment were implanted into myocardial infarction for muscle regeneration. At 6 weeks after ischemic injury, control hearts (without cells, injected with serum-free medium) showed significant amounts of dense scar tissue and thinning of the ventricular wall (Figure 8.7). The hearts implanted with

116

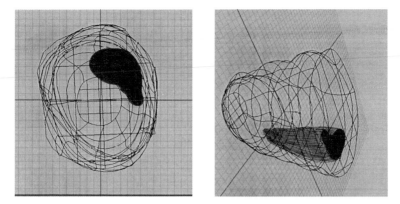

Figure 8.6 *Three-dimensional reconstruction of scanned data for quantification of scar tissue or regenerated myocardium.*

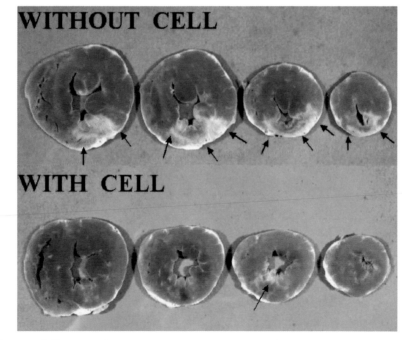

Figure 8.7 *Slices of canine myocardium at 6 weeks after myocardial infarction with and without autologous myogenic cardiac fibroblast implantation. Thinning of the left ventricular wall with massive dense scarring was observed in the heart without cell therapy. Transplantation of myogenic cardiac fibroblasts restored the normal morphology of myocardium and drastically reduced the amount of scar tissue. (a) Injected with serum-free culture medium after heart injury. (b) Implanted with autologous myogenic cardiac fibroblasts after heart injury.*

117

autologous myogenic cardiac fibroblasts showed muscle formation replacing scar tissue with normal ventricular morphology.

Discussion

Adult mammalian ventricular myocytes are terminally differentiated cells that cannot multiply to meet increased physiologic demands or replace lost myocytes. Myocardium does not contain myogenic stem cells, and damaged heart is repaired by scar formation, hypertrophy of surviving myocytes and hyperplasia of non-muscle cells. 5-Azacytidine has been reported to produce striated muscle cells from non-myoblast precursors such as fibroblasts, keratinocytes, mesenchymal stem cells and bone marrow stromal cells. It has been suggested that the conversion of 5-azacytidine into 5-aza-2'-deoxycytidine and incorporation into DNA to covalently trap the DNA methyltransferase subsequently resulting in hypomethylation of DNA and regulation of gene expression, are the mechanisms of myogenic transdifferentiation of non-muscle cells.

Myocardial infarction was induced in dogs by occluding both the left anterior descending coronary artery and vein for 4 h before reperfusion. Hemodynamic functions were determined before and after ischemic injury as well as 6 weeks after surgery. The ischemic area defined by cyanosis and hypokinesis was marked by epicardial sutures surrounding the field. After restoration of coronary flow and stabilization of cardiac function, labeled (AAV-hrGFP) and treated (5-aza-2'-deoxycytidine) cardiac fibroblasts were transplanted into the ischemic area, while serum-free culture medium was used for control animals. Six weeks after the surgical procedure, hearts from a group of treated animals and a group of control animals were obtained for pathologic evaluations. Transplantation of autologous myogenic cardiac fibroblasts restored LV function to normal levels, significantly reduced scar tissue by neomyocardial formation, and maintained normal morphology of the hearts.

Our findings suggest that myogenic conversion of cardiac fibroblasts by 5-aza-2'-deoxycytidine is a possible treatment for myocardial regeneration after a heart attack. If pharmacologic or molecular interventions can be established to transform scar into viable myocardium, the therapy can be administered by a catheter into the coronary vessel or the heart muscle. The advantages of this approach compared to cellular cardiomyoplasty using autologous satellite cells are as follows: (1) it does not require muscle biopsy, and thus eliminates a surgical procedure; (2) it will not require cell culture and therefore avoids possible contamination during the culture procedure; (3) the therapy can be given during percutaneous transluminal coronary angioplasty (PTCA) or during cardiac catheterization; (4) the treatment can be given without waiting for cell proliferation; and (5) this procedure is much simpler and easier than cellular cardiomyoplasty.

Our data have demonstrated that myocardial regeneration can be achieved by converting autologous cardiac fibroblasts into myogenic cells in the injured heart for replacing, repairing, maintaining and enhancing cardiac function. The hypothesis is that 5-aza-2'-deoxycytidine can induce myogenic transdifferentiation of cardiac fibroblasts, which can be used to turn the scar into viable myocardium. Although other types of fibroblasts (dermal or skeletal muscle) or bone marrow stromal cells can be obtained more easily than cardiac fibroblasts, we selected cardiac fibroblasts because of the possibility of developing pharmacologic or molecular interventions to transform scar into viable myocardium. If the therapy can be established, the treatment can be given to patients during cardiac catheterization or PTCA, or intramyocardial administration can be carried out using an injectable catheter.

Acknowledgment

Our studies were supported by NIH grant HL72138, American Heart Association grant 0051458B, and a VA Merit Review Grant.

References

1. American Heart Association. 2002 heart and stroke statistical update. Dallas, TX: American Heart Association, 2001.

2. Cleutjens JPM, Blankesteijn WM, Daemen MJAP, Smits JFM. The infarcted myocardium: simply dead tissue, or a lively target for therapeutic interventions. Cardiovasc Res 1999; 44: 232–41.

3. Sun Y, Kiani MF, Postlethwaite AE, Weber KT. Infarct scar as living tissue. Basic Res Cardiol 2002; 97: 343–7.

4. Eghbali-Webb M. Cardiac fibroblasts: important players in cardiac muscle and vascular regeneration. Cardiac Vasc Regen 2000; 1: 133–43.

5. Powell DW, Mifflin RC, Valentich JD et al. Myofibroblasts. I. Paracrine cells important in health and disease. Am J Physiol 1999; 277: C1–19.

6. Constantinides PG, Jones PA, Gevers W. Functional striated muscle cells from non-myoblast precursors following 5-azacytidine treatment. Nature 1977; 267: 364–6.

7. Taylor SM, Jones PA. Multiple new phenotypes induced in 10T1/2 and 3T3 cells treated with 5-azacytidine. Cell 1979; 17: 771–9.

8. Taylor SM, Jones PA. Changes in phenotypic expression in embryonic and adult cells treated with 5-azacytidine. J Cell Physiol 1982; 111: 187–94.

9. Boukamp P, Chen J, Gonzales F et al. Progressive stages of 'transdifferentiation' from epidermal to mesenchymal phenotype induced by MyoD1 transfection, 5-aza-2'-deoxycytidine treatment, and selection for reduced cell attachment in the human keratinocyte line HaCaT. J Cell Biol 1992; 116: 1257–71.

10. Makino S, Fukuda K, Miyoshi S et al. Cardiomyocytes can be generated from marrow stromal cells in vitro. J Clin Invest 1999; 103: 697–705.

11. Blau HM, Brazelton TR, Weimann JM. The evolving concept of a stem cell: entity or function? Cell 2001; 105: 829–41.

12. Goodell MA, Jackson KA, Majka SM et al. Stem cell plasticity in muscle and bone marrow. Ann NY Acad Sci 2001; 938: 208–18.

13. Eghbali M, Tomek R, Woods C et al. Cardiac fibroblasts are predisposed to convert into myocyte phenotype: specific effect of transforming growth factor beta. Proc Natl Acad Sci USA 1991; 88: 795–9.

14. Robertson KD, Jones PA. DNA methylation: past, present and future directions. Carcinogenesis 2000; 21(3): 461–7.

15. Jones PA, Taylor SM. Cellular differentiation, cytidine analogs and DNA methylation. Cell 1980; 20: 85–93.

16. Glover AB, Leyland-Jones B. Biochemistry of azacytidine: a review. Cancer Treat Rep 1987; 71: 959–64.

17. Jackson-Grusby L, Laird RW, Magge SN et al. Mutagenicity of 5-aza-2'-deoxycytidine is mediated by the mammalian DNA methyltransferase. Proc Natl Acad Sci USA 1997; 94: 4681–5.

18. Davis RL, Weintraub H, Lasser AB. Expression of a single transfected cDNA converts fibroblasts to myoblasts. Cell 1987; 51: 987–1000.

19. Lattanzi L, Salvatori G, Coletta M et al. High efficiency myogenic conversion of human fibroblasts by adenoviral vector-mediated MyoD transfer. An alternative strategy for ex vivo gene therapy of primary myopathies. J Clin Invest 1998; 101: 2119–28.

20. Pownall ME, Gustafsson MK, Emerson CP Jr. Myogenic regulatory factors and the specification of muscle progenitors in vertebrate embryos. Annu Rev Cell Dev Biol 2002; 18: 747–83.

120

21. Pye D, Watt DJ. Dermal fibroblasts participate in the formation of new muscle fibers when implanted into regenerating normal mouse muscle. J Anat 2001; 198: 163–73.

22. Etzion S, Barbash IM, Feinberg MS et al. Cellular cardiomyoplasty of cardiac fibroblasts by adenoviral delivery of MyoD ex vivo: an unlimited source of cells for myocardial repair. Circulation 2002; 106(suppl I): I-125–30.

23. Kao RL, Chin TK, Ganote CE et al. Satellite cell transplantation to repair injured myocardium. Cardiac Vasc Regen 2000; 1: 31–42.

24. Kao RL, Chiu RC-J. Satellite cell implantation. In: Kao RL, Chiu RC-J, eds. Cellular cardiomyoplasty: myocardial repair with cell implantation. Austin, TX: Landes, 1997: 129–62.

9. STRATEGIES TO ENHANCE THE EFFICACY OF MYOBLAST TRANSPLANTATION TO THE HEART

Bari Murtuza, Ken Suzuki and Magdi H Yacoub

In considering the optimal strategy for cell therapy to treat myocardial dysfunction, the first issue to be resolved is the donor cell type. Implantation of proliferative skeletal myogenic precursor cells (MPCs; myoblasts) into the heart has yielded consistently beneficial functional results in both small and large animal models.[1–5] In contrast to the limited regenerative capacity of adult myocardium, these proliferative MPCs (derived from activated satellite cells) are normally responsible for the postnatal growth and repair of skeletal muscle. Although the precise mechanism of functional improvement following MPC transplantation to the heart remains uncertain, the cardiac microenvironment is permissive for differentiation of these cells – at least along the skeletal myogenic lineage.[2,3] MPCs can be harvested autologously from patients; they form stable vehicles for gene therapy; and they do not have the associated ethical implications of embryonic stem cells or fetal cardiac myocytes.[4]

Previous use of dynamic skeletal cardiomyoplasty has shown the ability of skeletal muscle to adopt a fatigue-resistant phenotype with expression of slow-twitch myosins and cardiac-specific calcium regulatory proteins under conditions of chronic electrical stimulation.[6] This showed the capacity of skeletal muscle cells to adapt to a new functional environment. In addition, recent phase I clinical trials have suggested the feasibility and safety of using MPCs in patients.[7] The success of myoblast therapy depends upon the survival, proliferation, differentiation and integration of cells within the myocardium. Integration, in turn, could occur at three levels: mechanical, electrical and metabolic. Optimizing long-term results of MPC transplantation to the heart will depend critically on understanding these basic cellular processes and enhancing their efficacy. In this chapter, we discuss strategies aimed at: improving the quality, purity and number of donor cells; modulating their behavior within the myocardium (by physical/chemical or genetic manipulation); and optimizing the means of cell delivery.

Preparation, manipulation and delivery of cells

The single-fiber system

The conventional method of preparing cells for MPC transplantation involves enzymatic disaggregation of limb muscles. Cells are then expanded in vitro prior to implantation into the host tissue.[8] This technique has inherent disadvantages with respect to purity and change in phenotype imposed by culture conditions. The cell preparations are contaminated to varying degrees by fibroblasts and probably other cell types, and many procedures have been employed to purify the cells, such as preplating and differential gradient centrifugation.[8] As an alternative method of cell isolation and preparation with several major potential advantages, our laboratory has utilized the in vitro single-fiber (SF) system. In this protocol, muscles explanted from an animal are gently dissociated in vitro following a limited digestion and plated out as individual fibers. Satellite cells undergo activation and migrate off the fibers within a few hours as proliferating MPCs.[9] Purity is confirmed by immunocytochemistry for the muscle-specific protein α-sarcomeric actin, and differentiation capacity is confirmed by fusion into myotubes in vitro following reduction in the serum content of culture medium (Figure 9.1). Recently, we have exploited this system and hypothesized that implantation of isolated SFs themselves may be a more efficient means to deliver myogenic cells to the myocardium that would not entail prolonged periods of culture.[10]

Initial studies were performed to investigate the feasibility and efficiency of this approach. Following isolation as described above, SFs were immediately implanted into syngeneic, rat myocardium in which heart failure had been induced by either doxorubicin administration, as a model for idiopathic dilated cardiomyopathy, or following coronary artery ligation as an ischemic model. Surprisingly, implantation of only four isolated SFs in these models resulted in a significant improvement in global systolic cardiac function as measured by Langendorff perfusion. Diastolic compliance of engrafted hearts in both heart failure models was also increased with less left ventricular dilatation compared with medium-injected controls. There were no adverse effects on animal survival. On histologic examination of the engrafted hearts, we found evidence of skeletal myotube formation in vivo at 28 days as multiple foci of branching myotubes at individual loci of fiber injection. Every heart examined showed evidence of new myofiber formation, with an engraftment efficiency of approximately 65% of all implantation sites. This suggested that the parent fibers acted as platforms to deliver satellite cells, which then probably proliferated to some extent prior to differentiating in vivo. The mean number of satellite cells on the SFs isolated prior to implantation was estimated to be 20 from M-cadherin immunocytochemistry

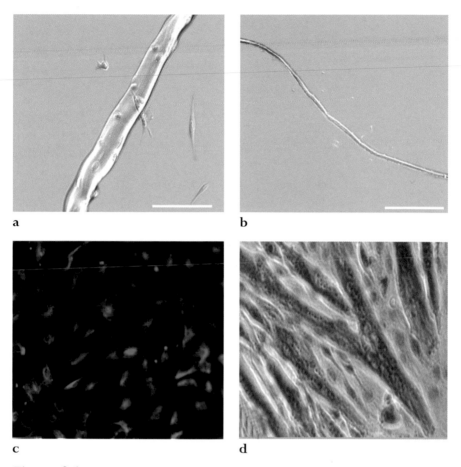

Figure 9.1 *(a,b) Isolated rat extensor digitorum longus (EDL) myofibers and derived MPCs (reverse-phase microscopy). (c) The majority of MPCs derived from the isolated fibers stain positive for α-sarcomeric actin (fluorescein isothiocyanate (FITC)); nuclei are counterstained blue with diamidino-phenylindole (DAPI). (d) Isolated MPCs show a high capacity for differentiation in vitro. Scale bars: 50 μm in (a); 250 μm in (b).*

(an accepted satellite cell marker). Therefore, transplantation of less than 100 satellite cells resulted in a global improvement in cardiac function. To explain this striking efficiency, we have begun to study the dynamics of the implanted fibers and of any derived cells using transgenic donor fibers which express nuclear ß-galactosidase under control of the skeletal myogenic fast myosin 1F/3F locus.[10] Interestingly, the parent fibers appeared to degenerate within 24 h, and evidence of cells derived from the fibers was seen by 72 h.[10] This implied that fibers did, indeed, act as a platform for delivery of these

125

cells, which were then able to proliferate and initiate the process of myogenic differentiation in vivo within a cardiac microenvironment.

Further studies to examine the mechanisms underlying the above observed effects are required. It is possible that delivery of cells associated with the parent fiber and an intact basal lamina affords some degree of endogenous self-protection against environmental stress during and immediately after implantation. We also hypothesize, however, that this technique may deliver a population of cells that is normally lost or compromised by the usual prolonged tissue culture methods. In particular, SFs may deliver a more primitive stem cell type with greater potential plasticity. The differences in phenotype between different subpopulations of MPCs in vitro have been previously described, as have the adverse phenotypic effects of prolonged tissue culture.[8,9] In addition, the parent fiber and/or its population of associated cells may release beneficial growth factors important for enhancing cardiac function. We therefore investigated the degree of angiogenesis in SF-engrafted hearts in an ischemic model and did indeed find evidence of enhanced angiogenesis in these hearts versus medium-injected hearts (capillary density of 4.1 ± 0.5 versus 2.3 ± 0.2 vessels per high-powered microscopic field).[10] This has also been described by our group and others following implantation of a myoblast suspension. Furthermore, we have found that implantation of a suspension of myoblasts transiently overexpressing vascular endothelial growth factor-165 ($VEGF_{165}$) isoform results in enhanced angiogenesis in vivo and an associated enhanced improvement in cardiac function in a myocardial infarct model, as described below.[11] Other studies have used minced or sliced muscle grafts as an alternative to implantation of cell suspensions.[12,13] Physical constraints within the myocardium compared with a recipient skeletal muscle bed, however, mean that these approaches are unlikely to be successful in the present context. The use of individual single skeletal muscle fibers is not subject to these limitations, and the fibers can be delivered in a minimal volume of carrying medium (about $3 \mu l$ in our studies) and therefore incite less of an inflammatory response. This may be another important factor in influencing the fate of the SF-derived cells in this system.

Physical manipulation of donor cells: heat shock treatment

Grafted MPCs are subject to environmental stress prior to, during and immediately after the implantation procedure. As a result, the majority of the cells undergo apoptosis and necrosis within the first 24 h.[14,15] Relative hypoxia just prior to grafting and an acute inflammatory response within the host myocardium following transplantation result in cell damage. Cytokines and free radicals are likely to be important mediators in this regard.[15] We have therefore investigated the effects of a strategy to improve graft cell number

126

in the heart following engraftment by intracoronary infusion (see below). An L6 rat skeletal myoblast cell line expressing nuclear-localized ß-galactosidase (n-ßgal-L6 clone) was subjected to in vitro heat shock treatment (42°C for 1 h) 24 h prior to grafting into the heart.[15] In vitro studies of the heat-shocked cells confirmed upregulation of the heat shock 70 family of proteins. These cells demonstrated an enhanced in vitro tolerance to hypoxia–reoxygenation as an apoptosis-inducing stimulus designed to mimic relative hypoxia of cells in the perigrafting period. The heat shock proteins consist of a family of related species which act as molecular chaperones during protein assembly.[16,17] Under conditions of increased heat stress, when the incidence of protein misfolding would normally be expected to increase, their expression is upregulated to reduce post-translational errors in protein assembly. In vivo delivery of L6 cells treated in this way resulted in an up to 60% improvement in cell number – both at early stages and at 28 days following grafting into the heart.[15] Although we did not examine the apoptosis of cells in vivo in this instance, this simple treatment must have had a beneficial effect on the survival and/or proliferation of cells in the early phase following implantation. The duration of upregulation of heat shock proteins in these cells in vitro was of the order of 5 days, although the duration may be different in vivo.

Genetic manipulation of donor cells: enhancing paracrine effects within the myocardium

Skeletal MPCs have been shown to be vehicles for stable transgene expression and, in particular, can effect appropriate post-translational modifications for processing of secreted peptide molecules.[18] MPCs modified in this way have been used to deliver peptides both locally and systemically into the circulation. In one study, ex vivo retroviral transduction of primary murine MPCs with cDNA for human factor IX (hFIX) protein resulted in stable circulating levels of hFIX for up to 10 months following limb muscle implantation in SCID recipients.[19] Human primary myoblasts have also been effectively transduced in vitro, and reporter gene expression has been demonstrated following grafting into immunodeficient mice.[20] Further, non-transformed MPCs may be manipulated by gene-targeting strategies involving homologous recombination.[21] We and others have investigated the possibility of enhancing the angiogenic effects of MPCs implanted into the heart by overexpressing $VEGF_{165}$ isoform in donor cells.[11,20] In our protocol, primary rat MPCs were transfected in vitro using the hemagglutinating virus of Japan (HVJ)–liposome system and implanted into infarcted rat hearts. This resulted in high-level VEGF expression within the myocardium of syngeneic recipients for 2 weeks and was associated with a significant increase in capillary density

127

in infarct border zones at the sites of cell implantation. Infarct size was reduced and cardiac function improved in the VEGF–MPC-engrafted hearts at 28 days without evidence of tumor formation. It is important to note that the duration and level of VEGF expression in this setting is critical to avoid angioma genesis. This deleterious effect of poorly regulated VEGF expression within the heart following MPC transfer has been reported by other investigators.[22] MPC-mediated gene delivery strategies could be further refined by the use of regulatable transgene expression cassettes. In one study, Bohl and co-workers successfully used a tetracycline-inducible system to regulate levels of erythropoietin expression in vivo by primary murine MPCs implanted into limb muscle.[23]

Intracoronary cell delivery

The most conventional method for delivery of exogenous cells to the myocardium in vivo is direct intramuscular injection into the left ventricular free wall.[1–5] This has the benefit of being an easy approach at the time of open surgical procedures and allows for well-defined sites of cell delivery – particularly in the case of infarcted hearts, in which cells may be targeted to peri-infarct zones. Unfortunately, direct injection inevitably results in a marked acute inflammatory response that kills both grafted cells and host cells. Indeed, studies on the survival of cells delivered by this method suggest that the majority of grafted cells die within 72 h.[14] Furthermore, the development of scar tissue following this inflammatory response may not be beneficial with regard to achieving maximal functional benefits, due to isolation of the graft – electrically, mechanically and for the delivery of putative paracrine mediators. As an alternative approach, intracoronary delivery of cells could potentially result in global dissemination of MPCs to the ventricular myocardium throughout all cardiac layers.[24] An in vivo rat model has been developed in our laboratory that involves explantation of the heart, ex vivo perfusion of the coronary arterial supply with a cell suspension under carefully defined conditions and heterotopic transplantation into a recipient animal's abdomen. This is a useful system for experimental delivery of cells and as a model of a therapeutically relevant method of cell delivery, as discussed elsewhere in this book.

We have found that cells migrate from the vasculature into the myocardial interstitium within 24 h of intracoronary delivery. The exact mechanism by which this occurs is unknown, although increased incubation pressure is likely to be an important factor. The volume and cell density infused also appear to be important factors for success. With the rat system, having more than a critical density of cells (10^7–10^8/ml) results in occlusion of the coronary capillaries with gross edema and abrupt cessation of contraction following reperfusion. Up to 1 million cells in a total volume of 1 ml can, however, be safely delivered by this approach. Using a rat L6 cell line with nuclear-localized ß-galactosidase expression (n-ßgal-L6), we have been able to follow the fate of MPCs delivered by this route. We have found that cells disseminate within the heart and appear to proliferate rapidly in the initial phase following transplantation.[24] By 28 days, easily discernible multinucleate myotubes were found in all hearts examined (Figure 9.2). Importantly, delivery of cells by this route did not result in a significant acute inflammatory response and did not result in the isolation of grafted cells by scar tissue. Indeed, the cells formed myotubes, which aligned with the

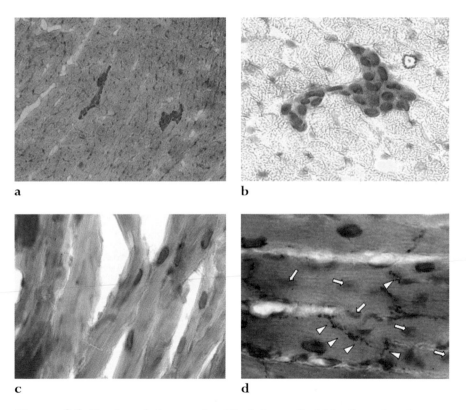

a

b

c

d

Figure 9.2 *Histologic findings at day 28 of clone n-ßgal-L6 cells implanted into the myocardium of adult Sprague Dawley rats via the coronary arteries. (a,b) At some loci, there were colonies of undifferentiated MPCs (a: ×100; b: ×400). (c,d) In contrast, at other loci, there was evidence of differentiation of donor cells into multinucleate myotubes (blue nuclei), which had aligned with the cardiac fiber axis. (d) Connexin 43 expression (arrowheads) was seen at the interfaces between grafted myotubes and host cardiac myocytes (arrow = unstained nuclei).*

129

cardiac fiber axis. Other studies have also suggested that delivery of cells by the intravascular route results in improved alignment of cells with the cardiac fiber axis and lack of formation of scar tissue.[25,26] Interestingly, we and others have found evidence of in vivo gap junction coupling between donor-derived myotubes and host cardiac myocytes, as shown by connexin 43 (Cx43) expression at the interfaces between the two cell types (Figure 9.2).[24,25] One might therefore postulate that this would be better for functional effects – particularly if mechanical contribution from the graft-derived myotubes is important.

More recently, we have demonstrated the feasibility of using the intracoronary delivery system to engraft MPCs in a rodent model of global cardiomyopathy induced by doxorubicin administration.[27] Using primary rat MPCs derived from muscle fibers of a fast-twitch lower limb muscle, we have found that similar cell number and density to those in the above L6 studies result in differentiation of graft cells within host myocardium, again with evidence of alignment with the cardiac fiber axis. Furthermore, a significant improvement was found in the systolic and diastolic function of the engrafted hearts as determined by ex vivo Langendorff perfusion. Interestingly, no evidence of tumor-like formation was found in these hearts, suggesting that this phenomenon may be related to the use of the immortalized L6 cell line.

Further work will be needed to examine serial changes in cardiac morphology and function following intracoronary cell delivery, using non-invasive techniques such as echocardiography. In addition, extensive large animal studies, without heterotopic transplantation, should be performed to determine the optimal cell number and density prior to further clinical trials. Interestingly, we have recently begun to investigate a retrograde technique of intravascular cell delivery to the myocardium by using the coronary venous system in rats. Preliminary results suggest that this is an efficacious method for engrafting MPCs that may have fewer potential risks compared with anterograde intracoronary delivery (K. Suzuki and B. Murtuza, unpublished observations).

As well as effects on angiogenesis, implanted MPCs could be modified to directly attenuate or reverse pathways implicated in adverse remodeling of the failing heart. One interesting possibility that we have begun to explore is the modulation of extracellular matrix metabolism within infarcted murine myocardium by implantation of MPCs modified to secrete an interleukin-1 inhibitor. Preliminary data from this study suggest that these modified MPCs may attenuate remodeling by influencing both collagen and matrix metalloproteinase gene expression (B. Murtuza and K. Suzuki, unpublished observations). While MPCs may be manipulated to enhance their survival or

130

secrete beneficial molecules such as VEGF within the host myocardium, it is not clear to what extent coupling between the donor cells and host myocardium is important for the functional effects observed. As an initial step in the investigation of this problem, we examined the importance of the gap junction protein Cx43 in the differentiation and intercellular communication of skeletal myoblasts in vitro.

Enhancing differentiation and functional integration of grafts

The relevance of connexin 43 in myoblast transplantation to the heart

Functional coupling between grafted skeletal muscle-derived cells and the host myocardium may be a critical component in effecting the functional improvement that is seen in experimental models as described. This could occur at three levels – electrical, mechanical and metabolic. Our initial studies and that of Robinson et al suggested expression of Cx43 at the interface between grafted skeletal myotubes and host cardiac myocytes following implantation by the intra-arterial route.[24,25] Cx43 is one of the major proteins involved in gap junctional intercellular communication in the heart. This transmembrane molecule forms channels composed of hexamers (connexons), and hemichannels of these hexamers on adjacent cells can align to form complete channels for communication (Figure 9.3).[28] The channels permit the exchange of ions, metabolites and other small molecules between cells and enable electrical coupling. In the myocardium, this functional coupling is required for the normal electrical and mechanical activity of the myocardium as a syncitium. Cx43 is also expressed in many other cell types, such as smooth muscle cells, endothelial cells and astrocytes, and is also of significance in cancer cells, where it has been shown to be downregulated.[28,29] Cx43 is known to enhance differentiation of cells, and in this regard may also act as a tumor suppressor. We have generated a Cx43-overexpressing L6 skeletal myoblast cell line to examine the influence of Cx43 on the properties of these cells and myotubes in vitro, with a view to establishing its relevance to in vivo grafting of muscle cells to the heart.

Normally, Cx43 is expressed at early stages of myogenesis, although it is downregulated and not expressed in mature muscle.[30] We found that Cx43-overexpressing L6 cell lines demonstrate decreased proliferation rates, but enhanced differentiative capacity in vitro as measured by creatine kinase expression.[31] This is consistent with the above-described effects of this protein. We then studied the intercellular communication between these cells

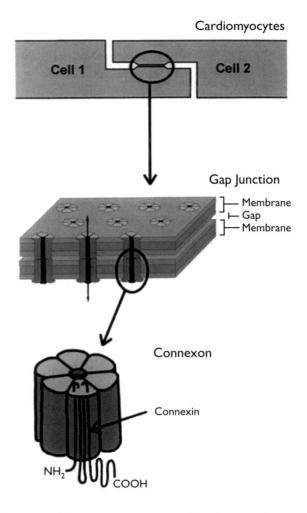

Figure 9.3 *Diagram illustrating components and localization of gap junction channels between two cardiac myocytes. Gap junctions are formed by the apposition of two hemichannels (connexons) on adjacent cell surfaces – each composed of hexamers of the protein connexin 43.*

in vitro. Studies using micro-dye injection or scrape-loading protocols to load target cells with fluorescent dyes clearly showed an enhanced transfer of these small molecules in the cell lines overexpressing Cx43 as compared with control myoblasts (Figure 9.4). These properties may be useful for the functional integration of grafts in the myocardium in vivo. In another study,

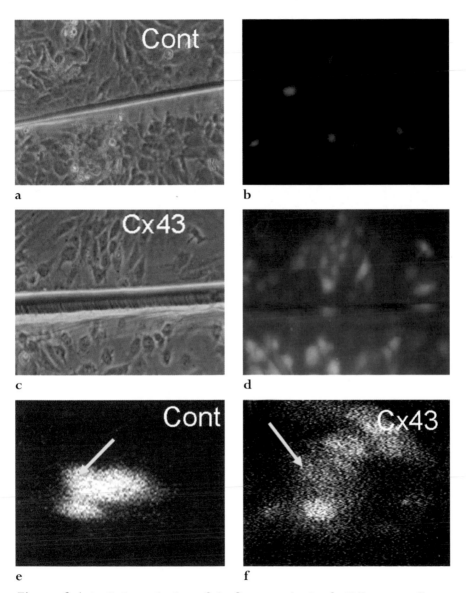

Figure 9.4 *(a–d) Scrape loading of the fluorescent dye Lucifer Yellow onto cell monolayers in culture. There is a clear enhancement of the intercellular communication in the Cx43-overexpressing L6 cell line (d) as shown by dye transfer up to nine cell diameters distant from the site of dye loading compared with control cells (b). Further studies using micro-dye injection of 6-carboxyfluorescein also showed enhanced intercellular communication in the Cx43-L6 cells (f) compared with control cells (e). (a) and (b) are reverse-phase microscopic images.*

133

Reinecke et al examined the electrical coupling between cardiac myocytes and skeletal myoblasts in vitro and found evidence of coupling as determined by synchronous calcium transients.[32] The potential of Cx43-overexpressing MPCs in vivo remains to be established and will be difficult to prove, due to technical limitations, although novel techniques, such as high-resolution optical mapping, which allow the study of cells in the intact, beating heart could help.[33] Theoretically, however, although enhanced differentiation capacity could be considered beneficial, the consequent reduction in proliferative potential may be a significant limitation, particularly following direct intramyocardial injection, which usually results in the death of the majority of the cells at the outset. With respect to electrical coupling, the effects of Cx43-overexpressing MPCs on the incidence of cardiac arrhythmias following implantation remains to be determined.

Recently, many phase I clinical trials of myoblast transplantation to the heart have been initiated to determine the safety and feasibility of this approach. The major adverse events related to the procedures appear to be arrhythmias, as reported by the group who had the initial experience in patients.[7] Indeed, many patients in this study have undergone implantation of automatic implantable ventricular defibrillator devices. These effects do appear, however, to be at least partly related to the cell density and/or number implanted, as other groups who have implanted far fewer cells into patients report a much lower incidence of arrhythmias following direct injection.[34] Clinical trials of intravascular delivery using myoblasts and bone marrow-derived precursor cells are also in progress, although, due to the worrying phenomenon of coronary capillary occlusion that we have clearly demonstrated in an experimental model, we would suggest that many more small and large animal studies be undertaken prior to embarking upon such procedures.

Summary and conclusions

In this chapter, we have discussed strategies for the preparation, manipulation and delivery of MPCs aimed at optimizing their functional properties within the heart. We have highlighted the benefits of the SF system in terms of cell quality and purity and have shown that the survival and proliferation of MPCs may be enhanced by physical manipulation (heat shock treatment) or by genetic manipulation leading to the expression of beneficial paracrine molecules such as VEGF. In addition, we have suggested the potential relevance of Cx43-overexpressing MPCs in enhancing integration with host cardiac myocytes. While mechanistic studies will be required to define exactly how cell implantation improves cardiac function, enhancement of these properties of the grafted cells is likely to enhance the results obtained, if, as appears to be likely, the degree of improvement can be correlated with the success of grafting as defined by these parameters. There is thus an urgent need for further experimental work in parallel with clinical trials to clarify the mechanism by which cell implantation improves cardiac function in heart failure.

References

1. Taylor DA, Atkins BZ, Hungspreugs P et al. Regenerating functional myocardium: improved performance after skeletal myoblast transplantation. Nat Med 1998; 4: 929–33.

2. Murry CE, Wiseman RW, Schwartz SM, Hauschka SD. Skeletal myoblast transplantation for repair of myocardial necrosis. J Clin Invest 1996; 98: 2512–23.

3. Koh GY, Klug MG, Soonpaa MH, Field LJ. Differentiation and long-term survival of C2C12 myoblast grafts in heart. J Clin Invest 1993; 92: 1548–54.

4. Koh GY, Soonpaa MH, Klug MG et al. Stable fetal cardiomyocyte grafts in the hearts of dystrophic mice and dogs. J Clin Invest 1995; 96: 2034–42.

5. Koh GY, Kim SJ, Klug MG et al. Targeted expression of transforming growth factor-beta 1 in intracardiac grafts promotes vascular endothelial cell DNA synthesis. J Clin Invest 1995; 95: 114–21.

6. Kass DA, Baughman KL, Pak PH et al. Reverse remodeling from cardiomyoplasty in human heart failure. External constraint versus active assist. Circulation 1995; 91: 2314–18.

7. Menasche P, Hagege AA, Scorsin M et al. Myoblast transplantation for heart failure. Lancet 2001; 357: 279–80.

8. Qu Z, Balkir L, van Deutekom JC et al. Development of approaches to improve cell survival in myoblast transfer therapy. J Cell Biol 1998; 142: 1257–67.

9. Rosenblatt JD, Lunt AI, Parry DJ, Partridge TA. Culturing satellite cells from living single muscle fiber explants. In Vitro Cell Dev Biol Anim 1995; 31: 773–9.

10. Suzuki K, Murtuza B, Heslop L et al. Single fibers of skeletal muscle as a novel graft for cell transplantation to the heart. J Thorac Cardiovasc Surg 2002; 123: 984–92.

11. Suzuki K, Murtuza B, Smolenski RT et al. Cell transplantation for the treatment of acute myocardial infarction using vascular endothelial growth factor-expressing skeletal myoblasts. Circulation 2001; 104: I207–12.

12. Pouzet B, Vilquin JT, Hagege AA et al. Intramyocardial transplantation of autologous myoblasts: can tissue processing be optimized? Circulation 2000; 102: III-210–15.

13. Fan Y, Beilharz MW, Grounds MD. A potential alternative strategy for myoblast transfer therapy: the use of sliced muscle grafts. Cell Transplant 1996; 5: 421–9.

14. Zhang M, Methot D, Poppa V et al. Cardiomyocyte grafting for cardiac repair: graft cell death and anti-death strategies. J Mol Cell Cardiol 2001; 33: 907–21.

15. Suzuki K, Smolenski RT, Jayakumar J et al. Heat shock treatment enhances graft cell survival in skeletal myoblast transplantation to the heart. Circulation 2000; 102: III-216–21.

16. Mosser DD, Caron AW, Bourget L et al. Role of the human heat shock protein hsp70 in protection against stress-induced apoptosis. Mol Cell Biol 1997; 17: 5317–27.

17. Suzuki K, Sawa Y, Kaneda Y et al. In vivo gene transfection with heat shock protein 70 enhances myocardial tolerance to ischemia–reperfusion injury in rat. J Clin Invest 1997; 99: 1645–50.

18. Springer ML, Blau HM. High-efficiency retroviral infection of primary myoblasts. Somat Cell Mol Genet 1997; 23: 203–9.

19. Wang JM, Zheng H, Blaivas M, Kurachi K. Persistent systemic production of human factor IX in mice by skeletal myoblast-mediated gene transfer: feasibility of repeat application to obtain therapeutic levels. Blood 1997; 90: 1075–82.

20. Salvatori G, Ferrari G, Mezzogiorno A et al. Retroviral vector-mediated gene transfer into human primary myogenic cells leads to expression in muscle fibers in vivo. Hum Gene Ther 1993; 4: 713–23.

21. Arbones ML, Austin HA, Capon DJ, Greenburg G. Gene targeting in normal somatic cells: inactivation of the interferon-gamma receptor in myoblasts. Nat Genet 1994; 6: 90–7.

22. Lee RJ, Springer ML, Blanco-Bose WE et al. VEGF gene delivery to myocardium: deleterious effects of unregulated expression. Circulation 2000; 102: 898–901.

23. Bohl D, Naffakh N, Heard JM. Long-term control of erythropoietin secretion by doxycycline in mice transplanted with engineered primary myoblasts. Nat Med 1997; 3: 299–305.

24. Suzuki K, Brand NJ, Smolenski RT et al. Development of a novel method for cell transplantation through the coronary artery. Circulation 2000; 102: III-359–64.

25. Robinson SW, Cho PW, Levitsky HI et al. Arterial delivery of genetically labelled skeletal myoblasts to the murine heart: long-term survival and phenotypic modification of implanted myoblasts. Cell Transplant 1996; 5: 77–91.

26. Taylor DA, Silvestry SC, Bishop SP et al. Delivery of primary autologous skeletal myoblasts into rabbit heart by coronary infusion: a potential approach to myocardial repair. Proc Assoc Am Physicians 1997; 109: 245–53.

27. Suzuki K, Murtuza B, Suzuki N et al. Intracoronary infusion of skeletal myoblasts improves cardiac function in doxorubicin-induced heart failure. Circulation 2001; 104: I-213–17.

28. Goodenough DA, Goliger JA, Paul DL. Connexins, connexons, and intercellular communication. Annu Rev Biochem 1996; 65: 475–502.

29. Yamasaki H, Naus CC. Role of connexin genes in growth control. Carcinogenesis 1996; 17: 1199–213.

30. Balogh S, Naus CC, Merrifield PA. Expression of gap junctions in cultured rat L6 cells during myogenesis. Dev Biol 1993; 155: 351–60.

31. Suzuki K, Brand NJ, Allen S et al. Overexpression of connexin 43 in skeletal myoblasts: relevance to cell transplantation to the heart. J Thorac Cardiovasc Surg 2001; 122: 759–66.

32. Reinecke H, MacDonald GH, Hauschka SD, Murry CE. Electromechanical coupling between skeletal and cardiac muscle. Implications for infarct repair. J Cell Biol 2000; 149: 731–40.

33. Eloff BC, Lerner DL, Yamada KA et al. High resolution optical mapping reveals conduction slowing in connexion 43 deficient mice. Circulation 2000; 102: II-3 (abstract).

34. Dib N, McCarthy P, Campbell A et al. Safety and feasibility of autologous myoblast transplantation in patients with ischaemic cardiomyopathy: interim results from the United States experience. Circulation 2002; 106: II-463 (abstract).

10. STEM CELLS AND MYOCARDIAL REGENERATION

E Michael Molnar

Introduction

Cardiomyocytes lose their ability to proliferate soon after birth, and therefore heart muscle fibers cannot regenerate. For this reason, myocardial injury, such as myocardial infarction (MI), heals by replacement of contractile heart muscle fibers by fibrotic tissue scar, which not only is unable to participate in the pumping of blood, but does not even contribute to the passive mechanics of the heart. Massive loss of cardiomyocytes post-MI is a common cause of heart failure (HF), which is a consequence of many other cardiovascular diseases, and a serious public health problem.

An abundance of experimental data regarding the ability of implanted myoblastic cells to restore the function of damaged cardiomyocytes encouraged cardiovascular surgeons and interventional cardiologists in Paris, France and Dusseldorf, Germany to treat patients with extensive MI by cell transplantation (CT).[1,2] Owing to the paucity of suitable donors for orthotopic heart transplantation, as well as the severity and risks of such an undertaking, the success of cell transplantation in the prevention of massive damage of heart muscle after MI has been encouraging.

The cell transplants used in the above clinical trials were autologous: skeletal myoblasts in Paris[1] and mononuclear bone marrow cells in Dusseldorf.[2]

Strauer et al reported the clinical data of 10 patients after MI treated with their method of cell transplantation plus standard therapy, compared with the parameters of 10 patients receiving standard therapy only. After 3 months' follow-up, the post-MI scar, measured by left ventriculography, was decreased significantly in size within the CT group, and was significantly smaller than in the standard therapy group. Infarction wall movement velocity increased significantly in the CT group only. Dobutamine stress echocardiography, radionuclide ventriculography and catheterization of the right heart all showed a significant improvement in stroke volume index, left ventricular end-systolic volume, contractility and myocardial perfusion of the infarct region.[3]

Owing to the limited availability of human fetal cardiomyocytes, alternative sources of suitable cell transplants for treatment of MI, congestive HF, dilated cardiomyopathy and other heart diseases have been looked for.

A single fiber of skeletal muscle retains skeletal myoblasts beneath the basal lamina throughout life. From these myoblasts, skeletal muscle regenerates in the case of injury. In two rat models of HF, allogeneic skeletal myoblasts were injected into four myocardial sites. Within 3 days, donor single skeletal fibers disappeared, while their myoblasts began to differentiate into multinucleated myotubes. This process took 4 weeks, and resulted in significant improvement in cardiac function.[4]

In a group of rats that received intramyocardial injection ex vivo for 7 days, expanded autologous skeletal myoblasts 7 days after infarct had significantly better left ventricular function than controls at 2 months' follow-up, and somewhat better function than the group treated with ACE inhibitors alone, as assessed by two-dimensional echocardiography. The best results were seen in the group that received CT and ACE inhibitors simultaneously.[5]

In a rat model of MI, an intra-infarct injection of allogeneic skeletal myoblasts 7 days after MI improved post-MI in vivo exercise capacity and ex vivo global ventricular dilatation and septum-to-free wall diameter, as determined by pressure–volume curves obtained from isolated, red cell-perfused, balloon-in-left ventricle hearts, 3 and 6 weeks after cell transplantation. As many as 13 out of 14 hearts showed evidence of survival of transplanted myoblasts.[6]

In a pig model of MI, 2 weeks after MI an intra-infarct injection of autologous mesenchymal stem cells from bone marrow was given. Two weeks after transplantation, a robust engraftment in all treated animals, with expression of muscle-specific proteins, attenuation of contractile dysfunction and marked reduction of the extent of wall thinning measured by piezoelectric crystals placed in the myocardium before MI was observed.[7]

As an alternative to skeletal myoblasts, allogeneic fetal cultured stomach smooth muscle cells were transplanted in a rat model of MI. All animals were immunosuppressed by cyclosporin A. Transplants formed smooth muscle tissue in the infarcted myocardium and improved contractile function as compared with controls. Angiogenesis was also apparent.[8]

Embryonic cells injected into infarcted myocardium of a rat model of MI demonstrated their new cardiomyocyte phenotype by strong positive staining to sarcomeric α-actin, cardiac α-myosin heavy chain, and troponin I, 6 weeks after cell transplantation, at which time significantly improved cardiac function was also measured.[9]

Clonal stem cell line WB-F344 from a male adult rat liver was injected as a cell xenogeneic transplant into the left ventricle of adult female nude mice. Male WB-F344 cells with the same genotype were identified within the implantation site 6 weeks later. The phenotype of these new 'stem cell-derived cells' was that of cardiomyocytes. Thus adult liver-derived stem cells responded in vivo to the tissue environment of adult heart and differentiated into mature cardiomyocytes.[10]

Autologous skeletal myoblasts have been favored in clinical practice to date because of easy availability. In reality, due to lack of connexin 43, a gap junction protein, skeletal myoblast transplants should not be as effective as cardiomyocytes in the treament of MI. Only connexin 43-containing cardiomyocyte transplants build intercellular connections with host myocardial fibers, such as gap junctions and desmosomes, and thereby act synchronously with the host heart.

Neonatal cardiomyocytes of 3-day-old rats were injected into the border zone of infarct 10 days after injury. Subsequently, 4–14 days later, the treated hearts were studied by immunohistochemistry. Antibodies against connexin 43, desmoplakin and cadherin, identifying gap junctions, desmosomes and adherens junctions, respectively, were found between grafted cardiomyocytes, as well as between grafted and host cardiomyocytes. Grafted cardiomyocytes were seen aligning parallel to, and establishing electrical pathways with, the host cardiomyocytes.[11]

In two adult X-linked muscular dystrophy dogs lacking expression of dystrophin in both cardiac and skeletal muscles, fetal canine atrial cardiomyocytes, including sinus nodal cells, were injected into the left ventricle. Four weeks later, catheter ablation of the arterioventricular (AV) node was carried out. Immediately thereafter, a ventricular escape rhythm emerged, which originated from a new pacemaker within the labeled cell transplantation site. This was the first in vivo evidence of electrical and mechanical coupling between allogeneic donor cardiomyocytes and host myocardium.[12]

A comparison of fetal cardiomyocyte and skeletal myoblast transplantation in a rat model of MI showed no difference in left ventricular ejection fraction, but it was significantly lower in a control group of untreated animals. All animals were immunosuppressed.[13]

In a comparative study of the effects of transplantation of fetal ventricular cardiomyocytes, enteric smooth muscle cells and skin fibroblasts in a rat model of MI, 4 weeks after injury the above cell transplants were injected into myocardial scar. End-diastolic volume, $+dP/dt$, and $-dP/dt$, were all significantly higher in the group of rats receiving fetal cardiomyocytes. All animals were immunosuppressed.[14]

The results of autologous skeletal myoblast and dermal fibroblast transplantation were compared in a rabbit chronically injured heart model: both contractile skeletal myoblasts and non-contractile fibroblasts improved the structural properties of injured heart, as reflected in diastolic performance, but only skeletal myoblasts enhanced the systolic performance of the terminally injured heart.[15]

How soon after MI should CT be done? The following two studies are not in full agreement but indicate that CT should be carried out no later than 6 days after MI. When carried out by selective coronary catheterization and infusion of myoblasts, rather than injection into infarcted myocardium, CT can take place at the time of initial balloon angioplasty, stenting or other invasive procedure.

In a rat model of MI, fetal cardiomyocytes were transplanted immediately at 2 and 4 weeks after myocardial injury. At 8 weeks, studies of heart function, planimetry and histology were carried out. The inflammatory reaction was greatest during the first week and subsided during the second week after MI. Scar size increased for up to 8 weeks after MI. Cardiomyocytes transplanted immediately after MI were absent at 8 weeks, and the scar size and heart function were as in the untreated group. Cardiomyocyte transplantation should be carried out immediately after the inflammatory reaction is over, but before scar expansion.[16]

Ultrastructural analysis of infarcted myocardium in a murine model of MI showed a complete loss of damaged cardiomyocytes within 2 days and healing by scar within 7 days after MI. Implanted cardiomyocytes were already engrafted throughout the wall of infarct 2 weeks after MI, with their excitability intact, and their differentiation proceeding at a fast pace.[17]

The fate of cardiomyocytes injected into infarcted myocardium of an adult rat model of MI, 7 days after injury, was followed by a quantitative TaqMan PCR and histology, and heart function was evaluated by biplane angiography. Grafted neonatal cardiomyocytes were still present 6 months after transplantation; they thickened the left ventricular wall, significantly increased ejection fraction, and reduced paradoxical systolic bulging of the infarcted area.[18]

Previous studies with bone marrow stromal cells engrafted into xenogeneic fetal recipients were repeated: the recipients were fully immunocompetent adults, and no immunosuppression was used. Bone marrow stromal cells were taken from C57B1/6 mice and injected into adult Lewis rats. One week later the recipients underwent coronary artery ligation and they were sacrificed 1–12 weeks thereafter. Labeled mouse cells were engrafted into bone marrow cavities for the duration of the experiment. Circulating mouse cells were found only in rats with 1-day-old MI. Mouse cells were found in the damaged myocardium by immunohistochemistry. This study proved that adult stem cells engraft into a xenogeneic live being, without immunosuppression, without difficulty. Simultaneously, they can home to injured myocardium, differentiate into cardiomyocytes and create a stable chimera in the heart.[19]

Human mesenchymal xenogeneic stem cells were injected into the left ventricle of CB17 SCID beige adult mice without immunosuppression. After 7 days, de novo expression of desmin, ß-myosin heavy chains, α-actinin, cardiac troponin T and phospholamban, all typical of cardiomyocytes, could be detected. Human adult xenogeneic mesenchymal stem cells engrafted in the myocardium and differentiated into cardiomyocytes.[20]

Embryonic cardiac cells were cultured for 3 days, and then implanted 7 days after extensive MI into the myocardium of a rat model, without immunosuppression. Engraftment of cell xenotransplants was observed 1, 4 and 7 weeks after CT. Differentiation of embryonic cells into cardiomyocytes was demonstrated by antibodies against α-SMA, connexin-43, and fast and slow myosin heavy chain. Serial echocardiography revealed that CT prevented scar thinning, left ventricular dilatation and dysfunction as compared with controls.[21]

Some reports on the experimental use of stem cell transplantation list angiogenesis as one of the benefits. In a rat model of MI, allogeneic aortic endothelial cells were injected into myocardial scar 2 weeks after infarct. The transplanted cells stimulated angiogenesis and increased perfusion in the myocardial scar, but there was no improvement in overall heart function.[22]

Early experiences

For years, transplantation of placental cells has played a major role in therapy for arteriosclerotic vascular disease, because placenta cells cause generalized vasodilatation, overall circulatory improvement and increased budding of capillary collaterals.

While developing corneal transplantation, Filatov searched for a method to avoid postoperative clouding of corneal transplants. Once, during such an operation, he implanted tissue fragments of placenta subcutaneously. Corneal clouding did not occur, and implantation of placental cells became a major topic of Soviet research institutes, soon spreading to the West as the 'Filatov treatment'.

An experimental study on the treatment of arteriosclerotic vascular disease by placenta cell transplantation reported on the clinical application of the same treatment.[23]

The scientific reason why placenta cells have been the most widely used cell transplants to date is not entirely clear. Embryonic stem cell research will undoubtedly provide answers because of the close relationship between embryonic stem cells and trophoblastic cells.

Without trophoblasts an embryo could never become a newborn. At the beginning of conception trophoblasts are indistinguishable from 'embryonic stem cells'. Only at the 58-cell human blastocyst stage can the outer cells, destined to produce trophoblasts of placenta, be recognized as different from the inner cells, which will form the embryo. In a 107-cell human blastocyst, eight embryo-producing cells are surrounded by 99 trophoblastic cells, a 12 : 1 ratio.[24]

Advances in the therapy of MI and HF, as well as other heart diseases, based on the initial experimental work of Chiu (1995), Li (1996) and Menasche (1996), were preceded by several decades of clinical experience of German practitioners of cell therapy and Soviet cell transplantologists.

From 1953, there were yearly national symposia in Germany, where theoreticians and practitioners of cell therapy exchanged ideas and discussed results. In 1954, 'Therapiewoche' in Karlsruhe attracted 5000 physicians practicing cell therapy. Since 1953, German medical journals have published upwards of 2000 articles on cell therapy. The summary of the most important ones was published in 1975 by the International Research Association for Cell Therapy in Frankfurt: 'Literaturverzeichnes der Internationalen Forshungsgesellschaft fur Zelltherapie'.

In the USSR there were biannual all-USSR cell transplantation symposia from 1976 until 1990 and many publications; however, reports prior to the 1970s are hard to find.

The sole publication in English[25] (a translation of the same book in German of 4 years earlier[26]) presents the scientific basis of cell therapy. This book includes a report on the treatment of 251 cardiac patients with cell therapy; only one patient's condition worsened. The rest were improved or unchanged. In 35 patients, 3–6 months post-MI the success rate was 51%; in 76 patients with various types of myocardial damage, the success rate was 53%; in 41 patients with 'myodegeneratio cordis', the success rate was 72%; and in 9 patients with conduction block of the Adams–Stokes type, the success rate was 55%.[27]

This was before the era of routine heart catheterization and interventional cardiology, and other modern technologies: none of the above patients received cell transplants via injection into damaged myocardium or via balloon catheter in the branch of the coronary artery. Fetal cell xenotransplants were implanted deeply subcutaneously, counting on homing of these fetal progenitor cells into injured tissue, and their differentiation into cardiomyocytes and vascular cells. The concept of homing was proved in the 1950s in Germany in isotope and intravital dye studies,[25,26,28,29] and since 1993 in the US and other Western countries as well.[30–32]

Publications on the treatment of diabetes mellitus and its microangiopathic complications by islet cell transplantation are more numerous than for any other illness in which CT is indicated. It is remarkable that no-one has ever thought to transplant islet cells directly into the pancreas of a diabetic patient. Usually the implantation was into the liver, directly (very rarely), indirectly via the portal vein (used only in urgent situations), or indirectly into the liver via the portal vein–vena cava anastomotic system above the umbilicus (commonly used). The liver is the most immunoprotective organ in the body: no live cell implanted directly into the liver is ever rejected. This well-established scientific fact has never been explained. In islet cell transplantation for diabetes mellitus, the idea of homing has been accepted for decades.

In 1993 the author gained his first clinical experience with CT in cardiology. In a cooperative study by the International Institute of Biological Medicine in Moscow and the Russian Research Institute of Pediatrics of the Russian Academy of Medical Sciences, seven terminal patients with dilated cardiomyopathy, aged 4–14 years, were treated by human fetal cell transplantation. Cell transplants of myocardium, liver and placenta were implanted under the aponeurosis of the rectus abdominis muscle above the umbilicus. One patient 10 years of age died 4 days after CT: on autopsy, it was found that dilated cardiomyopathy was secondary to an anomalous origin of the coronary arteries. The remaining patients benefited from the procedure and were able to return home in improved condition, which was entirely unexpected. One of the patients became worse 1 month later at home, was admitted to the Coronary Care Unit of the local hospital and subsequently died.

Besides homing, cell therapy in Germany and CT in the USSR has been based on the following concepts. Only fetal cells are used for transplantation (with the exception of cell transplants of various endocrine glands, where neonatal cells have been utilized). The following are the major reasons for preferring fetal cells: (1) their ability to undergo change in response to environmental or genetic factors; (2) their easy adaptability (growth, migration, mobility, creation of cell-to-cell contacts); (3) their more frequent and faster cell division and differentiation; (4) their production of large amounts of various growth factors; (5) their lowered immunogenicity; (6) their ability to survive on energy supplied by glycolysis and on lower amounts of oxygen; and (7) their lack of cell extensions that could be easily damaged during the processing of cell transplants.

In addition, fetal stem cells are much more numerous than rare adult stem cells, so that no special cell isolation procedures have to be utilized in the preparation of cell transplants. Fetal stem cells live in a milieu of various already differentiated cells, and fetal stem transplants contain other cells of the same family, of various generations and in cell-to-cell contact.

The primary benefit of CT is direct stimulation of the regeneration of damaged cells of the recipient rather than replacement of destroyed cells.

Only small children in the early stages of their illness are treated by one cell transplant only. The usual chronically ill patient requires transplantation of cells of all those organs or tissues which are involved in the pathophysiology of their disease(s). The more exact the pathophysiologic and biochemical diagnosis, the more accurate will be the choice of cell transplants for treatment. Cardiac patients have usually received, in addition to transplantation of myocardial cells, cells of liver and placenta (and lungs in cases of left-side HF with pulmonary congestion and hypertension), unless additional malfunctions are discovered which could be corrected by transplants of cells with necessary compensatory functions.

No immunosuppression is required in the clinical application of CT. Of the estimated 5–25 million patients treated by CT worldwide, 99.99% underwent allogeneic or xenogeneic transplantation without immunosuppression. In its approbation of islet cell transplantation for clinical practice in 1984, the Ministry of Health of the USSR stated under '4/' that no immunosuppression is necessary, provided that guidelines for preparation of cell transplants are followed: namely the use of primary cell culture. Of 22 recent studies described in this chapter,[1–22] in five dealing with cell xenotransplantation no immunosuppression was required, and of 12 studies on allogeneic CT the authors utilized immunosuppresssion in three studies only.

Cell transplants can be prepared for patient treatment from any vertebrate, from *Homo sapiens* to fish. The sole exception is the frontal lobe of the brain, which animals lack, so frontal lobe cell transplants have to be of human fetal origin. For obvious ethical, moral, religious and practical reasons, only cell xenotransplantation has been used in Germany and other Western European countries until recently. In the USSR, human fetal tissue transplantation was abandoned after 1988 in favor of xenotransplantation. The scientific basis for the use of cell xenotransplantation has been the principle of 'organospecificity'.

Key cells of the same organ or tissue are the same in nature, regardless of the species of origin, i.e. they are organ-specific (or tissue-specific) and not species-specific, and the same applies to any of over 200 kinds of cell found in the human or animal body. In 1898, Wilson described his observation that in various genera the same organs always originated from the same group of cells, e.g. organospecificity.[33]

There are no antigenic differences between the corresponding cells of identical organs of different animal species (and humans), and cell surface antibodies are organ-specific (or tissue-specific) and non-species-specific. This is another proof of organospecificity.[34–36] Organospecificity has been *res ipsa loquitur* for German and USSR cell transplantologists.

The development of molecular cell biology during the last century was based on the fact that all eukaryotic cells in nature develop and function according to the same laws. The great majority of proteins from different organisms (including humans) are similar over the entire amino acid sequence, e.g. they are homologous to each other.[37]

Since 1987, the author has used solely fetal cell xenotransplants of rabbit origin, prepared by primary organ culture. Figure 10.1 shows photomicrographs of: (a) rabbit adult myocardium; (b) histology of primary organ culture of rabbit fetal cardiomyoblasts after 48 h; and (c) the same

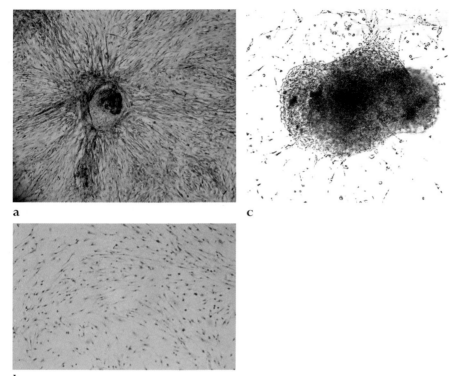

a

c

b

Figure 10.1 *(a) Histology of adult rabbit heart; stained by the May–Grunwald–Giemsa method. (b) Histology of primary organ culture of fetal rabbit myocardium, duration 48 h, stained as a monolayer in a Leighton vial by the May–Grunwald–Giemsa method. (c) Live unstained primary organ culture of fetal rabbit myocardium from explants, duration 96 h, as seen under the inverted microscope. Comparison of (a) and (b) reveals cytologic similarities between adult rabbit cardiomyocytes and fetal rabbit cardiomyoblasts, as well as a clear tendency of cardiomyoblasts to become aligned parallel to each other in order to become cardiac muscle fibers. Primary organ culture appears to consist of only cardiomyoblasts, as most of the other cells found in the heart have been eliminated by tissue culture. The inverted microscope is utilized for continuous daily observation of growth characteristics of primary organ cultures and cytologic details during the preparation of cell xenotransplants, as seen in (c). With the passage of time, cardiomyoblasts assume the phenotypic features of cardiomyocytes and the structure of myocardial fibers. Two-dimensional digital photography cannot reproduce the visual image stored in the memory of the tissue culture expert, in particular the day-to-day 'slow-motion' changes taking place during the preparation of cell xenotransplants. The lack of a three-dimensional image is particularly noticeable in (c), despite computer modifications to increase plasticity (the inverted microscope presents a much lighter, and less sharp, picture).*

147

primary organ culture as seen live unstained under the inverted microscope, after 96 h. If you compare pictures of adult and fetal myocardium in any standard histology and embryology textbook, you may be surprised by the morphologic similarities between human and rabbit myocardium.

Future perspectives

Autologous cell transplantation of skeletal myoblasts, or mononuclear bone marrow stem cells, directly into damaged myocardium is a reliable treatment for patients with serious MI or HF who do not need CT immediately to save their life and are hospitalized in a top hospital, with qualified invasive cardiologists and an excellent tissue culture laboratory.

If this therapeutic method is to become important for the healthcare system worldwide, stem cell xenotransplantation will probably have to be utilized. Stem cell xenotransplants can be delivered to any hospital without delay, at all times, and transplanted indirectly into the liver if an interventional cardiologist is not at hand, without immunosuppression. Subsequently, such patients can be transferred to the higher-level hospital for more specialized care.

Acknowledgments

I would like to acknowledge the help of Dr. D. Elias for photographing the micrographs and Ing. A. Matas for the help in the preparation of this manuscript.

References

1. Menasche P, Hagege A, Scorsin M et al. Autologous skeletal myoblast transplantation for cardiac insufficiency. First clinical case. Arch Mal Coeur Vaiss 2001; 94: 180–2.

2. Strauer BE, Brehm M, Zeus T et al. Intracoronary, human autologous stem cell transplantation for myocardial regeneration following myocardial infarction. Dtsch Med Wochenschr 2001; 126: 932–8.

3. Strauer BE, Brehm M, Zeus T et al. Repair of infarcted myocardium by autologous intracoronary mononuclear bone marrow cell transplantation. Circulation 2002; 106: 1913–16.

4. Suzuki K, Murtuza B, Heslop L et al. Single fibers of skeletal muscle as a novel graft for cell transplantation to the heart. J Thorac Cardiovasc Surg 2002; 123: 984–92.

5. Pouzet B, Ghostine S, Vilquin JT et al. Is skeletal myoblast transplantation clinically relevant in the era of angiotensin-converting enzyme inhibitors? Circulation 2001; 104(suppl 1): 1223–8.

6. Jain M, DerSimonian H, Brenner DA et al. Cell therapy attenuates deleterious ventricular remodeling and improves cardiac performance after myocardial infarction. Circulation 2001; 103: 1920–7.

7. Shake JG, Gruber PJ, Baumgartner WA et al. Mesenchymal stem cell implantation in a swine myocardial infarct model: engraftment and functional effect. Ann Thorac Surg 2002; 73: 1919–25.

8. Li RK, Jia ZQ, Weisel RD et al. Smooth muscle cell transplantation into myocardial scar tissue improves heart function. J Mol Cell Cardiol 1999; 31: 513–22.

9. Min YI, Yang Y, Converso KL et al. Transplantation of embryonic stem cells improves cardiac function in postinfarcted rats. J Appl Physiol 2002; 92: 288–96.

10. Malouf NN, Coleman WB, Grisham JW et al. Adult-derived stem cells from the liver become myocytes in the heart in vivo. Am J Pathol 2001; 158: 1929–35.

11. Matsushita T, Oyamada M, Kurata H et al. Formation of cell junctions between grafted and host cardiomyocytes at the border zone of rat myocardial infarction. Circulation 1999; 19(suppl II): 262–8.

12. Ruhparwar A, Tebbeenjohans J, Niehaus M et al. Transplanted fetal cardiomyocytes as cardiac pacemaker. Eur J Cardiothorac Surg 2002; 21: 853–7.

13. Scorsin M, Hagege A, Vilquin JT et al. Comparison of the effects of fetal cardiomyocytes and skeletal myoblasts transplantation on postinfarction left ventricular function. J Thorac Cardiovasc Surg 2000; 119: 1169–75.

14. Sakai T, Li RK, Weisel RD et al. Fetal cell transplantation: a comparison of three cell types. J Thorac Cardiovasc Surg 1999; 118: 714–24.

15. Hutcheson KA, Atkins BZ, Hueman MT et al. Comparison of benefits on myocardial performance of cellular cardiomyoplasty with skeletal myoblasts and fibroblasts. Cell Transplant 2000; 9: 359–68.

16. Li RK, Mickle DA, Weisel RD et al. Optimal time for cardiomyocyte transplantation to maximize myocardial function after left ventricular injury. Ann Thorac Surg 2001; 72: 1957–63.

17. Roell W, Lu ZJ, Bloch W et al. Cellular cardiomyoplasty improves survival after myocardial injury. Circulation 2002; 105: 2435–41.

18. Muller-Ehmsen J, Peterson KL, Kedes L et al. Rebuilding a damaged heart: long-term survival of transplanted neonatal rat cardiomyocytes after myocardial infarction and effect on cardiac function. Circulation 2002; 105: 1720–6.

19. Saito T, Kuang JQ, Bittira B et al. Xenotransplant cardiac chimera: immunotolerance of adult stem cells. Ann Thorac Surg 2002; 74: 19–24.

20. Toma C, Pittenger MF, Cahill KS et al. Human mesenchymal stem cells differentiate to a cardiomyocyte phenotype in the adult murine heart. Circulation 2002; 105: 93–8.

21. Etzion S, Battler A, Barbash IM et al. Influence of embryonic cardiomyocyte transplantation on the progression of heart failure in a rat model of extensive myocardial infarction. J Mol Cell Cardiol 2001; 33: 1321–30.

22. Kim EJ, Li RK, Weizel RD et al. Angiogenesis by endothelial cell transplantation. J Thorac Cardiovasc Surg 2001; 122: 963–71.

23. Dornbusch S. The effect of placenta on experimental cholesterinsclerosis. In: Schmid F, Stein J, eds. Cell-research and cellular therapy. Thun: Ott Publishers, 1967: 134–40.

24. Cunningham FG, MacDonald PC, Leveno KJ et al. Williams obstetrics, 19th edn. Appleton & Lange, 1993.

25. Schmid F, Stein J. Cell-research and cellular therapy. Thun: Ott Publishers, 1967.

26. Schmid F, Stein J. Zellforschung und zelltherapie. Bern, Stuttgart: Verlag H. Huber, 1963.

27. Oetzmann HJ. Cell therapy for diseases of organs. In: Schmid F, Stein J, eds. Cell-research and cellular therapy. Thun: Ott Publishers, 1967: 149–85.

28. Schmid F. Zelltherapie-Grundlagen-Klinik-Praxis. Thun: Ott-Verlag, 1981.

29. Schmid F. Cell therapy, a new dimension of medicine. Thun: Ott Publishers, 1983.

30. Hendricks PJ, Martens A, Hagenbeek A et al. Homing of fluorescently labeled murine hematopoietic stem cells. Exp Hematol 1996; 24: 129–40.

31. Zanjani E, Ascensao J, Tavassoli M. Liver-derived hematopoietic stem cells selectively and preferentially home to the fetal bone marrow. Blood 1993; 81: 399–404.

32. Hardy C. The homing of hematopoietic stem cells to the bone marrow. Am J Med Sci 1995; 309: 260–6.

33. Gilbert SF. Developmental biology, 4th edn. Sunderland, MA: Sinauer Associates, 1994.

34. Lenmark A, Freedman ZR, Hofmann C. Islet-cell-surface antibodies in juvenile diabetes mellitus. N Engl J Med 1978; 299: 375–80.

35. Kondrat'ev YaYu, Sadovnikova NV, Liozner AL, Fedotov VP. Antibodies to the surface of pancreatic islet cells: immunoenzymatic determination with rat target cells. Problemi Endokrinologii 1986; 32: 39–43.

36. Hopf U, Meyer zum Buschenfelde KH, Freudenberg J. Liver-specific antigens of different species. Clin Exp Immunol 1974; 16: 117–24.

37. Lodish H, Baltimore D, Berk A et al. Molecular cell biology, 3rd edn. New York: Scientific American Books, 1995.

11. Angiogenic Effects of Endothelial Precursor Cells: Implications for Development of Cell Therapy Protocols for Myocardial Infarction

Silviu Itescu, Alfred A Kocher and Michael D Schuster

Introduction

Congestive heart failure remains a major public health problem, with recent estimates indicating that end-stage heart failure with 2-year mortality rates of 70–80% affects over 60 000 patients in the USA each year.[1] In Western societies, heart failure is primarily the consequence of previous myocardial infarction.[2] As new modalities have emerged which have enabled significant reductions in early mortality from acute myocardial infarction, affecting over 1 million new patients in the USA annually, there has been a paradoxical increase in the incidence of post-infarction heart failure among the survivors. Current therapy of heart failure is limited to the treatment of already established disease and is predominantly pharmacologic in nature, aiming primarily to inhibit the neurohormonal axis that results in excessive cardiac activation through angiotensin- or norepinephrine-dependent pathways. For patients with end-stage heart failure, treatment options are extremely limited, with less than 3000 being offered cardiac transplants annually due to the severely limited supply of donor organs,[3,4] and implantable left ventricular assist devices (LVADs) being expensive, not proven for long-term use and associated with significant complications.[5–7] Clearly, approaches that prevent heart failure after myocardial infarction would be preferable to those that simply ameliorate or treat already established disease.

Heart failure after myocardial infarction results from progressive ventricular remodeling

Heart failure after myocardial infarction occurs as a result of a process termed myocardial remodeling. This process is characterized by myocyte

151

apoptosis, cardiomyocyte replacement by fibrous tissue deposition in the ventricular wall,[8–10] progressive expansion of the initial infarct area and dilatation of the left ventricular lumen.[11,12] Another integral component of the remodeling process appears to be the development of neoangiogenesis within the myocardial infarct scar,[13,14] a process requiring activation of latent collagenase and other proteinases.[15] Under normal circumstances, the contribution of neoangiogenesis to the infarct bed capillary network is insufficient to keep pace with the tissue growth required for contractile compensation and is unable to support the greater demands of the hypertrophied, but viable, myocardium. The relative lack of oxygen and nutrients reaching the hypertrophied myocytes may be an important etiologic factor in the death of otherwise viable myocardium, resulting in progressive infarct extension and fibrous replacement. Since late reperfusion of the infarct vascular bed in both humans and experimental animal models significantly benefits ventricular remodeling and survival,[16–18] we have postulated that methods to successfully augment vascular bed neovascularization might improve cardiac function by preventing loss of hypertrophied, but otherwise viable, cardiac myocytes.

Endothelial precursors and formation of vascular structures during embryogenesis

In order to develop successful methods for inducing neovascularization of the adult heart, one needs to understand the process of definitive vascular network formation during embryogenesis. In the prenatal period, hemangioblasts derived from the human ventral aorta give rise to cellular elements involved in both vasculogenesis, or formation of the primitive capillary network, and hematopoiesis.[19,20] In addition to hematopoietic lineage markers, embryonic hemangioblasts are characterized by expression of the vascular endothelial cell growth factor receptor-2 (VEGFR-2), and have high proliferative potential with blast colony formation in response to VEGF.[21–24] Under the regulatory influence of various transcriptional and differentiation factors, embryonic hemangioblasts mature, migrate and differentiate to become endothelial lining cells and create the primitive vasculogenic network. The differentiation of embryonic hemangioblasts to pluripotent stem cells and to endothelial precursors appears to be related to co-expression of the GATA-2 transcription factor, since GATA-2 knockout embryonic stem cells have a complete block in definitive hematopoiesis and seeding of the fetal liver and bone marrow.[25] Moreover, the earliest precursor of both hematopoietic and endothelial cell lineage to have diverged from embryonic ventral endothelium has been shown to express VEGF receptors as well as GATA-2 and α-integrins.[26] Subsequent to capillary tube formation, the newly created vasculogenic vessels undergo sprouting, tapering, remodeling and regression under the direction of VEGF, angiopoietins and other factors, a process termed angiogenesis. The final component required for definitive vascular network formation to sustain embryonic organogenesis is influx of mesenchymal lineage cells to form the vascular supporting structures such as smooth muscle cells and pericytes.

Endothelial precursors in adult bone marrow and postnatal vasculogenesis

In an intriguing report several years ago, Isner and co-workers demonstrated that endothelial progenitor cells can, on occasion, be identified in the peripheral circulation, that such cells can be induced to differentiate into endothelial cells under specific conditions in vitro and that they can be incorporated into the walls of pre-existing vascular structures within ischemic tissues.[27] These findings were in contrast to those of a number of studies using various animal models of peripheral ischemia which showed the potential of bone marrow-derived elements to induce neovascularization of ischemic tissues.[27–33] Although the nature of the bone marrow-derived endothelial progenitors was not precisely identified in these studies, the cumulative reports indicated that this site may be an important source of endothelial progenitors which could be useful for augmenting collateral vessel growth in ischemic tissues, a process termed therapeutic angiogenesis.

Phenotypic characterization of endothelial precursors, or angioblasts, in human adult bone marrow

In more recent studies, our group has identified such endothelial progenitors in human adult bone marrow.[34] By employing both in vitro and in vivo experimental models, we have sought to precisely identify the surface characteristics and biological properties of these bone marrow-derived endothelial progenitor cells. Following granulocyte colony-stimulating factor (G-CSF) treatment, mobilized mononuclear cells were harvested and CD34[+] cells were separated using anti-CD34 monoclonal antibody (mAb) coupled to magnetic beads. Of the CD34[+] cells, 90–95% co-expressed the hematopoietic lineage marker CD45, 60–80% co-expressed the stem cell factor receptor CD117, and <1% co-expressed the monocyte/macrophage lineage marker

153

CD14. Among double-positive CD34⁺CD117⁺ cells, CD117 expression was dim in 75–85% and bright in 15–25%. Both CD34⁺CD117^{dim} and CD34⁺CD117^{bright} populations contained cells of endothelial lineage, as defined by expression of the vascular endothelial growth factor receptor VEGFR-2 (Flk-1). VEGFR-2 expression was detected at high density on 20–30% of CD117^{dim} cells and at lower density on 10–15% of CD117^{bright} cells. By quadruple-parameter analysis, the VEGFR-2-positive cells within the CD34⁺CD117^{dim} population displayed phenotypic characteristics of mature, vascular endothelium, including high-level expression of Tie-2, ecNOS, von Willebrand factor (vWF), E-selectin (CD62E) and ICAM (CD54). In contrast, the VEGFR-2-positive cells within the CD34⁺CD117^{bright} subset displayed phenotypic characteristics of endothelial progenitors, including co-expression of Tie-2, as well as AC133, but not markers of mature endothelium such as ecNOS, vWF, E-selectin and ICAM. These cells were additionally identified as expressing proteins characteristic of primitive hemangioblasts arising during waves of murine and human embryogenesis, including the transcription factors GATA-2 and GATA-3. Intracellular staining of CD34⁺ cells sorted on the basis of CD117 bright or dim expression demonstrated that GATA-2 protein levels, as determined by mean channel fluorescence, were approximately 25% higher in the CD34⁺CD117^{bright} than in the CD34⁺CD117^{dim} population. This was confirmed by quantitative mRNA measurement, with GATA-2 mRNA levels found to be 58% higher in CD34⁺ cells expressing CD117 brightly compared with those expressing CD117 dimly. Since surface expression of VEGFR-2, Tie-2 and AC133 was also detected on a subset of CD117^{dim} cells which had low levels of GATA-2 mRNA and protein activity, we conclude that identification of an embryonic bone marrow-derived angioblast phenotype requires concomitant CD117^{bright} surface expression and cellular GATA-2 activity in addition to expression of VEGFR-2, Tie-2 and AC133.

Human angioblasts proliferate in response to vascular endothelial growth factor and differentiate into endothelial cells

Since the frequency of circulating endothelial cell precursors in animal models has been shown to be increased by either VEGF[35] or regional ischemia,[27–30] we next examined the proliferative responses of phenotypically defined angioblasts to VEGF and to factors in ischemic serum. CD117^{bright}GATA-2^{high}angioblasts demonstrated significantly higher proliferative responses relative to CD117^{dim}GATA-2^{low} bone marrow-derived cells from the same

donor following culture for 96 h with either VEGF or ischemic serum. The
expanded angioblast population consisted of large blast cells, defined by
forward scatter, which continued to express immature markers, including
GATA-2, GATA-3 and CD117[bright], but not markers of mature endothelial
cells, including eNOS or E-selectin, indicating blast proliferation without
differentiation under these culture conditions. However, culture on
fibronectin with endothelial growth medium resulted in outgrowth of
monolayers with endothelial morphology and functional and phenotypic
features characteristic of endothelial cells, including uniform uptake of
acetylated low-density lipoprotein (LDL), and co-expression of CD34, factor
VIII and eNOS (Figure 11.1). Thus, G-CSF treatment of adult humans
mobilizes into the peripheral circulation a bone marrow-derived population
with phenotypic and functional characteristics of embryonic angioblasts, as
defined by specific surface phenotype, high proliferative responses to VEGF
and cytokines in ischemic serum, and ability to differentiate into endothelial
cells by culture in medium enriched with endothelial growth factors.

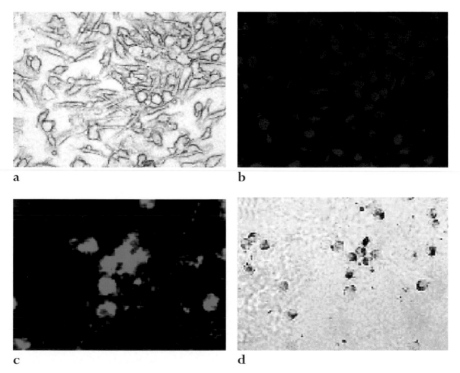

a   b

c   d

Figure 11.1 Angioblasts differentiate into new blood vessels in vitro. (a) and (b)
demonstrate typical cobblestone morphology with uptake of acetylated LDL following 2
weeks of culture. The cells also stain positive for CD31 and factor VIII (c,d).

Human angioblasts induce neovascularization of the myocardial infarct zone

Intravenous injection of freshly obtained human angioblasts into athymic nude rats who had undergone ligation of the left anterior descending coronary artery (LAD) resulted in infarct zone infiltration within 48 h. Few human cells were detected in unaffected areas of hearts with regional infarcts or in myocardium of sham-operated rats. Histologic examination at 2 weeks post-infarction revealed that injection of human angioblasts was accompanied by a significant increase in infarct zone microvascularity, cellularity and numbers of capillaries, and by reduction in matrix deposition and fibrosis in comparison to controls. Neovascularization was significantly increased within both the infarct zone and in the peri-infarct rim in rats receiving angioblasts compared with controls receiving saline or other cells which infiltrated the heart (e.g. CD34⁻ cells or saphenous vein endothelial cells (SVECs). The neovascularization induced by human angioblasts was due to increases in capillaries of both human and rat origin, as defined by monoclonal antibodies with specificity for human or rat CD31 endothelial markers. Capillaries of human origin, defined by co-expression of dialkylcarbocyanine (DiI) fluorescence and human CD31, but not rat CD31, accounted for 20–25% of the total myocardial capillary vasculature, and was located exclusively within the central infarct zone of collagen deposition (Figure 11.2). In contrast, capillaries of rat origin, as determined by expression of rat, but not human, CD31, demonstrated a distinctively different pattern of localization, being absent within the central zone of collagen deposition and abundant both at the peri-infarct rim between the region of collagen deposition and myocytes, and between myocytes.

Human angioblasts protect hypertrophied cardiomyocytes against apoptosis and prevent ventricular remodeling

We next sought to relate the early infarct zone neovascularization observed after angioblast infusion to cardiomyocyte apoptosis and size, and to left ventricular scar formation and function. After concomitant staining of rat tissues for the myocyte-specific marker desmin and the performance of DNA end-labeling using the TUNEL technique, temporal examinations demonstrated that the infarct zone neovascularization induced by injection of human angioblasts prevented an eccentrically extending pro-apoptotic process evident in saline controls. Thus, at 2 weeks post-infarction, myocardial tissue

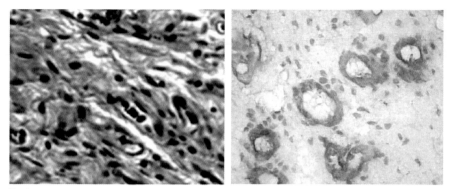

Trichrome   Human CD31

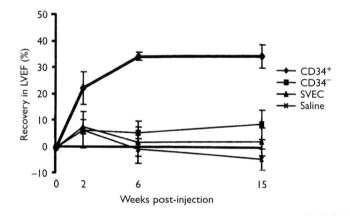

2×10^5
Angioblast concentration (cells/mm³)

CD34+
CD34⁻
SVEC
Saline

Figure 11.2 *Angioblasts differentiate into new blood vessels in vivo, resulting in
improved cardiac function.*

of LAD-ligated rats who received saline demonstrated six-fold higher numbers
of apoptotic myocytes compared with that from rats receiving intravenous
injections of human angioblasts. Moreover, these myocytes had distorted
appearance and an irregular shape. In contrast, myocytes from LAD-ligated rats
who received human angioblasts had a regular, oval shape and were significantly
larger than myocytes from control rats (diameter $0.036 \, mm \pm 0.004$ versus
$0.019 \, mm \pm 0.001$, $P < 0.01$). By 15 weeks post-infarction, rats receiving human
angioblasts demonstrated markedly smaller scar sizes together with increased
mass of viable myocardium within the anterior free wall. The increased left
ventricular mass comprised myocytes exclusively of rat origin, expressing rat
but not human MHC molecules, confirming intrinsic myocyte salvage rather

157

than myocyte regeneration from human stem cell precursors. Whereas collagen deposition and scar formation extended almost throughout the entire left ventricular wall thickness in controls, with aneurysmal dilatation and typical ECG abnormalities, the infarct scar extended to only 20–50% of the left ventricular wall thickness in rats receiving CD34[+] cells. Moreover, pathologic collagen deposition in the non-infarct zone was markedly reduced in rats receiving CD34[+] cells. At 15 weeks, the mean proportion of scar/normal left ventricular myocardium was 13% in rats receiving CD34[+] cells compared with 36–45% for each of the other groups studied (saline, CD34[-], SVEC) ($P < 0.01$). Together, these results strongly indicate that the reduction in peri-infarct myocyte apoptosis observed at 2 weeks resulted in prolonged survival of hypertrophied, but viable, myocytes and prevented myocardial replacement with collagen and fibrous tissue by 15 weeks.

Neovascularization of acutely ischemic myocardium by human angioblasts causes sustained improvement in cardiac function

We next compared the effects of injecting angioblasts or other cellular fractions on the myocardial function of rats following infarction. Remarkably, by 2 weeks after injection of human angioblasts, and in parallel with the observed neovascularization, left ventricular ejection fraction (LVEF) recovered by a mean of 22%. This effect was long-lived, with LVEF recovering by a mean of 34% at the end of follow-up, 15 weeks post-injection. Neither CD34[-] cells nor SVECs demonstrated similar effects. At 15 weeks post-infarction, the mean cardiac index in rats injected with human angioblasts was only reduced by 26% relative to normal rats, whereas for each of the other groups it was reduced by 48–59%. Together, these results indicate that the neovascularization and reduction in peri-infarct myocyte apoptosis observed at 2 weeks after injection of human angioblasts resulted in prolonged survival of viable myocytes, prevented myocardial replacement with collagen and fibrous tissue by 15 weeks (Figure 11.3), and caused sustained improvement in myocardial function.

Role of non-endothelial lineage stem cells in myocardial repair/regeneration

Over the past several years, several studies have suggested that stem cells can be used to generate cardiomyocytes ex vivo for potential use in a range of cardiovascular diseases.[36-40] Multipotent bone marrow-derived mesenchymal

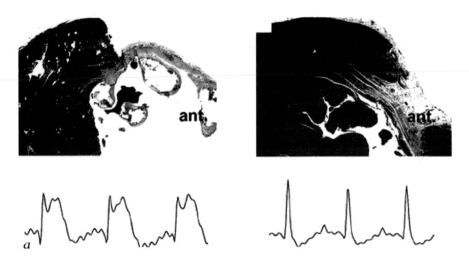

Figure 11.3 *Neovascularization by human angioblast prevents remodeling and subsequent long-term loss of myocardium. (a) A representative control animal 15 weeks after myocardial infarction demonstrating significant collagen deposition and ECG abnormalities. (b) In contrast, a representative animal receiving angioblasts has significantly less scar deposition and improved cardiac function.*

stem cells have been identified in adult murine and human bone marrow, and shown to differ from endothelial lineage progenitors by lack of expression of hematopoietic lineage markers such as CD34 or CD45,[38] and by their ability to differentiate to lineages of diverse mesenchymal tissues, including bone, cartilage, fat, tendon, and both skeletal and cardiac muscle,[39] under appropriate culture conditions. Recently, Kehat et al were able to demonstrate that human embryonic stem cells can also differentiate in vitro into cells with characteristics of cardiomyocytes.[40] Irrespective of whether the stem cells are from adult bone marrow or embryonic sources, the newly generated cardiomyocytes appear to resemble normal cardiomyocytes in terms of phenotypic properties, such as expression of actinin, desmin and troponin I, and function, including positive and negative chronotropic regulation of contractility by pharmacologic agents and production of vasoactive factors such as atrial and brain natriuretic peptides.

In vivo evidence for functional cardiac improvement following cardiomyocyte regeneration by mesenchymal stem cells has been exceedingly difficult to show to date. In part this may be because the signals required for cardiomyocyte differentiation and functional regulation are complex and poorly understood. For example, phenotypic and functional differentiation of mesenchymal stem cells to cardiomyocyte lineage cells in vitro requires

159

culture with exogenously added 5-azacytidine.[36,37] An alternative explanation may be that in order for exogenous cardiomyocytes to permanently engraft and become fully functional, there is a requirement for generation of new capillary vasculature to provide the implanted cells with oxygenation and nutrients. Indeed, in a recent study which did demonstrate significant improvement in cardiac function after direct myocardial injection of syngeneic bone marrow-derived mesenchymal stem cells into the hearts of mice who had previously undergone LAD ligation, cardiomyocyte survival was accompanied by prominent neovascularization.[41] Since the bone marrow inoculum contained a mixture of cellular elements, including CD117-positive angioblasts, one may speculate that the observed improvement in cardiac function was due to the combined effects of increased cardiomyocyte numbers and improved perfusion following angioblast-dependent neovascularization. This raises the intriguing possibility that angioblast co-administration and subsequent neovascularization may be a necessary prerequisite for long-term in vivo viability and functional integrity of transplanted stem cell-derived cardiomyocytes.

Potential for use of angioblasts in combination with cardiomyocyte progenitors for repair and regeneration of ischemic myocardium

While increasing capillary density as a result of angioblast-dependent vasculogenesis is a promising approach for preventing the apoptotic death of at-risk hypertrophied myocytes following acute myocardial infarction, the role of angioblast therapy for the treatment of congestive heart failure following chronic ischemia is at present unknown. It is reasonable to anticipate that cellular therapies for congestive heart failure due to ischemic cardiomyopathy will need to address two interdependent processes: (1) a renewable source of proliferating, functional cardiomyocytes, and (2) development of a network of capillaries and larger blood vessels for supply of oxygen and nutrients to both the chronically ischemic, endogenous myocardium and the newly implanted cardiomyocytes. To achieve these endpoints, it is likely that co-administration of angioblasts and mesenchymal/cardiomyocyte stem cells will be needed in order to develop regenerating cardiomyocytes, vascular structures and supporting cells such as pericytes and smooth muscle cells. Future studies will need to address the timing, relative concentrations and source and route of delivery of each of these cellular populations in animal models of acute and chronic myocardial ischemia.

160

In addition to synergistic cellular therapies, it is likely that optimal regimens for the treatment of acute and chronically ischemic hearts will require a combined approach employing additional pharmacologic strategies. For example, augmentation in myocardial function might be achieved by combining infusion of human angioblasts and cardiomyocyte progenitors with beta-blockade, angiotensin-converting enzyme inhibition or AT_1-receptor blockade to reduce angiotensin II-dependent cardiac fibroblast proliferation and collagen secretion.[42-45] Understanding the potential of defined lineages of stem cells or undifferentiated progenitors, and their interactions with pharmacologic interventions, will lead to better and more focused clinical trial designs using each cell type independently or in combination, depending on which particular clinical indication is being targeted.

References

1. Effects of enalapril on mortality in severe congestive heart failure. Results of the Cooperative North Scandinavian Enalapril Survival Study (CONSENSUS) Trial Study Group. N Engl J Med 1987; 316(23): 1429–35.

2. Mahon NG, O'Roke C, Codd MB et al. Hospital mortality of acute myocardial infarction in the thrombolytic era. Heart 1999; 81: 478–82.

3. Hogness JR. The artificial heart: prototypes, policies and patients. Washington, DC: National Academy Press, 1991.

4. Annual Report of the US Scientific Registry for Organ Transplantation and the Organ Procurement and Transplantation Network – 1990. Washington, DC: US Department of Health and Human Services, 1990.

5. Frazier OH, Rose EA, Macmanus Q et al. Multicenter clinical evaluation of the HeartMate 1000 IP left ventricular assist device. Ann Thorac Surg 1992; 53: 1080–90.

6. McCarthy PM, Rose EA, Macmanus Q et al. Clinical experience with the Novacor ventricular assist system. Bridge to transplantation and the transition to permanent application. J Thorac Cardiovasc Surg 1991; 102: 578–87.

7. Oz MC, Argenziano M, Catanese KA et al. Bridge experience with long-term implantable left ventricular assist devices. Are they an alternative to transplantation? Circulation 1997; 95(7): 1844–52.

8. Colucci WS. Molecular and cellular mechanisms of myocardial failure. Am J Cardiol 1997; 80(11A): 15L–25L.

9. Ravichandran LV, Puvanakrishnan R. In vivo labeling studies on the biosynthesis and degradation of collagen in experimental myocardial infarction. Biochem Int 1991; 24: 405–14.

10. Agocha A, Lee H-W, Eghali-Webb M. Hypoxia regulates basal and induced DNA synthesis and collagen type I production in human cardiac fibroblasts: effects of TGF-beta, thyroid hormone, angiotensin II and basic fibroblast growth factor. J Mol Cell Cardiol 1997; 29: 2233–44H.

11. Pfeffer JM, Pfeffer MA, Fletcher PJ, Braunwald E. Progressive ventricular remodeling in rat with myocardial infarction. Am J Physiol 1991; 260: H1406-14.

12. White HD, Norris RM, Brown MA et al. Left ventricular end systolic volume as the major determinant of survival after recovery from myocardial infarction. Circulation 1987; 76: 44–51.

13. Nelissen-Vrancken H, Debets J, Snoeckx L et al. Time-related normalization of maximal coronary flow in isolated perfused hearts of rats with myocardial infarction. Circulation 1996; 93: 349–55.

14. Kalkman EAJ, Bilgin YM, van Haren P et al. Determinants of coronary reserve in rats subjected to coronary artery ligation or aortic banding. Cardiovasc Res 1996; 32: 1088–95.

15. Heymans S, Luutun A, Nuyens D et al. Inhibition of plasminogen activators or matrix metalloproteinases prevents cardiac rupture but impairs therapeutic angiogenesis and causes cardiac failure. Nat Med 1999; 5: 1135–42.

16. Hochman JS, Choo H. Limitation of myocardial infarct expansion by reperfusion independent of myocardial salvage. Circulation 1987; 75: 299–306.

17. White HD, Cross DB, Elliot JM et al. Long-term prognostic importance of patency of the infarct-related coronary artery after thrombolytic therapy for myocardial infarction. Circulation 1994; 89: 61–7.

18. Nidorf SM, Siu SC, Galambos G et al. Benefit of late coronary reperfusion on ventricular morphology and function after myocardial infarction. J Am Coll Cardiol 1992; 20: 307–13.

19. Tavian M, Coulombel L, Luton D et al. Aorta-associated CD34 hematopoietic cells in the early human embryo. Blood 1996; 87: 67–72.

20. Jaffredo T, Gautier R, Eichmann A, Dieterlen-Lievre F. Intraaortic hemopoietic cells are derived from endothelial cells during ontogeny. Development 1998; 125: 4575–83.

21. Kennedy M, Firpo M, Choi K et al. A common precursor for primitive erythropoiesis and definitive haematopoiesis. Nature 1997; 386: 488–93.

22. Choi K, Kennedy M, Kazarov A et al. A common precursor for hematopoietic and endothelial cells. Development 1998; 125: 725–32.

23. Elefanty AG, Robb L, Birner R, Begley CG. Hematopoietic-specific genes are not induced during in vitro differentiation of scl-null embryonic stem cells. Blood 1997; 90: 1435–47.

24. Labastie M-C, Cortes F, Romeo P-H et al. Molecular identity of hematopoietic precursor cells emerging in the human embryo. Blood 1998; 92: 3624–35.

25. Tsai FY, Keller G, Kuo FC et al. An early hematopoietic defect in mice lacking the transcription factor GATA-2. Nature 1994; 371: 221–5.

26. Ogawa M, Kizumoto M, Nishikawa S et al. Expression of alpha4-integrin defines the earliest precursor of hematopoietic cell lineage diverged from endothelial cells. Blood 1999; 93: 1168–77.

27. Asahara T, Murohara T, Sullivan A et al. Isolation of putative progenitor cells for endothelial angiogenesis. Science 1997; 275: 964–7.

28. Folkman J. Therapeutic angiogenesis in ischemic limbs. Circulation 1998; 97: 108–10.

29. Takahashi T, Kalka C, Masuda H et al. Ischemia- and cytokine-induced mobilization of bone marrow-derived endothelial progenitor cells for neovascularization. Nat Med 1999; 5: 434–8.

30. Kalka C, Masuda H, Takahashi T et al. Transplantation of ex vivo expanded endothelial progenitor cells for therapeutic neovascularization. Proc Natl Acad Sci USA 2000; 97: 3422–7.

31. Rafii S, Shapiro F, Rimarachin J et al. Isolation and characterization of human bone marrow microvascular endothelial cells: hematopoietic progenitor cell adhesion. Blood 1994; 84: 10–19.

32. Shi Q, Rafii S, Wu MH-D et al. Evidence for circulating bone marrow-derived endothelial cells. Blood 1998; 92: 362–7.

33. Lin Y, Weisdorf DJ, Solovey A, Hebbel RP. Origins of circulating endothelial cells and endothelial outgrowth from blood. J Clin Invest 2000; 105: 71–7.

34. Kocher AA, Schuster MD, Szabolcs MJ et al. Neovascularization of ischemic myocardium by human bone-marrow-derived angioblasts prevents cardiomyocyte apoptosis, reduces remodeling and improves cardiac function. Nat Med 2001; 7: 430–6.

35. Asahara T, Takahashi T, Masuda H et al. VEGF contributes to postnatal neovascularization by mobilizing bone marrow-derived endothelial progenitor cells. EMBO J 1999; 18: 3964–72.

36. Makino S, Fukuda K, Miyoshi S et al. Cardiomyocytes can be generated from marrow stromal cells in vitro. J Clin Invest 1999; 103: 697–705.

37. Tomita S, Li R-K, Weisel RD et al. Autologous transplantation of bone marrow cells improves damaged heart function. Circulation 1999; 100: II-247.

38. Pittenger MF, Mackay AM, Beck SC et al. Multilineage potential of adult human mesenchymal stem cells. Science 1999; 284: 143–7.

39. Liechty KW, MacKenzie TC, Shaaban AF et al. Human mesenchymal stem cells engraft and demonstrate site-specific differentiation after in utero transplantation in sheep. Nat Med 2000; 6: 1282–6.

40. Kehat I, Kenyagin-Karsenti D, Snir M et al. Human embryonic stem cells can differentiate into myocytes with structural and functional properties of cardiomyocytes. J Clin Invest 2001; 108: 407–14.

41. Orlic D, Kajstura J, Chimenti S et al. Bone marrow cells regenerate infarcted myocardium. Nature 2001; 410: 701–5.

42. McEwan PE, Gray GA, Sherry L et al. Differential effects of angiotensin II on cardiac cell proliferation and intramyocardial perivascular fibrosis in vivo. Circulation 1998; 98: 2765–73.

43. Kawano H, Do YS, Kawano Y et al. Angiotensin II has multiple profibrotic effects in human cardiac fibroblasts. Circulation 2000; 101: 1130–7.

44. Pfeffer MA, Braunwald E, Moye LA et al. Effect of captopril on mortality and morbidity in patients with left ventricular dysfunction after myocardial infarction. Results of the survival and ventricular enlargement trial. The SAVE investigators. N Engl J Med 1992; 327: 669–77.

45. Pitt B, Segal R, Martinez FA et al. Randomised trial of losartan versus captopril in patients over 65 with heart failure (Evaluation of Losartan in the Elderly Study, ELITE). Lancet 1997; 349: 747–52.

12. CELL TRANSPLANTATION FOR THERAPEUTIC ANGIOGENESIS

Paul WM Fedak, Hao Zhang and Ren-Ke Li

Introduction

Ischemic heart disease is the leading cause of mortality in North America. Approximately 465 000 new cases are diagnosed in the USA each year, and 15 million new cases are diagnosed worldwide.[1,2] Standard treatments for coronary artery disease include percutaneous coronary interventions and coronary artery bypass grafting.[3,4] However, approximately 10% of patients are not ideal candidates for conventional revascularization procedures, because of diffuse coronary disease. These patients may have no therapeutic options other than cardiac transplantation. Newer experimental therapies involve a 'biological bypass' without intraluminal or surgical interventions. In the last 10 years, two treatments have become available for no-option patients with diffuse atherosclerotic coronary disease: transmyocardial laser revascularization and angiogenic gene or protein therapy.

Transmyocardial laser revascularization involves the creation of transmural myocardial channels with a laser to deliver blood from the left ventricle cavity to the surrounding myocardium.[5-7] These sinusoids are believed to function as in reptilian hearts. Despite controversial data indicating improved myocardial perfusion in animals,[6,8-10] clinical studies were instituted. Since 1990, more than 6000 patients worldwide have undergone transmyocardial laser revascularization for the treatment of ischemic cardiomyopathy (reviewed by Horvath[11]). Several randomized controlled trials have demonstrated that transmyocardial laser revascularization provides significant relief of angina when compared to medical management.[12] Although angina was reduced significantly (patients felt better), most studies did not demonstrate improved myocardial perfusion by nuclear scans. The relief of anginal symptoms following the transmyocardial laser revascularization procedure may have resulted from denervation of the heart, rather than improved angiogenesis.[13] Therefore, other novel experimental approaches to create new blood vessels have been examined.

Therapeutic angiogenesis by way of gene or protein therapy is a strategy to amplify the native angiogenic process and enhance the reperfusion of ischemic tissues.[14] The expression of angiogenic growth factors in ischemic myocardium with targeted gene or protein therapy has been used clinically with variable success. Local expression of these factors may restore perfusion to the ischemic region, recruiting surviving hibernating cardiomyocytes in the scar or the infarct zone and potentially reducing angina and improving regional contractility.[15] Angiogenic growth factor therapy has been shown to enhance vascular ingrowth and collateral formation in both experimental animal models and in patients with ischemic heart disease.[15–17]

Two angiogenic growth factors, basic fibroblast growth factor (bFGF) and vascular endothelial growth factor (VEGF), have been studied extensively.[18] Significant beneficial effects of angiogenic factors on the ischemic myocardium of animal hearts encouraged clinical trials. Both the proteins and genes of angiogenic factors have been injected into ischemic myocardium at the time of bypass surgery (as adjunctive treatment) or through a mini-thoracotomy as the sole therapy. The safety of angiogenic factor treatment has been reported by a number of studies, and the encouraging data led to the approval of several phase II clinical trials.[16,17,19]

Side-effects caused by the delivered VEGF gene or viral vector have received much attention. Schwarz et al reported that VEGF resulted in angioma-like structures at the site of gene delivery in rat hearts.[20] Lee et al obtained similar results.[21] The regulation of gene expression after delivery can be difficult to control, and excessive levels of growth factors may be detrimental. In addition, Celletti et al reported in 2001 that VEGF might enhance the development of atherosclerosis.[22] Other side-effects may occur outside the heart. Systemic delivery of angiogenic factor genes or proteins may cause problematic angiogenesis in the brain or retina, or potentiate tumor growth.[18] Also, the delivery of angiogenic genes, either as naked DNA or in viral vectors, is subject to difficulties with DNA stability or vector immunogenicity and tumorigenicity, respectively.

Cell transplantation to induce blood vessel formation

The two major phase II clinical trials using angiogenic protein therapy were less successful than anticipated, but were important early attempts at therapeutic angiogenesis with growth factors.[18] These human trials support the idea that regulation of the process of angiogenesis is probably far more complex than any single protein factor alone. Cell transplantation may offer a novel approach to establish a 'biological bypass' for patients that may be superior to laser and gene/protein therapies.[23] Cell transplantation involves the injection of healthy muscle cells into damaged myocardium to stimulate new tissue formation and improve functional recovery. Heart cells, skeletal muscle cells, bone marrow cells, smooth muscle cells, endothelial cells and fibroblasts have all been implanted into ischemic hearts, with varied effects.[23,34] Cell transplantation studies have demonstrated that donor muscle cells can engraft and survive within the injured myocardial region. Angiogenesis was increased in the area of transplantation and cardiac function was improved as compared to controls. The extent and type of angiogenesis was determined by the phenotype of the cells implanted in the ischemic region.

Endothelial progenitor cells

Angiogenesis is a complex cascade of events, and definitions with respect to the process of angiogenesis can differ dramatically. The classic definition refers to new capillary vessels sprouting from pre-existing capillary structures. A more general concept of angiogenesis includes both vasculogenesis and arteriogenesis. Vasculogenesis involves the process by which pluripotent endothelial cell precursors are recruited and then differentiate into mature endothelial cells to form primitive blood vessels.[19] Vasculogenesis was once believed to occur only during embryonic development. Many recent studies have shown that vasculogenesis may be involved in the rebuilding of a functional new blood vessel network in postnatal tissues as a response to injury, such as coronary insufficiency and myocardial infarction.

In 1997, Asahara et al[35] isolated a cell population from human peripheral blood that shares many protein markers with endothelial cells, such as CD34 and factor VIII (Figure 12.1). These cells can differentiate into endothelial cells and form blood vessel networks both in vitro and in vivo. Accordingly, these cells were named 'endothelial progenitor cells'.[35,36] Importantly, these novel findings reshaped the well-established concept of angiogenesis in adult tissues. A new hypothesis emerged to suggest that cytokines released after tissue injury stimulate local endothelial cells to migrate from the pre-existing vessel walls and form new blood vessels. In addition, pluripotent endothelial cell precursors are also recruited from the circulation. These stem cells differentiate into mature endothelial cells to form primitive blood vessels.[19] Most circulating endothelial progenitor cells are derived from the bone marrow.[37,38] These cells have an enhanced capacity to proliferate, localize and incorporate into injured tissues, and hence they contribute substantially to the process of angiogenesis.

Gene or protein therapy aims to introduce angiogenic growth factors to recruit endothelial cells to migrate into the ischemic region and induce regional angiogenesis. However, the cells required to build the new vasculature may be limited in number, particularly in injured regions with ongoing cell death. The concept of cell transplantation is to locally deliver both the growth factors and cells needed to build new blood vessels in an injured region.

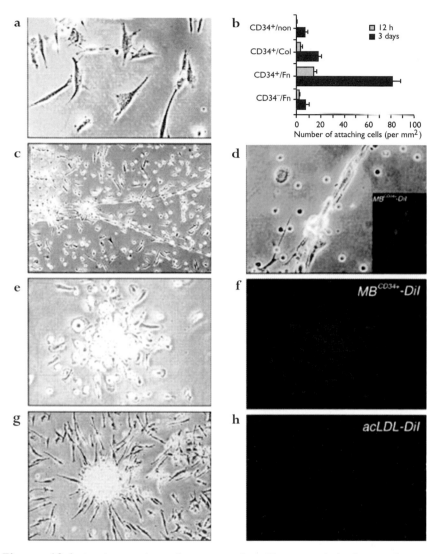

Figure 12.1 *Attachment, cluster formation and capillary network development by endothelial progenitor cells in vitro. (a) Spindle-shaped attaching cells (AT^CD34+) 7 days after plating MB^CD34+ (50 cells/mm²) on fibronectin in standard medium. (b) Number of AT^CD34+ cells 12 h and 3 days after culture of MB^CD34+ on plastic alone (CD34+/non), collagen coating (CD34+/Col), or fibronectin (CD34+/Fn), and MB^CD34- on fibronectin (CD34-/Fn). Network formation (c) and cord-like structures (d) were observed 48 h after plating co-culture, MB^CD34+, labeled with dialkylcarbocyanine (DiI), with unlabeled MB^CD34- cells (ratio 1 : 100) on fibronectin. At 12 h after co-culture, MB^CD34+ -derived cells formed multiple clusters (e and f). After 5 days, uptake of acLDL–DiI was detected in AT^CD34+ cells at the periphery but not the center of the cluster (g and h). (Reproduced with permission from Science 1997; 275(5302): 964–7.)*

The donor cells can be implanted in a target area of myocardium either by systemic delivery or by direct injection. Kalka et al injected human endothelial progenitor cells into the circulation of the nude mouse after the induction of hindlimb ischemia.[39] The implanted cells survived in the ischemic tissue, increased blood vessel density and improved regional perfusion within the damaged area. Limb loss was significantly reduced by the neovascularization. Kawamoto et al also evaluated the ability of circulating progenitor cells to contribute to myocardial angiogenesis.[40] These investigators intravenously injected ex vivo expanded human endothelial progenitor cells into adult nude rats at 3 h after myocardial infarction. Myocardial injury recruited progenitor cells into the damaged myocardium, and progenitor cells were involved in the neovascularization.[40] This process increased regional perfusion and had beneficial effects on heart function. Since angiogenesis can be enhanced by the administration of vascular endothelial growth factors,[41] local signals after tissue damage are thus capable of recruiting progenitor cells. After myocardial infarction, cytokines are released from the site of injury that can attract endothelial progenitor cells to migrate into the ischemic region. However, the quantity of progenitor cells capable of being recruited from the circulation is limited. Transplanting an expanded population of progenitor cells after myocardial injury may have a greater potential to reverse ischemic damage in the setting of acute myocardial ischemia.

In the case of end-stage heart failure and chronic complete myocardial infarctions without ongoing ischemia, the signals to recruit progenitor cells may be absent. In this case, systemic transplantation of endothelial progenitor cells may not enhance the angiogenesis process and thus may not influence myocardial perfusion. Local and direct injection of donor cells into ischemic myocardium may be more effective. Direct injection cell transplantation may have an advantage in these situations, given that poor perfusion in these regions will limit the ability to deliver cells and growth factors systemically.

Endothelial cells

While endothelial progenitor cells may be beneficial, their clinical utility is hampered by the excessive amounts of blood required for their isolation. Given the right environmental cues, such as the presence of angiogenic growth factors, endothelial cells in the blood vessels will proliferate and migrate to create new vessels. Implantation of differentiated endothelial cells may also enhance new blood vessel formation. We transplanted aortic endothelial cells into the myocardial scar tissue of adult rats.[42] The implanted cells enhanced blood vessel density as early as 1 week after injury. At 6 weeks, blood vessel density in the transplanted area was significantly greater

169

than in the non-cell-transplanted area and groups. By labeling the donor cells with markers, we identified the transplanted cells in the endothelium of the newly forming blood vessels (Figure 12.2). Microsphere perfusion studies showed that the neovascularization increased regional bloodflow after cell transplantation compared to controls. The increased angiogenesis did not result in an improvement in global heart function in this animal model. Compared with our previous studies of muscle cell transplantation, endothelial cells do not have the elastic elements necessary to modify ventricular remodeling and prevent dilatation. Although the adult endothelial cell transplantation stimulated angiogenesis, it cannot replace lost cardiomyocytes in the damaged heart and would probably not have significant benefits for patients with extensive, transmural myocardial infarctions with depressed cardiac function. In contrast, if the endothelial cells are implanted into ischemic myocardial tissue, the enhanced perfusion might recover the contractile function of hibernating muscle cells and improve global heart

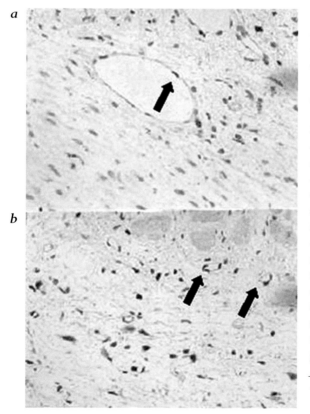

Figure 12.2
Photomicrograph (×400) of bromodeoxyuridine (BrdU)-labeled cells transplanted into the myocardial scar. The scar was stained 6 weeks after transplantation, using hematoxylin and antibodies against BrdU. Some endothelial cells in both the large (a) and small (b) blood vessels stained positively (brown-colored nuclei, arrows), indicating that some of the transplanted endothelial cells were incorporated into the newly formed capillaries. (Reproduced with permission from J Thorac Cardiovasc Surg 2001; 122(5): 963–71.)

function. In support of this, Chekanov et al generated ischemic cardiomyopathy in sheep by placing an ameroid constrictor on the circumflex artery.[43] Autologous endothelial cells isolated from jugular veins were implanted into the damaged area. Eight weeks after cell implantation, regional perfusion was significantly improved in the cell-transplanted group, but not in controls. Cardiac function in the cell-transplanted hearts was much better than in controls. Importantly, these data suggest that endothelial cells isolated from adults can also be used for cell transplantation to relieve myocardial ischemia by angiogenesis. Although these studies are promising, cells harvested from large vessels such as the aorta may be difficult to apply in the clinical arena. Future studies will be required to confirm that smaller peripheral arteries and veins, such as the radial arteries and greater saphenous veins, can afford similar benefits when harvested for cells.

Bone marrow cells

Multiple studies have demonstrated that peripheral blood endothelial progenitor cells originate from the bone marrow. Accordingly, bone marrow is a promising alternative cell source for cells that may be capable of inducing angiogenesis after cell transplantation. Tomita et al implanted fresh isolated bone marrow cells, cultured bone marrow cells and bone marrow cells pretreated with 5-azacytidine into myocardial scar tissue.[32] Five weeks following transplantation, blood vessel density in the transplanted scar area in all cell groups was significantly greater than in controls injected with the vehicle alone (culture medium). In some animals, cells prelabeled with bromodeoxyuridine (BrdU) prior to transplantation were later found as mature endothelial cells in the capillary wall of newly formed vessels. Thus, bone marrow cells are capable of transforming into useful endothelial cells in the formation of new vessels after transplantation (Figure 12.3). Similar results have been observed in the ischemic myocardium of adult rats.[44,45]

These impressive findings have been extended into a large animal model of ischemic cardiomyopathy. Hamano et al determined that implanted autologous canine bone marrow cells increased the blood vessel density in the transplant region almost two-fold compared to controls.[46] In addition, Fuchs et al reported that freshly isolated bone marrow cells from adult swine induced angiogenesis in ischemic myocardium after autologous transplantation.[47] Cultured bone marrow cells also increase regional perfusion after injection into porcine myocardium 4 weeks after occlusion of the left anterior descending coronary artery.[48]

Mononuclear cells isolated from bone marrow have also been examined for their capacity to induce angiogenesis. In a rabbit model of hindlimb ischemia, Shintani et al[49] showed 4 weeks after transplantation that mononuclear cell transplantation enhanced collateral vessel formation, capillary density and blood

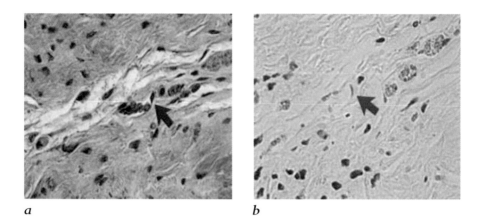

a   *b*

Figure 12.3 *Transplanted bone marrow-derived endothelial cells incorporate into the capillary walls in myocardial scar tissue (×400). Bone marrow cells were labeled with BrdU before transplantation into myocardial scar tissue. The arrow in (a) indicates a capillary with some erythrocytes in its lumen after bone marrow transplantation. In (b), an adjacent tissue slice was stained for BrdU.*
The arrow points at a BrdU-labeled endothelial cell, which is part of a newly formed capillary wall. (Reproduced with permission from Circulation 1999; 100(19 suppl): II-247–56.)

perfusion index compared to media-injected controls and fibroblast transplantation. Kamihata et al implanted bone marrow mononuclear cells into the ischemic myocardium of miniature swine.[50] They found that the implanted cells increased blood vessel density significantly in the cell-transplanted area as compared with control groups. These studies all suggest that the bone marrow might provide an important source of stem cells that could give rise to therapeutic vasculogenesis after transplantation into ischemic myocardium.

While bone marrow cell transplantation can stimulate angiogenesis and increase the capillary density, the question remains whether global heart function can be improved by these stem cells, particularly without prior induction of the cells in vitro into a muscle cell lineage. Interestingly, freshly isolated or cultured bone marrow cells transplanted in rats after myocardial cryoinjury did not result in improved cardiac function.[32] Only bone marrow cells pretreated to form muscle-like cells resulted in improved heart function after implantation into the myocardial scar tissue. In addition, using a canine model of chronic coronary occlusion, Shake et al locally injected bone marrow cells into the injured heart.[51] One month later, despite significantly

172

greater wall thickening in the area of cell transplantation, there was no corresponding improvement of heart function. These data suggested that angiogenesis induced by bone marrow transplantation would not improve heart function if there were no muscle in the defect area (transmural scar). Both myogenesis and angiogenesis may be required to restore cardiac function in patients with transmural scar tissue. Thus, endothelial progenitor cell transplantation alone may be inadequate to reverse cardiac dysfunction in patients with transmural scars.

Further work will be required to maximize the enormous potential of bone marrow-derived cells for transplantation. Transplantation of freshly isolated bone marrow cells is clinically feasible, but may not be desirable unless sufficient cell numbers of the appropriate cell types can be obtained from the unprocessed aspirate. More research directed at the development of culture media and culture conditions to promote bone marrow cells to differentiate into myogenic cells or endothelial progenitor cells needs to be performed. Recently, after depleting the CD45+ and glycophorin A+ cells from bone marrow cells, Reyes et al isolated a multipotent adult progenitor cell line from human postnatal bone marrow that produced large numbers of functional, differentiated endothelial cells capable of producing in vivo angiogenesis.[52] These cells may reflect an important bone marrow-derived source of endothelial cells for therapeutic angiogenesis by cell transplantation.

In summary, bone marrow cells comprise an important source of easily obtainable stem cells that are capable of significant angiogenesis and vasculogenesis after transplantation into ischemic tissues. Clinical trials are currently underway.[53]

Other cells

Like peripheral blood and bone marrow, umbilical cord blood is a rich source of hematopoietic stem cells and endothelial progenitor cells. Cord blood is a novel source for isolating cells for transplantation to induce angiogenesis. With CD34 as a marker to isolate endothelial progenitor cells, the number of CD34+ mononuclear cells in cord blood was almost 10 times greater than that in adult peripheral blood.[54] In addition, the progenitor cells isolated from cord blood have a greater proliferative capacity than equivalent cells from adult peripheral blood. However, the disadvantage of allogenic cord blood-derived endothelial progenitor cells for therapeutic angiogenesis is the potential for rejection. Use of cryopreservation of patients' own umbilical cord blood for later use may reduce this complication, and until this becomes routine, the clinical utilization of cord blood-derived progenitor cell transplantation may be limited.

In addition to the progenitor cells, other cell types may also contribute to blood vessel formation after being implanted into the ischemic myocardium. For example, we transplanted vascular smooth muscle cells into myocardial scar tissue as well as the dilated cardiomyopathic heart.[55,56] We found increased angiogenesis in the cell-transplanted scar as compared to the control scar. There were more blood vessels observed in the myocardial scar tissue implanted with cardiomyocytes than in the non-cell-transplanted group. There was a trend for more arteriole formation in the smooth muscle cell-transplanted group than in the endothelial cell-transplanted group. The optimal cell type and tissue source for stimulating both angiogenesis and vasculogenesis to improve regional myocardial perfusion and overall contractile function remain to be determined.

Possible mechanisms underlying cell transplantation angiogenesis

Although the mechanism by which transplanted cells stimulate angiogenesis in damaged myocardium is unknown, we believe that the mechanism by which cell transplantation improves angiogenesis is three-fold. First, the transplanted cells themselves become incorporated into new vessels and thus provide the building blocks needed for new vessels to form. In areas of injury with ongoing cell losses, angiogenesis may be limited by a poor supply of cells to form new vessels. The addition of healthy endothelial and smooth muscle cells in an ischemic area may increase the rate at which the natural process of angiogenesis occurs. We and others have observed that transplanted endothelial cells incorporated into the newly formed blood vessels and transplanted smooth muscle cells are involved in large blood vessel formation during vasculogenesis. Second, transplanted cells are capable of significant growth factor secretion, particularly the angiogenic factors such as VEGF and FGF. These molecular cues probably aid in coordinating the angiogenesis process. Different cell types in the body may produce different amounts or types of angiogenic factors, which may favor arteriole, capillary and venule formation, depending on the distribution, abundance and timing of the secreted factors. Third, a local inflammatory reaction to the injection process and the implanted cells may also contribute to angiogenesis. After cell implantation, both damaged and dead cells result from mechanical stresses and hypoxia, and these cells may induce lymphocyte infiltration. The cytokines and angiogenic factors secreted by lymphocytes would also contribute to new blood vessel formation.

174

Gene-enhanced cell transplantation for therapeutic angiogenesis

These observations suggest that cell transplantation might be a means, other than gene therapy, to induce angiogenesis. The advantage of this technique is that fewer side-effects are expected in cell-induced angiogenesis than in gene therapy, especially if autologous cells are selected and implanted for angiogenesis, as the cells will not be harmful to the host tissue. Cell transplantation may be an effective strategy for therapeutic angiogenesis, as it provides the necessary signals and the required cellular substrate for new vessel formation, which may offer a novel approach for the development of safe and effective therapeutic angiogenesis.

The difficulty for gene therapy lies in the technique to introduce the genes to the defective myocardium. The immunity induced by repeating adenovirus infection and low transfection efficiency limit the ability of the angiogenic growth factor to efficiently induce neovascularization. Since cell implantation can introduce the cells into the defective area, the combination of gene transfer and cell transplantation strategies may enhance the angiogenic and vasculogenic response elicited by the implanted cells while increasing the survival of cells transplanted into a hypoperfused infarct zone. Our initial studies of transplantation of VEGF-transfected heart cells have demonstrated increased vascular densities and regional bloodflow (Figure 12.4) compared to rat hearts transplanted with untransfected cells.[57] Iwaguro et al transfected endothelial progenitor cells with an adenovirus encoding the murine VEGF gene to achieve phenotypic modulation of the progenitor cells.[58] They found that genetically modified progenitor cells stimulated cell proliferation, adhesion and incorporation into endothelial cell monolayers in culture. After the cells were implanted into ischemic tissue, the VEGF gene-modified cells augmented naturally impaired neovascularization. These studies suggested that the ability to deliver specific angiogenic genes to the ischemic myocardium can be achieved with ex vivo gene transfection of the transplanted cells. Given the number and complexity of angiogenic factors involved in the process of angiogenesis and vasculogenesis, a flexible and targeted approach to their replacement in ischemic tissues may be facilitated by gene-enhanced cells.

Clinical application of cellular therapeutic angiogenesis for ischemic cardiomyopathy

The effective delivery of angiogenic cells can be a considerable challenge.[59] The strategy is two-fold. First, an adequate number of cells must engraft in

175

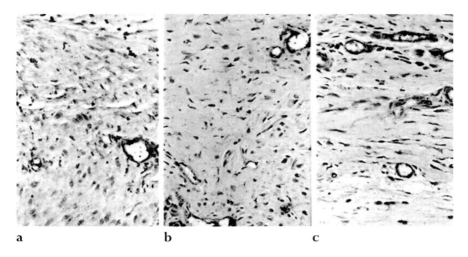

a   b   c

Figure 12.4 *Photomicrographs of adult rat hearts transplanted (a) with culture medium alone (control), (b) untransfected heart cells, or (c) transfected heart cells. Sections have been stained with antibodies against factor VIII to facilitate counting of vessels. Control hearts were relatively avascular. Hearts transplanted with untransfected cells had greater capillary density, and vascular densities were highest in hearts transplanted with VEGF-transfected cells (×400). (Reproduced with permission from Circulation 2001; 104(12 suppl 1): I-218-22.)*

the ischemic region. Second, trauma to the recipient heart and donor cells should be minimized during the process of cell delivery. These tenets must be met by the techniques used for cell delivery, either direct epicardial injection, or coronary arterial or systemic intravenous.

Systemic administration (intravenous delivery) is a simple technique for cell implantation. Several studies successfully demonstrated that implanted cells were recruited into the damaged area and were involved in neovascularization. Intravenous delivery methods would require the cells to recognize the ischemic regions and then migrate into them. This process may occur naturally when endothelial progenitor cells mobilize from the bone marrow into the systemic circulation and then into areas of ischemia. These signaling events, which are probably mediated by cytokines and chemokines, are enhanced in patients with ischemic injury or myocardial infarction. Therefore, in all the successful studies, cell transplantation was performed immediately prior to or soon after myocardial injury. If the signals to recruit progenitor cells can be amplified, the efficiency of cell transplantation to induce angiogenesis will be improved significantly. Takahashi and colleagues

176

used exogenous cytokine therapy with granulocyte–macrophage colony-stimulating factor to mobilize endothelial progenitor cells from the bone marrow into the systemic circulation.[60] The abundance of circulating endothelial progenitor cells was increased and neovascularization was improved in response to ischemia.

However, the recruiting signals may be complex in their timing, distribution and number. They can be different in acute and chronic ischemia. Most patients with ischemic cardiomyopathy are chronic and lack these recruiting signals. It is unclear how many cells can actually be mobilized from the bone marrow or peripheral blood into ischemic myocardium and whether the number is adequate to repair ischemic myocardium. We believe that the number of migrated cells will be limited (otherwise there will be no ischemic cardiomyopathy). In addition, systemic infusions of large amounts of cells may be inefficient and has the potential for serious systemic complications, including progression of occult tumors, exacerbation of retinopathy, angioma formation, neointimal proliferation, arrhythmia and coronary plaque rupture.

A recent novel approach involves the coronary arterial system. Suzuki et al successfully delivered skeletal myoblasts with an intracoronary delivery technique in an animal model.[61] Strauer et al transplanted autologous bone marrow cells into patients through the coronary arterial system and demonstrated that the transplanted cells improved regional perfusion and cardiac function.[62] The prospect of cell delivery via a non-invasive catheter-based approach is conceivable. However, it is unclear if the cells will be adequately delivered to ischemic areas, given that coronary flow will be absent or impaired within these regions. The ability of the donor cells to mobilize into the myocardium and then engraft is also a concern. It has been assumed that implanted cells will deposit at the damaged area, migrate out of blood vessels and repair the injured myocardium. Given the clinical utility of such a technique, further studies should investigate endothelial progenitor cell delivery with a coronary catheter.

For patients with chronic ischemic cardiomyopathy or myocardial infarction, the lack of recruiting signals for blood vessel formation will limit the beneficial effects of cell therapy if injected systemically or into the coronary arterial system. For these patients, myocardial cell injection holds the most promise, either by direct transepicardial injection or by percutaneous transendocardial routes. However, endoventricular delivery is 'blind' and may not be as effective as epicardial injections under direct vision. Direct epicardial injection has the advantage of easily identifying the infarct region and efficient delivery of the cells, and has been approved by clinical trials. The limitation of this technique is that it can only be combined with surgery.

Conclusion

In summary, cell transplantation to induce angiogenesis is a promising experimental therapy. Autologous cell transplantation offers the promise of delivering both the cellular substrate and the specific signaling factors necessary to effect significant and sustained myocardial revascularization. Through continued rigorous investigation, therapeutic angiogenesis, either by cell transplantation or gene-enhanced cell transplantation, may emerge as a valuable tool to provide complete and definitive revascularization for our most challenging patients.

Acknowledgments

P.W.M.F. and H.Z. contributed equally to this chapter.
P.W.M.F. is a Research Fellow of the Canadian Institute for Health Research (CIHR) and the Heart & Stroke Foundation of Canada (HSFC). R.K.L. is a Career Investigator of the HSFC. Funding was provided by the HSFO (NA4603) and CIHR (MT14795) to R.K.L.

References

1. Lefkowitz RJ, Willerson JT. Prospects for cardiovascular research. JAMA 2001; 285(5): 581–7.

2. Mann DL. Mechanisms and models in heart failure: a combinatorial approach. Circulation 1999; 100(9): 999–1008.

3. Cecere R, Latter D, Chiu RC, Fitchett D. An integrated approach to the surgical management of heart failure. Can J Cardiol 1995; 11(5): 407–14.

4. Massie BM, Shah NB. Evolving trends in the epidemiologic factors of heart failure: rationale for preventive strategies and comprehensive disease management. Am Heart J 1997; 133(6): 703–12.

5. Gassler N, Wintzer HO, Stubbe HM et al. Transmyocardial laser revascularization. Histological features in human nonresponder myocardium. Circulation 1997; 95(2): 371–5.

6. Kohmoto T, Fisher PE, Gu A et al. Physiology, histology, and 2-week morphology of acute transmyocardial channels made with a CO_2 laser. Ann Thorac Surg 1997; 63(5): 1275–83.

7. Krabatsch T, Schaper F, Leder C et al. Histological findings after transmyocardial laser revascularization. J Card Surg 1996; 11(5): 326–31.

8. Oberpriller JO, Oberpriller JC, Arefyeva AM et al. Nuclear characteristics of cardiac myocytes following the proliferative response to mincing of the myocardium in the adult newt, *Notophthalmus viridescens*. Cell Tissue Res 1988; 253(3): 619–24.

9. Whittaker P, Kloner RA, Przyklenk K. Laser-mediated transmural myocardial channels do not salvage acutely ischemic myocardium. J Am Coll Cardiol 1993; 22(1): 302–9.

10. Whittaker P, Rakusan K, Kloner RA. Transmural channels can protect ischemic tissue. Assessment of long-term myocardial response to laser- and needle-made channels. Circulation 1996; 93(1): 143–52.

11. Horvath KA. Results of prospective randomized controlled trials of transmyocardial laser revascularization. Heart Surg Forum 2002; 5(1): 33–9.

12. Horvath KA, Aranki SF, Cohn LH et al. Sustained angina relief 5 years after transmyocardial laser revascularization with a $CO(2)$ laser. Circulation 2001; 104(12 suppl 1): I-81–4.

13. Horvath KA. Shedding light on denervation and transmyocardial laser revascularization. J Thorac Cardiovasc Surg 2001; 122(4): 647–8.

14. Fedak PWM, Verma S, Weisel RD et al. Angiogenesis: protein, gene, or cell therapy? Heart Surg Forum 2001; 4(4): 301–4.

15. Banai S, Jaklitsch MT, Shou M et al. Angiogenic-induced enhancement of collateral blood flow to ischemic myocardium by vascular endothelial growth factor in dogs. Circulation 1994; 89(5): 2183–9.

16. Laham RJ, Sellke FW, Edelman ER et al. Local perivascular delivery of basic fibroblast growth factor in patients undergoing coronary bypass surgery: results of a phase I randomized, double-blind, placebo-controlled trial. Circulation 1999; 100(18): 1865–71.

17. Ruel M, Laham RJ, Parker JA et al. Long-term effects of surgical angiogenic therapy with fibroblast growth factor 2 protein. J Thorac Cardiovasc Surg 2002; 124(1): 28–34.

18. Epstein SE, Fuchs S, Zhou YF et al. Therapeutic interventions for enhancing collateral development by administration of growth factors: basic principles, early results and potential hazards. Cardiovasc Res 2001; 49(3): 532–42.

19. Simons M, Bonow RO, Chronos NA et al. Clinical trials in coronary angiogenesis: issues, problems, consensus: an expert panel summary. Circulation 2000; 102(11): E73–86.

20. Schwarz ER, Speakman MT, Patterson M et al. Evaluation of the effects of intramyocardial injection of DNA expressing vascular endothelial growth factor (VEGF) in a myocardial infarction model in the rat – angiogenesis and angioma formation. J Am Coll Cardiol 2000; 35(5): 1323–30.

50. Kamihata H, Matsubara H, Nishiue T et al. Implantation of bone marrow mononuclear cells into ischemic myocardium enhances collateral perfusion and regional function via side supply of angioblasts, angiogenic ligands, and cytokines. Circulation 2001; 104(9): 1046–52.

51. Shake JG, Gruber PJ, Baumgartner WA et al. Mesenchymal stem cell implantation in a swine myocardial infarct model: engraftment and functional effects. Ann Thorac Surg 2002; 73(6): 1919–25.

52. Reyes M, Dudek A, Jahagirdar B et al. Origin of endothelial progenitors in human postnatal bone marrow. J Clin Invest 2002; 109(3): 337–46.

53. Tateishi-Yuyama E, Matsubara H, Murohara T et al. Therapeutic angiogenesis for patients with limb ischaemia by autologous transplantation of bone-marrow cells: a pilot study and a randomised controlled trial. Lancet 2002; 360(9331): 427.

54. Murohara T, Ikeda H, Duan J et al. Transplanted cord blood-derived endothelial precursor cells augment postnatal neovascularization. J Clin Invest 2000; 105(11): 1527–36.

55. Li RK, Jia ZQ, Weisel RD et al. Smooth muscle cell transplantation into myocardial scar tissue improves heart function. J Mol Cell Cardiol 1999; 31(3): 513–22.

56. Yoo KJ, Li RK, Weisel RD et al. Smooth muscle cells transplantation is better than heart cells transplantation for improvement of heart function in dilated cardiomyopathy. Yonsei Med J 2002; 43(3): 296–303.

57. Yau TM, Fung K, Weisel RD et al. Enhanced myocardial angiogenesis by gene transfer with transplanted cells. Circulation 2001; 104(12 suppl 1): I-218–22.

58. Iwaguro H, Yamaguchi J, Kalka C et al. Endothelial progenitor cell vascular endothelial growth factor gene transfer for vascular regeneration. Circulation 2002; 105(6): 732–8.

59. Kornowski R, Fuchs S, Leon MB, Epstein SE. Delivery strategies to achieve therapeutic myocardial angiogenesis. Circulation 2000; 101(4): 454–8.

60. Takahashi T, Kalka C, Masuda H et al. Ischemia- and cytokine-induced mobilization of bone marrow-derived endothelial progenitor cells for neovascularization. Nat Med 1999; 5(4): 434–8.

61. Suzuki K, Murtuza B, Suzuki N et al. Intracoronary infusion of skeletal myoblasts improves cardiac function in doxorubicin-induced heart failure. Circulation 2001; 104(12 suppl 1): I-213–17.

62. Strauer BE, Brehm M, Zeus T et al. Repair of infarcted myocardium by autologous intracoronary mononuclear bone marrow cell transplantation in humans. Circulation 2002; 106(15): 1913–18.

13. TRANSPLANTATION OF AUTOLOGOUS ENDOTHELIAL CELLS TO INDUCE NEOVASCULARIZATION: EXPERIMENTAL FINDINGS

Valeri Chekanov, Victor Nikolaychik, Mykola Tsapenko and Nicholas N Kipshidze

Coronary artery disease is the most common cause of morbidity and mortality in industrialized countries. Despite many advances made in cardiovascular medicine in recent years, a significant number of patients are not optimal candidates for surgical revascularization or interventional procedures. The promotion of new vessel growth may be one of the most promising methods in the treatment of these patients with non-operable coronary artery disease.

The concept of new vessel growth induction is based on the fact that the formation of new blood vessels can be established by two processes: vasculogenesis, in which a primitive vascular supply is developed from endothelial cell precursors, e.g. angioblasts; and neovascularization (also called angiogenesis), in which pre-existing vessels serve as a source to produce new vessels by sending out capillary buds and sprouts.

Neovascularization involves a highly coordinated process that can be divided into several major steps. It begins with the activation of the endothelial cells in a parent vessel followed by proteolytic degradation of the base membrane (BM) to allow formation of a capillary sprout and subsequent endothelial cell migration towards the angiogenic stimulus. Proliferation of endothelial cells starts just behind the leading front of migrating cells. Subsequent steps include maturation of endothelial cells with inhibition of growth and remodeling into capillary tubes and recruitment of periendothelial cells, including pericytes, for small capillaries and vascular smooth muscle cells (SMCs) for larger vessels to support the endothelial tubes.[1] All these steps are initiated and controlled by interactions among growth factors, vascular cells and the extracellular matrix (ECM).

Inspired by seminal observations of Folkman,[2] many experimental studies have demonstrated that receptors of ischemic endothelial cells (ECs) accept endogenous and exogenous growth factors (GFs) or their DNA constructs. It has been considered as a primary mechanism for the intrinsic process of compensatory neovascularization. Among the growth factors involved in blood vessel growth and development, vascular endothelial growth factors (VEGFs) and fibroblast growth factors (FGFs) have been most extensively studied. Although FGF has powerful angiogenic properties, most evidence supports a primary role of VEGF in angiogenesis and vasculogenesis.[1,3] It is secreted by many mesenchymal and stromal cells, but its receptors are mainly restricted to endothelium. VEGF expression is stimulated by certain cytokines and growth factors (e.g. transforming growth factor-alpha (TGF-α), TGF-ß, platelet-derived growth factor (PDGF)) and by tissue hypoxia.[1,2] VEGF and FGF have been the most widely used angiogenic factors in experimental and human clinical trials. Preliminary animal experiments have been promising, with evidence of capillary formation at the target tissue after GF administration.[4,5] Improved myocardial perfusion and function after administration of angiogenic GFs has been also demonstrated in animal models of chronic myocardial ischemia. The modest results of the first clinical trials have significantly dampened the original enthusiasm for this new technique.[6-8] However, recent clinical trials using GF proteins or genes coding these angiogenic factors have demonstrated clinical and other objective evidence of relevant angiogenesis.[9,10] This might indicate the existence of different angiogenic phenotypes in humans as well as the fact that only some of the interactions between the angiogenic factors themselves and receptors are known.

Another expanding research area in promoting new vessel growth involves utilization of bone marrow cells and/or endothelial precursor cells.[11-13] Stump et al[14] in 1963 provided evidence that ECs could originate from the peripheral blood. Further studies confirmed the origin of the hematopoietic stem cells and EC precursor cells from hemangioblasts.[15-18] Endothelial progenitor cells isolated from peripheral blood could directly originate from monocytes/macrophages as well.[19] These data were the main reason for experimental studies suggesting that transplantation of blood-derived or bone marrow-derived progenitor cells can beneficially affect angiogenesis and postnatal vasculogenesis. Experimental studies[20-22] produced promising results. It was also suggested that major angiogenic effects are most likely mediated by GF secretion.[19] The first clinical trials[23-26] provided strong evidence that transplantation of blood-derived or bone marrow-derived progenitor cells appears to be a feasible and safe method of therapeutic neovascularization.

Heterotopic mature EC transplantation is another approach to induce revascularization in ischemic tissue, even though it is still unknown whether the technique causes enough vascular cell proliferation to form a functional capillary network.

Transplantation of mature cells has been proposed as a strategy for organ replacement or tissue repair for a variety of therapeutic needs, including the generation of bioengineered skin, blood vessels, liver, nerves, bone and

184

cartilage.[27–29] There is strong evidence that mature ECs, having a constant
supply of blood-borne multipotent endothelial-like cells, could undergo transdifferentiation itself and serve as a potential source of at least some mesenchymal
cells, which include SMCs as well.[30,31] Based on all these data, we investigated
the possibility of enhancing neovascularization in the ischemic myocardium of
sheep by heterotopic transplantation of ECs within a fibrin matrix.

A crucial component of this transplantation procedure is the formation of
a three-dimensional biodegradable matrix in which the neomorphogenic
processes take place. Such a matrix is generally needed for anchorage, guided
migration, proliferation and differentiation of the transplanted cells. The
matrices currently used in cardiovascular bioengineering are potentially
immunogenic; they show toxic degradation and provoke inflammatory
reactions and they act primarily as passive scaffolding for cell manipulations in
culture or for implantation as a film.

Rather than a passive matrix for EC transplantation, we needed a matrix
that had two essential characteristics: morphogenic activity that would direct
implanted cells to form vessel-like structures, and availability in the form of
an injectable liquid that would polymerize and solidify after administration
into the target territory. Fibrin-based materials have these and many other
characteristics beneficial for bioengineering a vascular bed. We also needed to
be able to generate a specific cellular signal that would direct the
morphogenesis of implanted cells to form a neovascular network that would
be connected to existing vessels.

The concept of using fibrin as an angiogenic substance either alone or with
the addition of proteins was invented by Fasol et al,[32] who demonstrated in a
rat model that significant site-directed formation of new blood vessel structures
could be induced by using a modified fibrin glue implant containing the basic FGF.

In previous experiments, we found that a fibrin-based sealant becomes
vascularized[33] and thus capable of delivering needed plasma proteins to perform
functions as an extracellular matrix to anchor ECs to the vessel wall.[34] We also
demonstrated clinically in patients with peripheral arterial disease that
exogenous VEGF and a fibrin-based sealant could accelerate angiogenesis.[29,35]

On the basis of previous studies showing that fibrin sealant can perform a
number of roles, including (1) a carrier for pharmaceutical agents to help in
wound healing and local delivery of angiogenic substance, (2) a matrix for GF
therapy, (3) a platform for endothelialization of vascular grafts and (4) in cell
transplantation,[32–39] we hypothesized that a fibrin platform would enhance the
viability of transplanted mature ECs, direct the morpho-functional process of
capillary formation, and accelerate neovascularization in ischemic myocardium.

In our pilot study, we investigated the feasibility and efficacy of autologous
EC transplantation using a fibrin matrix in the ischemic myocardium of

185

sheep. The strategy of mature EC transplantation that we implemented in this investigation contrasts with other approaches used before, including GF therapy, bone marrow cell transplantation and ex vivo expanded EC progenitor transplantation. The clinical relevance of these findings is based on obtaining autologous mature ECs directly in the operating room. For this purpose, EC were cultivated from the endothelium of the jugular veins of sheep. Four weeks after placement of an ameroid constrictor in the circumflex artery of 12 adult sheep (Figure 13.1), four animals were subjected to EC transplantation, four others were injected with saline with added inactivated cells and four animals served as controls.

Baseline left ventricular ejection fraction (LVEF) was 0.68 ± 0.08, left ventricular end-systolic volume (LVESV) was 26.4 ± 6.1 ml, and left ventricular end-diastolic volume (LVEDV) was 53.4 ± 10.4 ml. Four weeks after ameroid placement (before treatment), LVEF had decreased to 0.49 ± 0.05 ($P < 0.0001$), LVEDV increased to 68.1 ± 9.9 ml ($P < 0.01$) and LVESV increased to 42.4 ± 7.5 ml ($P < 0.001$).

Eight weeks after treatment, ventricular function was markedly improved in the EC transplant group, but had deteriorated in the saline and control group (Figure 13.2). In animals subjected to EC transplantation, LVEF increased to 0.56 ± 0.04 ($P < 0.05$ versus before treatment). In the control group with no

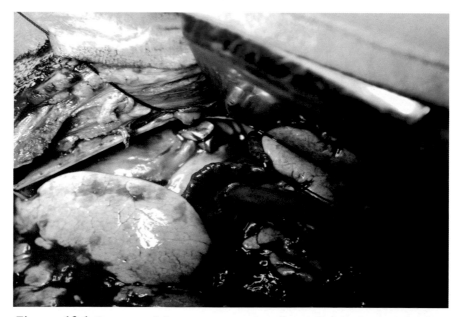

Figure 13.1 Experimental design: an ameroid constrictor (3.5 mm in diameter) is placed around the artery and the second branch of the circumflex artery.

treatment, LVEF decreased to 0.40 ± 0.08 ($P < 0.05$ versus EC treatment group), and in the saline treatment group it decreased to 0.39 ± 0.05 ($P < 0.05$ versus EC treatment group). LVEDV increased: to 81.3 ± 9.9 ml in the control group and to 76.1 ± 11.6 ml in the saline treatment group. In the EC treatment group, it was significantly lower, at 60.4 ± 2.7 ml ($P < 0.01$ versus control series). LVESV increased in both the control and saline treatment groups, to 51.1 ± 7.5 ml and to 53.8 ± 6.2 ml accordingly. It was significantly lower

Baseline

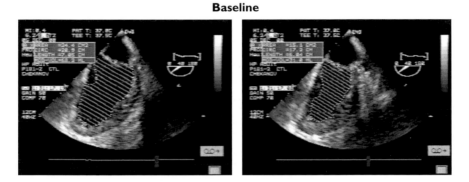

4 weeks after placement of ameroid

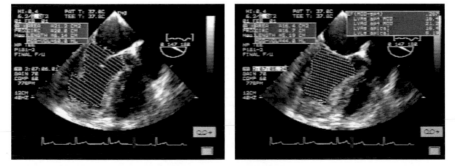

8-week F/U

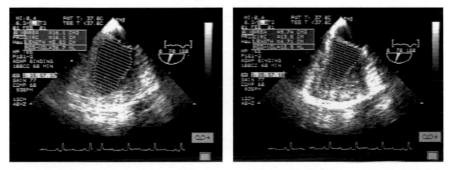

Figure 13.2 Echocardiogram of the sheep treated with EC–fibrin transplantation.

($P<0.05$ versus control group and $P<0.001$ versus saline-treated group) in the EC transplantation group, at 30.1 ± 4.1 ml.

Myocardial blood flow (MBF) was also increased in the EC group. Before placement of the ameroid constrictor, it was 0.59 ± 0.05 ml/min per g. Four weeks after ameroid constrictor placement, blood flow in the ischemic part of the myocardium decreased to 0.41 ± 0.07 ml/min per g ($P<0.001$ versus baseline). At the time when the animals were sacrificed (8 weeks after reoperation and the beginning of treatment), MBF decreased to 0.15 ± 0.03 ml/min per g in the control group ($P<0.001$ versus baseline, and 4 weeks) and to 0.18 ± 0.05 ml/min per g in the saline group ($P<0.001$ versus baseline, and $P<0.05$ versus 4 weeks). MBF in the EC group increased significantly to 0.66 ± 0.1 ml/min per g compared with 4 weeks after ameroid constrictor placement ($P<0.001$).

Histology and electron microscopy (Figures 13.3–13.7) revealed extensive neovascularization after EC transplantation. In normal non-ischemic myocardium, in all three groups, the capillaries occupied $5.6\pm0.43\%$ of the area. Twelve weeks after ameroid constrictor placement (and 8 weeks after

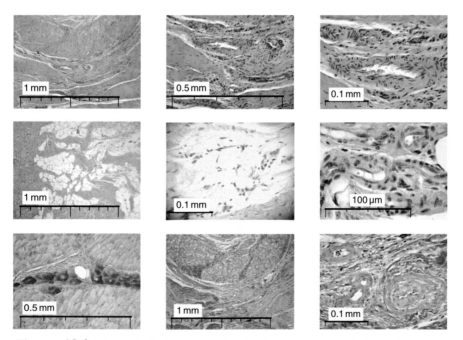

Figure 13.3 Histologic findings, control animal. The upper panel shows thick fibrocollagenous bands (H & N staining). The middle panel shows fibro-fatty tissue within the myocardium (H & N staining). The lower panel shows glycogen-rich hibernating myocardium (H & N and trichrome staining).

188

reoperation and beginning of treatment), the area had decreased to
$3.3 \pm 0.3\%$ ($P < 0.05$ versus baseline) in the control group and to $3.4 \pm 0.6\%$
($P < 0.01$ versus baseline) in the saline group. However, if in the control and
saline groups the area occupied by capillaries significantly decreased compared
with baseline, in the EC-treated group it increased to $8.4 \pm 1.3\%$ ($P < 0.001$)
and was considerably greater than in the control and saline groups
($P < 0.0001$) (Figures 13.3–13.5). According to transmission electron
microscopy, in both control and saline-treated animals, a typical pattern of
ischemic damage consisting of cytoplasmic foldings and projections into the
capillary lumen was found in the ECs of the ischemic vasculature. Capillary
structures were minimal or absent (Figure 13.6). However, in the border
areas of ischemic zones, a few ECs appeared to be normal and had no signs
of damage or injury. In contrast, tissue specimens obtained from animals in
the EC group at 30 days after intervention had capillary-like structures with
endoluminal openings and ECs forming an immature capillary meshwork
(Figure 13.7). At 60 days, however, functional arterioles and mature capillary
structures appeared (Figure 13.6).

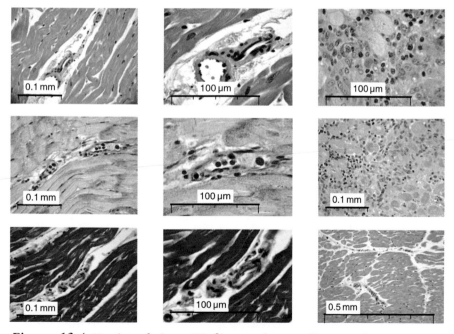

Figure 13.4 Histologic findings, EC–fibrin application. Upper panel: appearance
of normal myocardial vasculature with inflammatory infiltrates (H & N stain). Middle
panel: increased neovascularization with inflammatory cells (PAS and H & N stains).
Lower panel: vasculature of normal myocardium (trichrome and H & N stains).

Control

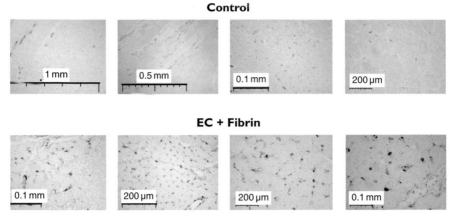

EC + Fibrin

Figure 13.5 *Immunohistochemical (von Willebrand factor) findings 60 days following EC transplantation, showing evidence of neovascularization. The control animal shows few EC between muscle fibers. With EC–fibrin transplantation, there is prominent EC staining.*

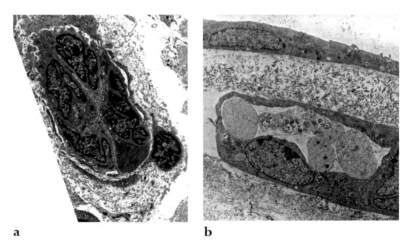

a   b

Figure 13.6 *(a) Transmission electronmicroscopy of myocardium at 30 days after treatment with EC transplantation shows a capillary-like structure with an endoluminal opening. The functional areas with extensive cellular overlaps. The pericapillary space is filled with rough and gentle fibrin fibers. (b) ECs and pericytes forming immature capillary structures. The endoluminal space is minimal. Webel–Palade bodies are visible.*

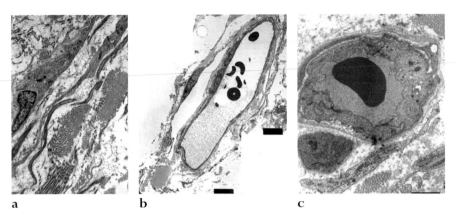

a   b   c

Figure 13.7 (a) Transmission electronmicroscopy of myocardium at 60 days after
treatment with saline injection. Capillary structures are absent. There is myocardial
tissue with large amounts of collagen fibers and fibroblasts. (b) Transmission
electronmicroscopy of myocardium at 60 days after treatment with EC transplantation
shows arterioles in the treated area with thin walls. Erythrocytes in the lumen
indicate that these are functional arterioles. (c) Capillaries formed in a fibrin matrix
enriched with fibroblasts. The lumen contains erythrocytes. The basement membrane is
well developed and includes SMCs and pericytes.

The results led us to conclude that heterotopic transplantation of ECs
within a fibrin matrix enhances neovascularization, increases MBF and
improves global left ventricular function in a sheep model of chronic
myocardial ischemia.

The present study has shown that ECs confined in a three-dimensional
fibrin matrix will form capillaries in ischemic myocardium. We have also
previously found two morphogenically distinct types of growth in
microvascular ECs.[40] Cultured in a two-dimensional matrix, ECs quickly
formed a cobblestone monolayer that had a density 2–2.5-fold higher than in
controls (i.e. those cultivated on a single-plane tissue culture surface). It was
also observed that the ionic strength of the ratio of these components enabled
the cells to 'recognize' minor spatial changes in fibrin meshwork
architecture.[40] Cultured in a three-dimensional matrix, ECs form 'true'
capillaries, while other vascular cells trapped in this matrix undergo
apoptosis.[41]

Because the direction in which capillaries form is generally determined by
the orientation of the administered angiogenic mixture, we needed to ensure
that the ECs would grow in the desired direction. On the other hand,
ischemic tissue itself produces many chemotactic factors that attract ECs or

EC precursors and will support capillary growth, suggesting that plasma proteins can perform some of the functions of the extracellular matrix involved in anchoring ECs to the myocardium.

Because it is well known that ischemia interrupts local circuit neurons, previous studies showing that fibrin enhances nerve regeneration[42,43] may point to another mechanism for improving left ventricular function after EC and fibrin intramyocardial injection.[44]

In the clinical setting, our proposed strategy would require that the patient donate autologous ECs and reagents for the fibrin matrix, thus avoiding potential immunologic rejection. As has been clearly demonstrated, transplantation of allogeneic cells, no matter how freshly prepared or viable, provokes a strong reaction with a spectrum of likely immunologic and inflammatory events that may lead to rejection.[45] Thus, autologous cell transplantation is a reasonable, if not mandatory, step, but it raises the problem of how to apply this laboratory technique clinically; namely, what source of autologous ECs should be used?

Certainly, patients who have cardiovascular disease cannot be autologous donors of ECs derived from jugular, cephalic or saphenous veins. Adipose tissue has been actively explored as an alternative source of ECs because it is abundant in the body, is easily accessible, and is composed primarily of two cell types, adipocytes and capillary ECs. In culture, these ECs demonstrate many of the functional and morphologic characteristics seen in ECs in large vessels, so large quantities of adipose tissue could be removed with minimal risk to the patient, and the inherent difference in density between adipocytes and capillary fragments means that they could be easily separated by simple centrifugation.

Once a human adipose tissue EC procurement protocol is developed, its use for high-density seeding would have to be validated by successive successful studies of the culturing of ECs derived from patients with cardiovascular diseases. One such study of the harvesting of adipose tissue ECs by means of liposuction has already reported a 100% success rate in 140 patients.[46]

Finally, we think that mature EC transplantation is more potent than GF therapy. Although it has been previously demonstrated that intramyocardial transplantation of bone marrow cells induces neovascularization of ischemic tissue,[11,12] it remains to be proved that these cells indeed differentiate into mature ECs and not into other types of cells such as fibroblasts and osteoblasts.

Recently, Kawamoto et al[13] demonstrated the therapeutic potential of ex vivo expanded endothelial progenitor cells in a small animal model; however, the safety of ex vivo culture expansion needs to be established.

However, for future investigations it will be important to consider some
of the unanswered questions. The mechanism of new collateral growth in our
experiments was not well defined, and may be caused by upregulation of GF
by ECs and/or fibrin or inflammatory reactions. Additional studies are
needed to address this issue, and it is difficult to differentiate the effect of
EC/fibrin transplantation upon neovasularization from the independent effect
of fibrin. Although EC transplantation induced capillary growth in the
myocardium and improved circulation in the ischemic muscle in a sheep
model, more experiments are needed to investigate the efficacy of this
intriguing technique.

We suggest that this technique or a similar one that uses EC
transplantation to accelerate the formation of collateral vasculature may be a
solution to one of the most challenging problems in contemporary cardiology:
how to treat small vessel pathology and disseminated lesions. Future
approaches may consist of delivering a 'cocktail' of angiogenic agents laced
with vasculogenic precursors and/or mature ECs in a temporally and spatially
coordinated fashion.

References

1. Cotran RS, Kumar V, Collins T. Robbins pathologic basis of disease, 6th edn.
    Philadelphia: WB Saunders, 1999.

2. Folkman J. Tumor angiogenesis: therapeutic implications. N Engl J Med 1971;
    285: 1182–6.

3. Ferrara N. Role of vascular endothelial growth factor in physiologic and
    pathologic angiogenesis: therapeutic implications. Semin Oncol 2002; 29(6
    suppl): 10–14.

4. Zakine G, Martinod E, Fornes P et al. Growth factors improve latissimus dorsi
    muscle vascularization and trophicity after cardiomyoplasty. Ann Thorac Surg
    2003; 75(2): 549–54.

5. Zhang R, Wang I, Zhang L et al. Nitric oxide enhances angiogenesis via the
    synthesis of vascular endothelial growth factor and cGMP after stroke in the
    rat. Circ Res 2003; 92(3): 308–13.

6. Laham RJ, Chronos NA, Pike M et al. Intracoronary basic fibroblast growth
    factor (FGF-2) in patients with severe ischemic heart disease: results of a phase
    I open-label dose escalation study. J Am Coll Cardiol 2000; 36: 2132–9.

7. Epstein SE, Fuchs S, Zhou YF et al. Therapeutic interventions for enhancing
    collateral development by administration of growth factors: basic principles,
    early results and potential hazards. Cardiovasc Res 2001; 49(3): 532–42.

8. Laham RJ, Simons M, Sellke F. Gene transfer for angiogenesis in coronary artery disease. Annu Rev Med 2001; 52: 485–502.

9. Henry TD, Annex BH, McKendall GR et al. The VIVA trail: vascular endothelial growth factor in ischemia for vascular angiogenesis. Circulation 2003; 107(10): 1359–65.

10. Shyu KG, Chang H, Wang BW et al. Intramuscular vascular endothelial growth factor gene therapy in patients with chronic critical leg ischemia. Am J Med 2003; 114(2): 85–92.

11. Kobayashi T, Hamano K, Li TS et al. Enhancement of angiogenesis by the implantation of self bone marrow cells in a rat ischemic heart model. J Surg Res. 2000; 89: 189–95.

12. Tomita S, Li RK, Weisel RD et al. Autologous transplantation of bone marrow cells improves damaged heart function. Circulation 1999; 100: II-247–56.

13. Kawamoto A, Gwon HC, Iwaguro H et al. Therapeutic potential of ex vivo expanded endothelial progenitor cells for myocardial ischemia. Circulation 2001; 103: 634–7.

14. Stump MM, Jordan GL, DeBakey ME et al. Endothelium grown from circulating blood on isolated intravascular Dacron. Am J Pathol 1963; 43: 361–7.

15. Gunsilius E. Evidence from a leukemia model for maintenance of vascular endothelium by bone marrow-derived endothelial cells. Adv Exp Med Biol 2003; 522: 17–24.

16. Asahara T, Masuda H, Takahashi T et al. Bone marrow origin of endothelial progenitor cells responsible for postnatal vasculogenesis in physiological and pathological neovascularization. Circ Res 1999; 85: 221–8.

17. Auerbach R, Huang H, Lu L. Hematopoietic stem cells in the mouse embryonic yolk sac. Stem Cells 1996; 14: 269–80.

18. Nishakawa S-I. Embryonic stem cells as a source of hematopoietic and vascular endothelial cells in vitro. J Allergy Clin Immunol 1997; 100: 102–4.

19. Rehman J, Li J, Orschell CM et al. Peripheral blood 'endothelial progenitor cells' are derived from monocyte/macrophages and secrete angiogenic growth factors. Circulation 2003; 107: 1164–9.

20. Nishuda M, Li TS, Hirata K et al. Improvement of cardiac function by bone marrow cell implantation in a rat hypoperfusion heart model. Ann Thorac Surg 2003; 75(3): 768–73.

21. Al-Khaldi A, Al-Sabti H, Galipeau J et al. Therapeutic angiogenesis using autologous bone marrow stromal cells: improved blood flow in a chronic limb ischemia model. Ann Thorac Surg 2003; 75(1): 204–9.

22. Yoshida M, Horimoto H, Mieno S et al. Intra-arterial bone marrow cell transplantation induces angiogenesis in rat hindlimb ischemia. Eur Surg Res 2003; 35(2): 86–91.

23. Tse HF, Kwong YL, Chan JK et al. Angiogenesis in ischemic myocardium by intramyocardial autologous bone marrow mononuclear cell implantation. Lancet 2003; 361(9351): 11–12.

24. Esato K, Hamano K, Li TS et al. Neovascularization induced by autologous bone marrow cell implantation in peripheral arterial disease. Cell Transplant 2002; 11(8): 747–52.

25. Tateishi-Yuyama E, Matsubara H, Murohara T et al. Therapeutic angiogenesis for patients with limb ischemia by autologous transplantation of bone marrow cells: a pilot study and a randomized controlled trial. Lancet 2002; 360: 427–35.

26. Assmus B, Schaechinger V, Teupe C et al. Transplantation of progenitor cells and regeneration enhancement in acute myocardial infarction (TOPCARE-AMI). Circulation 2002; 106: 3009–17.

27. Mikos AG, Bao Y, Cima LG et al. Preparation of poly(glycolic acid) bonded fiber structures for cell attachment and transplantation. J Biomed Mater Res 1993; 27(2): 183–9.

28. Chekanov V, Akhtar M, Tchekanov G et al. Transplantation of autologous endothelial cells induces angiogensis. Pacing Clin Electrophysiol 2003; 26(1): 496–9.

29. Kipshidze N, Johnson WD, Haudenschild CC. Therapeutic angiogenesis in patients with advanced coronary artery disease: hype or hope? J Invasive Cardiol 1999; 11(10): 589–99.

30. Frid MG, Kale VA, Stenmark KR. Mature vascular endothelium can give rise to smooth muscle cells via endothelial–mesenchymal transdifferentiation: in vitro analysis. Circ Res 2002; 90: 1189–96.

31. Brown CB, Boyer AS, Runyan RB et al. Requirement of type III TGF-ß receptor for endocardial cell transformation in the heart. Science 1999; 283: 2080–2.

32. Fasol R, Schumacher B, Schlaudraff K et al. Experimental use of a modified fibrin glue to induce site-directed angiogenesis from the aorta to the heart. J Thorac Cardiol Surg 1994; 107: 1432–9.

33. Chekanov V, Nikolaychik V, Tchekanov G. The use of biologic glue for better adhesion between the skeletal muscle flap and the myocardium and for increasing capillary ingrowth. J Thorac Cardiovasc Surg 1996; 111: 678–80.

34. Kipshidze N, Ferguson III JJ, Keelan MH et al. Endoluminal reconstruction of the arterial wall with endothelial cell/glue matrix reduces restenosis in an atherosclerotic rabbit. JACC 2000; 36(4): 1396–403.

35. Kipshidze N, Chekanov V, Chawla P et al. Angiogenesis in a patient with ischemic limb. Texas Heart Inst J 2000; 27(2): 196–200.

36. Byme DJ, Hardy J, Wood RA et al. Effect of fibrin glue on the mechanical properties of healing wounds. Br J Surg 1991; 78: 841–3.

37. Boyce ST, Holder IA, Supp AP et al. Delivery and activity of antimicrobial drugs released from human fibrin sealant. J Burn Care Rehab 1994; 15: 251–5.

38. Chekanov V, Akhtar M, Tchekanov G et al. Transplantation of autologous endothelial cells induces angiogenesis. 2003 Pacing Clin Electrophysiol; 26: 496–9.

39. Deutsch M, Meinhart J, Fischlein T, Preiss P. Clinical autologous in vitro endothelialization of infrainguinal ePTFE grafts in 100 patients: a 9-year experience. Surgery 1999; 126(5): 847–55.

40. Nikolaychik VV, Samet MM, Lelkes PI. A new, cryoprecipitate based coating for improved endothelial cell attachment and growth on medical grade artificial surfaces. ASAIO J 1994; 40(3): M846–52.

41. Wankowski DM, Samet MM, Nikolaychik VV, Lelkes PI. Endothelial cell seeding with rotation of a ventricular blood sac. ASAIO J 1994; 40(3): M319–24.

42. Sakiyama-Elbert SE, Hubbell JA. Controlled release of nerve growth factor from a heparin-containing fibrin-based cell ingrowth matrix. J Control Release 2000; 69(1): 149–58.

43. Robinson GA, Madison RD. Survival of adult rat retinal ganglion cells with regrown axons in peripheral nerve grafts: a comparison of graft attachment with suture of fibrin glue. J Neurosurg 2000; 93(2): 275–8.

44. Murphy DA, O'Blenes S, Hanna BD, Armour JA. Capacity of intrinsic cardiac neurons to modify the acutely autotransplanted mammalian heart. J Heart Lung Transplant 1994; 13: 847–56.

45. Adams PW, Lee HS, Ferguson RM, Orosz CG. Alloantigenicity of human endothelial cells. Transplantation 1994; 57: 115–22.

46. Williams SK, Rose DG, Jarrel BE. Microvascular endothelial cell seeding of ePTFE vascular grafts: improved patency and stability of cellular lining. J Biomed Mater Res 1994; 28: 203–13.

14. Intramyocardial Delivery of Autologous Bone Marrow: Experimental Justification and Early Clinical Experiences

Shmuel Fuchs, Tim Kinnaird and Eugenio Stabile

The natural growth of collateral blood vessels in response to physiologically significant arterial luminal narrowing is a complex process, involving multiple cells and growth factors acting in an orchestrated and time-dependent manner.[1-3] Local factors such as hypoxia, shear stress and inflammation stimulate angiogenesis, while systemic factors such as diabetes mellitus, aging and hypercholesterolemia have been clearly demonstrated to retard these reparative mechanisms.[4-8] Although collateral bloodflow can reduce myocardial ischemia and infarct size, typically less than half of the normal maximal bloodflow is restored and thus, in a substantial number of patients, anginal symptoms persist. Despite great progress in the treatment of cardiovascular disease, there are increasing numbers of patients with advanced symptomatic coronary artery disease not amenable to conventional revascularization techniques. Current estimates suggest that 5–10% of patients referred to tertiary centers for coronary interventions are currently considered as 'no-option' patients and hence are potential candidates for therapeutic angiogenesis.

Initial trials tested the hypothesis that a single angiogenic agent – such as vascular endothelial growth factor (VEGF) and fibroblast growth factor (FGF) proteins or genes – administered systemically or by the intracoronary route, or directly injected into the myocardium may improve patients' symptoms, exercise capacity and myocardial perfusion. However, the initial excitement, driven by several non-randomized small phase I studies, was hampered by the negative results of subsequent larger randomized trials.[9-17]

Given the complexity of the processes underpinning new blood vessel formation, these negative results suggest that a single growth factor approach may be too simplistic. One recent concept that may provide an alternative strategy is the utilization of combined growth factor/cell therapy, as provided by bone marrow (BM)-derived cells. This chapter summarizes the in vitro and small animal in vivo data, and the very preliminary clinical experience with BM-derived cells aimed at enhancing myocardial tissue perfusion.

197

Why bone marrow-derived cells?

The potential angiogenic activity of BM cells can be broadly divided into two types: (1) differentiation into cellular constituents that physically add to the developing collaterals – BM contains stem cells and progenitor endothelial cells that *may* differentiate into mature vascular endothelial cells and thereby contribute to new blood vessel formation; and (2) secretory – many growth factors required to stimulate and coordinate the complex processes involved in the remodeling of pre-existing small collaterals have been shown to be secreted by cultured BM cells.

BM-derived cell differentiation

In vitro studies have demonstrated that several BM-derived cells appear to differentiate into one or more of the cellular components of the vascular bed. The mechanisms by which the local milieu influences these possible stem cells to differentiate are as yet unknown. In addition, the signals that drive migration of cells out of the marrow cavity into the circulation, and ultimately to the vascular bed, are also largely unknown. However, it is agreed that several marrow cell subpopulations are the precursors of endothelial cells.[18–21] These cells probably represent a stage of stemness from multipotent progenitor cells through angioblasts to committed endothelial progenitor cells. Animal and human studies suggest that endothelial progenitor cells and angioblasts are present in the peripheral circulation in the resting state. However, similar cells resident in the marrow are preferentially released following tissue ischemia, migrate and actively participate in forming new capillaries.[22] Thus, direct administration of marrow cells into tissue can optimize the natural responses to ischemia. In addition, mesenchymal stem cells and multipotent progenitor cells have been demonstrated in vitro to differentiate into smooth muscle and endothelial cells, and subsequently therefore might also contribute to vessel remodeling.[23] Thus, transplantation of the whole marrow cell population theoretically donates cells with the ability to directly incorporate into new or remodeling blood vessels.

In addition, previous studies have also highlighted the potential importance of other hematopoietic cells – lymphocytes and monocytes – in mediating tissue responses to ischemia.[24–27] As BM mononuclear fractions contain significant numbers of mature and nearly mature populations of these cells, BM injection may contribute in an indirect way to enhance angiogenesis.

It is important to recognize that the magnitude of the actual incorporation of BM-derived cells into vascular structures varies substantially between studies (3.3–56%) and is the subject of continuing controversy. Differences in animal models (myocardial versus hindlimb ischemia, and coronary ligation versus

198

cryoinjury), number of injected cells and delivery mode preclude any meaningful comparison between studies. In addition, the issue of adult stem cell plasticity has recently been questioned. Several groups proposed that spontaneous cell fusion and generation of hybrid cells with subsequent adoption of recipient cell phenotype accounted for what was originally thought to be complete stem cell differentiation.[27,28] It is evident, therefore, that there are many unresolved issues in the field of BM-derived stem cells and angiogenesis.

Secretory

Despite evidence that BM-derived stem or progenitor endothelial cells incorporate into vascular structures, heterogeneous BM cell populations (i.e. BM-derived mononuclear cells and unfractionated BM) contain very small numbers of stem cells (<0.01% of total cells). Also, as discussed above, many studies suggest that only a small number of forming capillaries contain donated cells. Thus, the effects manifested by heterogeneous BM cell transplantation suggest the importance of secretory mechanisms.

BM cells are a source of an entire array of growth factors involved in the initiation and coordination of angiogenesis. These cytokines are secreted by several cellular components of the marrow population. For example, lymphocytes are a source of several cytokines, including FGF and epidermal growth factor.[29] With the use of immunoblotting, BM mononuclear cell extracts have been shown to contain VEGF, FGF, platelet-derived growth factor-AB and transforming growth factor proteins, while at a transcriptional level at least, angiopoietin-1 has been found.[30] Following direct myocardial delivery of these cells, increases in cardiac mRNA expression of VEGF, FGF and angiopoietin-1 were demonstrated, suggesting localized in vivo secretion of angiogenic growth factors by the injected cells. Other marrow cell subgroups such as megakaryocytes and platelets also release VEGF.[31]

One cell subgroup with potential importance in possible secretory mechanisms is the marrow stromal cell fraction. Placental growth factor, hepatocyte growth factor, insulin growth factors, VEGF, FGF, monocyte chemoattractant protein 1 (MCP-1) and metalloproteinases have all been found to be released by stromal cells.[32–35] In vivo, these cells support hematopoiesis, and several mediators secreted by stromal cells known to be involved in the maintenance of hematopoiesis may also regulate angiogenesis. These cytokines include interleukin-1, interleukin-6, colony-stimulating factors, erythropoietin and hepatocyte cell growth factor.[36] The humoral angiogenic potential of stromal BM cells was examined in a series of in vitro studies. The monocyte fraction of freshly aspirated and filtered porcine BM was cultured, and the effects of the conditioned medium on endothelial proliferation, migration and tube formation were measured. The results showed continuous secretion of VEGF and the arteriogenic cytokine MCP-1, and demonstrated enhanced endothelial proliferation and migration. Endothelial and smooth muscle cell tube formation, an integrative in vitro test to assess angiogenesis, was stimulated by BM-conditioned medium, suggesting effects on cells constituting capillaries and conductive vessels.[34]

Thus, the multipotentiality of BM-derived cells to affect local angiogenic and arteriogenic processes via transdifferentiation and coordinated secretion of multi-angiogenic cytokines make them highly attractive for interventions aimed at enhancing myocardial tissue perfusion.

Route of administration

There are several potential routes via which cell therapy may be administered. The least invasive – intravenous injection – allows repeated treatments with minimal risk. However, the rate and magnitude of cell incorporation depend on the transpulmonary first-pass effect on the cells, as well as on homing of the circulating stem and progenitor cells into the target tissue. Evidence suggests that these cells distribute widely following intravenous injection, although tissue ischemia may enhance localization.[37,38] Intracoronary delivery may improve tissue localization, and the feasibility of this approach was recently demonstrated in humans with the delivery of autologous mononuclear cells into a coronary artery following primary target vessel angioplasty.[39]

Direct intramyocardial delivery strategies are the most invasive, and include: (1) transepicardial injections as an adjunctive therapy to coronary bypass grafting; (2) transepicardial injections as a sole therapy during mini-thoracotomy or thoracoscopy; and (3) transendocardial injection using specially designed catheters. The main potential advantage of the surgical procedure is 'injection under visualization', allowing anatomic identification of the target area and even distribution of the injections. The limitations of this approach include difficulties in accessing septal and posterior segments, and an inability to perform multiple treatment sessions.

Transendocardial injection is a less invasive, catheter-based approach. The catheter is advanced retrogradely via an 8F arterial femoral sheath into the left ventricle (LV). Intraventricular manipulation of the catheter enables the operator to inject in multiple directions in all LV segments. Current clinical experience is greatest for the use of electromechanical mapping to generate three-dimensional LV reconstruction prior to the injection. The LV map serves as an anatomic navigation tool, allowing identification of catheter-tip location, annotation of each injection location, even injection distribution and avoidance of undesired zones such as the mitral valve apparatus or thinned myocardial walls. The

200

catheters of this and other systems incorporate an adjustable retractable needle, usually set to about half the thickness of the target wall (4–5 mm). With the use of fluoroscopic, electromechanical and electrocardiographic parameters to ensure catheter stability and needle penetration, the delivery efficiency is ~95%.[40] Intraventricular catheter manipulation, however, can irritate the myocardium, inducing ventricular premature beats and short runs of ventricular tachycardia. In certain cases, this precludes injection in the more arrhythmogenic zones, can extend significantly the duration of the procedure and should always be carefully monitored. Each catheter is tested for cell biocompatibility to ensure no mechanical and functional damage to cells being propelled under pressure through the catheter and injection needle.

Animal studies

Several small and large animal studies using multiple species have demonstrated the therapeutic potential of heterogeneous BM-derived cells. In a rat cardiac cryoinjury model, transepicardial injection of BM mononuclear cells improved ventricular function, induced angiogenesis and apparently contributed to myogenesis.[41] However, concerns regarding the extrapolation of data derived from a cryoinjury model led to studies utilizing more relevant ischemic hindlimb and myocardial infarction models. In a rat ischemic injury model, BM transplantation increased the number of visible capillaries, while intramuscular implantation of BM cells following femoral artery ligation in a further rat study improved exercise tolerance by 50% when compared to controls.[42,43] Of particular interest is the demonstration that ex vivo exposure of BM mononuclear cells to hypoxic stress for 24 h significantly enhanced the angiogenic benefit following transplantation into rat ischemic hindlimb, when compared to cells cultured under normoxia.[44]

Other groups have examined the role of more selected subpopulations of BM-derived cells. Particular interest has developed in the therapeutic potential of the putative angioblast – that is, cells lacking lineage markers, while expressing CD34 and c-kit surface antigens. Several elegant studies utilizing these cells isolated from human BM have demonstrated that, following injection into ischemic myocardium, these cells have the ability to incorporate into vascular structures, limiting the degree of cardiac fibrosis and scar formation, and ultimately resulting in improved cardiac function. In addition, significant plasticity of these cells was also suggested, with injected cells differentiated into myocytes and smooth muscle cells being noted in areas of regenerating myocardium.[45,46]

The first assessment of the safety and efficacy of transendocardial injection of autologous BM (ABM) cells to augment ischemic tissue perfusion was performed in a chronic ischemia pig ameroid model. The model leads to progressive total coronary artery occlusion and downstream myocardial ischemia with minimal (~10%) patchy infarction. Freshly aspirated and filtered unfractionated BM was injected transendocardially, with a catheter-based system, into the occluded left circumflex artery ischemic myocardial territory and its boundaries (12 injections, 0.2 ml each). Collateral flow, assessed by fluorescent microspheres (ischemic/normal zone × 100) improved at 4 weeks compared to pre-injection in ABM-treated pigs at rest (83 ±12% versus 98 ±12%) and during adenosine stress (78 ±12% versus 89 ±18%). Similarly, contractility (ischemic/normal zone × 100) increased in ABM-treated pigs at rest (60 ±32% versus 83 ±21%) and during atrial pacing (35 ±43% versus 91 ±44%). No improvement in either flow or regional function was observed in saline-injected controls. Interestingly, identical ABM injection into normal, non-ischemic regions induced no change in flow.[47] These observations underscore the importance of the local milieu in providing the vital signals for the BM cells to initiate angiogenesis.

Subsequently, these initial findings have been confirmed in other large animal models. In a porcine acute infarction model, injection of BM-derived mononuclear cells resulted in a five-fold increase in the numbers of angiographically visible collaterals, a three-fold increase in the number of capillaries, and an improvement in ejection fraction of 48%.[30] In a canine chronic coronary occlusion model, transepicardial injection of BM mononuclear cells following coronary occlusion led to a 50% increase in the number of microvessels observed and significant improvements in LV wall thickening.[48]

In the large animal studies conducted thus far, abnormal tissue development subsequent to injection (e.g. bone, cartilage, teratoma or medullary foci), increased cardiac fibrosis or adverse effects on atherosclerosis have not been demonstrated. Accordingly, the safety and suggestive potential efficacy results of these preclinical studies served as the basis for several ongoing clinical trials.

Preliminary clinical experience

The first human clinical study was performed in Japan in 1999.[49] The mononuclear fraction of ABM cells was injected into an ungraftable myocardial zone as adjunctive therapy to coronary artery bypass grafting in five patients. Postoperative evaluation revealed no adverse effects, and clinical follow-up was performed for at least 1 year. Flow in the target area improved in three of the five patients. It is important to recognize that while this study suggested the feasibility and potential safety of the transepicardial approach, no inferences can be drawn regarding tissue perfusion, as BM therapy was an adjunct to coronary bypass. Also, other softer endpoints such as the magnitude of creatine kinase MB fraction release and inflammatory reactions may be masked by the surgical intervention.

Intraoperative transepicardial injection of more selective BM-derived cell subpopulations was also recently examined in six patients.[50] In this study, patients with recent myocardial infarction who underwent routine coronary artery bypass graft (CABG) surgery received 10 direct intramyocardial injections of 1×10^5 AC133-positive cells. Patients were followed for 9–16 months after surgery. During this period, no malignant neoplasms or ventricular arrhythmias were noted. SPECT study revealed significant improvements in the previously non- or hypoperfused infarcted territory. The authors appropriately indicated that the cell transplantation was performed in conjunction with surgical revascularization, and the effectiveness of this stragegy, therefore, cannot be readily assessed. Nevertheless, the long follow-up provides additional safety for the BM-derived cell transplantation approach.

Transendocardial injection of autologous BM cells has been performed as part of several pilot and phase I safety and feasibility studies (Table 14.1). The target patient population, as in most previous myocardial angiogenic trials, comprises patients with symptomatic coronary artery disease not amenable to conventional coronary revascularization. At the time of writing, approximately 40 patients have been injected worldwide with ABM cells. All procedures were performed using the electromechanical-guided system (Figure 14.1), and only freshly aspirated and filtered BM or its isolated mononuclear fraction was injected. Preliminary and unpublished data of the first 20 patients enrolled in the first and largest ongoing study suggest the feasibility and potential safety of this approach.[51] At the time of writing of this chapter, a complete 3-month follow-up was available for the first 16 patients. The procedural success was 100%; the mean mapping and injection time were 32 ± 16 min and 28 ± 11 min, respectively. ABM injection was associated with no adverse effects; in particular there were no arrhythmias or clinical evidence of infection or myocardial inflammation. The post-procedural peak CK-MB was normal in 13 patients and < 2 times the upper limit of normal in the remainder. All patients completed a 3-month follow-up: three patients were readmitted for recurrent chest pain. The CCS angina score significantly improved (3.3 ± 0.9 versus 2.1 ± 0.8, $P = 0.001$), as did the quality of life score (26.0 ± 17 versus 44 ± 23, $P = 0.01$). Stress-induced ischemia occurring within the injected territories also improved (2.0 ± 0.8 versus 1.6 ± 0.8, $P < 0.001$). Treadmill exercise duration, available for 14 patients, improved in 10 and deteriorated in 4 patients. These encouraging results, however, should be interpreted as suggestive of safety (no

Table 14.1 Summary of phase I human trials of bone marrow cell therapy for angiogenesis

Author	No patients	Target myocardial region	Cell type	Route of administration	Concomitant procedures	Endpoints	Follow-up (months)	Outcomes
Strauer et al[39]	10	Recently infarcted, patent infarct artery	BMC	Intracoronary	PTCA	Ventriculography Dobutamine stress	3	Infarct region smaller Lower end-systolic volume Improvement in contractility
Hamano et al[49]	5	Infarcted, none bypassed	BMC	Direct intramyocardial	CABG	Scintigraphy	12	3/5 patients improved
Stamm et al[50]	6	Recently infarcted, none bypassed	AC133+	Direct intramyocardial	CABG	Echocardiography SPECT	3–10	Improved LVEF Smaller end-diastolic volume Improvement in 5/6 patients
Fuchs et al[51]	10	Ischemic, non-infarcted	UBM	Percutaneous intramyocardial	None	ETT SPECT	3	Trend for improved exercise time Reduction in stress-induced ischemia
Tse et al[52]	8	Ischemic, non-infarcted	BMC	Percutaneous intramyocardial	None	MRI perfusion	3	Improved wall thickening Reduction in mass of hypoperfused myocardium
Asmuss et al[53]	20	Recently infarcted, patent infarct artery	BMC or CPC	Intracoronary	PTCA	LV angiography Dobutamine stress PET scanning	4	Increase ejection fraction Fewer abnormal segments Increase in myocardial viability

BMC, bone marrow mononuclear cells; CPC, circulating progenitor cells; UBM, unfractionated bone marrow cells; PTCA, percutaneous transluminal coronary angioplasty; CABS, coronary artery bypass graft.

deterioration) rather than potential efficacy. The latter should only be evaluated in specifically designed, placebo-controlled studies, powered to detect differences between groups rather than within groups.

A similar transendocardial approach was also examined in eight patients who were injected with $1-2 \times 10^7$ BM-derived mononuclear cells.[51] At 3 months, a significant reduction in the number of angina episodes and nitroglycerin consumption was noted. Magnetic resonance imaging (MRI), performed in seven patients, revealed an $11.6 \pm 8.8\%$ improvement in target wall thickening and a $5.5 \pm 4.7\%$ improvement in target wall motion.

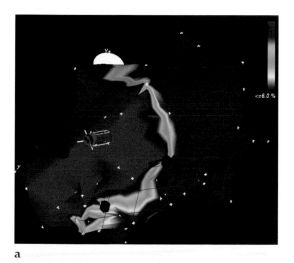

a

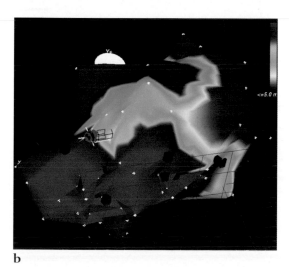

b

Figure 14.1 Left ventricular electromechanical maps (left oblique, bottom view projection) after intramyocardial injection of autologous bone marrow. Injections were delivered into an ischemic right coronary artery territory. Local shortening (a) and unipolar voltage (b) amplitudes are color-coded, and the exact location of each of the injection sites is tagged on the maps in real time (black dots).

205

Intracoronary injection of progenitor cells is potentially an attractive strategy, eliminating the need for special injection systems. Recently, 10 patients received autologous BM mononuclear cells in a coronary artery following primary angioplasty for acute myocardial infarction. Although the study was designed to investigate the role of these cells in myogenesis, improvements in myocardial perfusion were found, suggesting a contribution of these cells to neovascularization. Indices of myocardial performance also improved significantly at 3-month follow-up, while no change was observed in a control group of patients who underwent primary angioplasty alone.[39] A similar approach was examined in the Transplantation of Progenitor Cells and Regeneration Enhancement in Acute Myocardial Infarction (TOPCARE-AMI) study. In this study, the investigators assessed the safety and feasibility of intracoronary injection of BM-derived ($n = 10$) and peripheral blood-derived mononuclear cells ($n = 10$) 3–5 days after successful primary angioplasty. The primary analysis was performed at 4 months and included assessment of coronary flow reserve, myocardial viability and LV function indices. When patients with restenosis were excluded, flow reserve in the infarct related vessels improved substantially, with complete normalization relative to values measured in the reference vessels. Interestingly, the magnitude of the improvement was similar in the BM-derived and peripheral blood-derived mononuclear cell groups.[53]

Although encouraging, the preliminary data emerging from the early clinical experience should be cautiously interpreted. For example, the results can be extrapolated neither to the administration of larger volumes or higher injection density of ABMs, to injection of specific BM-derived cell populations, nor to BM injection into scar tissue for the purpose of myocardial repair. Similarly, the safety and feasibility should also be tested in higher-risk subpopulations, such as patients with severe LV dysfunction. Standardization of the number and quality of the injected cells may also be necessary to optimize this novel approach.

Conclusion

In conclusion, administration of freshly aspirated autologous BM cells is a potentially feasible and safe novel approach to enhance myocardial perfusion in patients not amenable to conventional revascularization. The current studies do not prove efficacy but they do warrant larger controlled blinded studies, and should stimulate further multidisciplinary investigational efforts to optimize this cell-based approach.

References

1. Risau W. Mechanisms of angiogenesis. Nature 1997; 86: 671–4.

2. Carmeliet P. Mechanisms of angiogenesis and arteriogenesis. Nat Med 2000; 6(4): 389–95.

3. Schaper W, Ito WD. Molecular mechanisms of coronary collateral vessel growth. Circ Res 1996; 79: 911–19.

4. Rivard A, Fabre JE, Silver M et al. Age-dependent impairment of angiogenesis. Circulation 1999; 99: 111–20.

5. Murayama T, Kalka C, Silver M et al. Aging impairs therapeutic contribution of human endothelial progenitor cells to post-natal neovascularization. Circulation 2001; 104: II-68 (abstract).

6. Panek R, Jung U, Lin Z et al. Age related impairment in microvascular outgrowth is associated with loss of VEGF, angiopoetin 1 and 2 expression. Circulation 2001; 104: II-68 (abstract).

7. Morishita R, Sakaki M, Yamamoto K et al. Impairment of collateral formation in lipoprotein(a) transgenic mice. Circulation 2002; 105: 1491–6.

8. Couffinhal T, Silver M, Kearney M et al. Impaired collateral development associated with reduced expression of vascular endothelial growth factor in ape E–/–mice. Circulation 1999; 99: 3188–98.

9. Grines CL, Watkins MW, Helmer G et al. Angiogenic Gene Therapy (AGENT) trial in patients with stable angina pectoris. Circulation 2002; 105: 1291–7.

10. Simons M, Annex BH, Laham RJ et al. Pharmacological treatment of coronary artery disease with recombinant fibroblast growth factor-2: double-blind, randomized, controlled clinical trial. Circulation 2002; 105: 788–93.

11. Losordo DW, Vale PR, Hendel RC et al. Phase 1/2 placebo-controlled, double-blind, dose-escalating trial of myocardial vascular endothelial growth factor 2 gene transfer by catheter delivery in patients with chronic myocardial ischemia. Circulation 2002; 105: 2012–18.

12. Udelson JE, Dilsizian V, Laham RJ et al. Therapeutic angiogenesis with recombinant fibroblast growth factor-2 improves stress and rest myocardial perfusion abnormalities in patients with severe symptomatic chronic coronary artery disease. Circulation 2000; 102: 1605–10.

13. Pecher P, Schumacher B. Angiogenesis in ischemic human myocardium: clinical results after 3 years. Ann Thorac Surg 2000; 61: 1414–19.

14. Losordo DW, Vale PR, Symes JF et al. Gene therapy for myocardial angiogenesis: initial clinical results with direct myocardial injection of phVEGF165 as sole therapy for myocardial ischemia. Circulation 1998; 98: 2800–4.

207

15. Unger EF, Goncalves L, Epstein SE et al. Effects of a single intracoronary injection of basic fibroblast growth factor in stable angina pectoris. Am J Cardiol 2000; 85: 1414–19.

16. Henry TD, Rocha-Singh K, Isner JM et al. Intracoronary administration of recombinant human vascular endothelial growth factor to patients with coronary artery disease. Am Heart J 2001, 142(5): 872 80.

17. Losordo DW, Vale PR, Hendel RC et al. Phase 1/2 placebo-controlled, double-blind, dose-escalating trial of myocardial vascular endothelial growth factor 2 gene transfer by catheter delivery in patients with chronic myocardial ischemia. Circulation 2002; 105: 2012.

18. Solovey A, Lin Y, Browne P et al. Circulating activated endothelial cells in sickle cell anemia. N Engl J Med. 1997; 337: 1584–90.

19. Asahara T, Murohara T, Sullivan A et al. Isolation of putative progenitor endothelial cells for angiogenesis. Science. 1997; 275: 964–7.

20. Kalka C, Masuda H, Takahashi T et al. Transplantation of ex vivo expanded endothelial progenitor cells for therapeutic neovascularization. Proc Natl Acad Sci USA 2000; 97: 3422–7.

21. Takahashi T, Kalka C, Masuda H et al. Ischemia- and cytokine-induced mobilization of bone marrow-derived endothelial progenitor cells for neovascularization. Nat Med 1999; 5: 434–8.

22. Jackon KA, Majka SM, Wang H et al. Regeneration of ischemic cardiac muscle and vascular endothelium by adult stem cells. J Clin Invest 2001; 107: 1395–402.

23. Jiang Y, Jahagirdar BN, Reinhardt RL et al. Pluripotency of mesenchymal stem cells derived from adult marrow. Nature 2002; 418: 41–9.

24. Stohlawetz P, Kolussi T, Kudlacej S et al. The effect of age on the transendothelial migration of human T lymphocytes. Scand J Immunol 1996; 44: 530–4.

25. Melter M, Reinders ME, Sho M et al. Ligation of CD40 induces the expression of vascular endothelial growth factor by endothelial cells and monocytes and promoted angiogenesis in vivo. Blood 2000; 96: 3801–8.

26. Arras M, Ito WD, Scholz D et al. Monocyte activation in angiogenesis and collateral growth in the rabbit hindlimb. J Clin Invest 1998; 101: 40–50.

27. Terada N, Hamazaki T, Oka M et al. Bone marrow cells adopt the phenotype of other cells by spontaneous cell fusion. Nature 2002; 416: 542–5.

28. Ying QL, Nichols J, Evans EP et al. Changing potency by spontaneous fusion. Nature 2002; 416: 545–8.

29. Blotnick S, Peoples G, Freeman M et al. T lymphocytes synthesize and export heparin binding epidermal growth factor-like growth factor and basic fibroblast growth factor, mitogens for vascular cells and fibroblasts. Proc Natl Acad Sci USA 1994; 91: 2890–4.

30. Kamihata H, Matsubara H, Nishiue T et al. Implantation of bone marrow mononuclear cells into ischemic myocardium enhances collateral perfusion and regional function via side supply of angioblasts, angiogenic ligands, and cytokines. Circulation 2001; 104: 1046–52.

31. Mohle R, Green D, Moore MA et al. Constitutive production and thrombin induced release of vascular endothelial growth factor by human megakaryocytes and platelets. Proc Natl Acad Sci USA 1997; 94: 663–8.

32. Weimar IS, Miranda N, Muller EJ et al. Hepatocyte growth factor is produced by human bone marrow stromal cells and promotes proliferation, adhesion and survival of human hematopoietic progenitor cells. Exp Hematol 1998; 26: 885–94.

33. Cheng SL, Zhang S, Mohan S et al. Regulation of insulin growth factors I and II and their binding proteins in human bone marrow stromal cells by dexamethasone. J Cell Biochem 1998; 17: 449–58.

34. Baffour R, Zhou YF, Fuchs S et al. Bone-marrow induced stimulation of endothelial and smooth muscle cell proliferation, migration, tube formation and production of growth factors. JACC 2001; 37: 232A.

35. Yoon SY, Tefferi A, Li C. Bone marrow stromal cell distribution of basic fibroblast growth factor in chronic myeloid disorders. Haematologica 2001; 86: 52–7.

36. Bikfalvi A, Han ZC. Angiogenic factors are hematopoietic factors and vice versa. Leukemia 1994; 8: 523–9.

37. Gao J, Dennis J, Muzic R et al. The dynamic in vivo distribution of bone marrow-derived mesenchymal stem cells after infusion. Cell Tissues Organs 2001; 169: 12–20.

38. Wiang JS, Shum-Tim D, Chedrawy E et al. The coronary delivery of marrow stromal cells for myocardial regeneration: pathophysiological and therapeutic implications. J Thorac Cardiovasc Surg 2001; 122: 699–705.

39. Strauer B, Brehmn M, Zeus T et al. Repair of infarcted myocardium by autologous intracoronary mononuclear bone marrow cell transplantation in humans. Circulation 2002; 106: 1913–18.

40. Kornowski R, Leon MB, Fuchs S et al. Electromagnetic guidance for catheter-based transendocardial injection: a platform for intramyocardial angiogenesis therapy. Results in normal and ischemic porcine models. J Am Coll Cardiol 2000; 35: 1031–9.

41. Tomita S, Ren-Ke Li, Weisel R et al. Autologous transplantation of bone marrow cells improves damaged heart function. Circulation 1999; 100: II-247–56.

42. Kobayashi T, Hamano K, Li T et al. Enhancement of angiogenesis by the implantation of self bone marrow cells in a rat ischemic heart model. J Surg Res 2000; 89: 189–95.

43. Ikenaga I, Hamano K, Nishida M et al. Autologous bone marrow implantation induced angiogenesis and improved deteriorated exercise capacity in a rat ischemic hindlimb model. J Surg Res 2001; 96: 277–83

44. Li TS, Hamano K, Suzuki K et al. Improved angiogenic potency by implantation of ex-vivo hypoxia pre-stimulated bone marrow cells in rats. Am J Physiol 2002; 283: H468–73.

45. Kocher AA, Schuster MD, Szabolcs MJ et al. Neovascularization of ischemic myocardium by human bone marrow derived angioblasts prevents cardiomyocyte apoptosis, reduces remodeling, and improves cardiac function. Nat Med 2001; 7: 430–6.

46. Orlic D, Kajstura J, Chimenti S et al. Bone marrow cells regenerate infarcted myocardium. Nature 2001; 410: 701–5.

47. Fuchs S, Baffour R, Zhou YF et al. Transendocardial delivery of autologous bone marrow enhances collateral perfusion and regional function in pigs with chronic experimental myocardial ischemia. J Am Coll Cardiol 2001; 37: 1726–32.

48. Hamano K, Li TS, Kobayashi T et al. Therapeutic angiogenesis induced by local autologous bone marrow cell implantation. Ann Thorac Surg 2002; 73: 1210–15.

49. Hamano K, Nishida M, Hirata K et al. Local implantation of autologous bone marrow cells for therapeutic angiogenesis in patients with ischemic heart disease: clinical trial and preliminary results. Jpn Circ J 2001; 65: 845–7.

50. Stamm C, Westphal B, Kleine HD et al. Autologous bone-marrow stem-cell transplantation for myocardial regeneration. Lancet 2003; 361: 45–6.

51. Fuchs S, Satler LF, Kornowski R et al. Catheter-based autologous bone marrow myocardial injection in no-option patients with advanced coronary artery disease – a feasibility study. J Am Coll Cardiol 2003; 41: 1721–4.

52. Tse HF, Kwong YL,Chan JKF et al. Angiogenesis in ischemic myocardium by intramyocardial autologous bone marrow mononuclear cell implantation. Lancet 2003; 361: 47–9.

53. Assmus B, Schachinger V, Teupe C et al. Transplantation of progenitor cells and regeneration enhancement in acute myocardial infarction (TOPCARE-AMI). Circulation 2002; 106: 3009–17.

15. LONG-TERM CLINICAL RESULTS OF CELLULAR CARDIOMYOPLASTY BY AUTOLOGOUS SKELETAL MYOBLASTS

Philippe Menasché

On 15 June 2000, we performed the first human autologous skeletal myoblast transplantation in a patient with severe post-infarction left ventricular dysfunction.[1] Nine additional patients were subsequently included in this phase I feasibility and safety trial, which ended in November 2001.[2] 'Medium term' is thus probably a more appropriate wording than long term for describing the effects of the procedure. Nevertheless, the data from this early experience as well as those subsequently reported by other groups allow us to draw some conclusions about the feasibility and safety of the procedure and, to a lesser extent, about its functional efficacy.

Database

In addition to our series of 10 patients, another group of 10 patients was reported by Siminiak et al at the 2002 annual meetings of the European Society of Cardiology and of the American Heart Association.[3] While these two series were physician-driven, an industry-sponsored trial has been initiated (and is still underway) in the USA, and the first 16 patients of this trial were reported during the last scientific sessions of the American Heart Association.[4] So far, the profiles of all the included patients have been fairly consistent; they consist of individuals with severe left ventricular dysfunction (the ejection fraction was usually below 30–35%), a history of infarct with a non-viable residual scar and an indication for surgical revascularization in remote ischemic areas. In all these cases, autologous skeletal myoblasts were grown from a peripheral muscular biopsy and subsequently reimplanted after a mean 2–4-week expansion period in multiple sites across the scarred area (including its borders) during a conventional coronary artery bypass operation (Figure 15.1), except for five patients of the US trial, who underwent placement of a left ventricular assist device at the time of cell transplantation with the objective of assessing the fate of the engrafted cells at the time of subsequent heart removal for transplantation. Other surgical cell implantations have been performed in different centers around the world, but the lack of

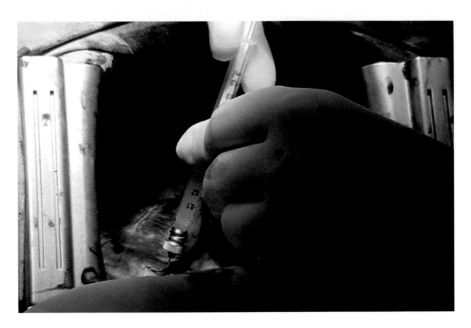

Figure 15.1 *Intraoperative injection of cells*

scientific reports precludes the use of these data in a comprehensive review. Finally, catheter-based cell transplantations through an endoventricular or transvenous approach have been performed in Europe as part of both physician-driven and industry-sponsored trials, and, based on the most recent report (before the study was temporarily halted because of serious adverse events), totalled 13 patients (P. Serruys, personal communication). Taken together, these figures show that the world experience is still limited (at least at the time of this writing), which mandates great caution in the interpretation of the data, in particular if one considers that there was a wide interinstitutional variability in the patient profile (some patients in Siminiak's series had dyskinesia rather than akinesia), the method used for assessing regional function data, cell-processing techniques, the final number of injected cells (from 10^6 in the lowest-dose group of the US dose-escalating safety trial to a maximum of 1 billion in our series) and the percentage of myogenic cells in the injectate.

On the assumption that this overall experience has unequivocally established the feasibility of the procedure and the efficacy of shipping logistics pertaining to the transportation of the biopsy from the transplant center to the cell therapy laboratory and that of the final cell yield in the opposite direction, this review will rather concentrate on the safety and efficacy issues.

Safety

Overall, the operation, by itself, has been shown to be safe, without specific procedural complications; in particular, bleeding through the multiple needle holes has not been reported and nor was there any documentation of postoperative systemic organ dysfunction that might have been attributed to cell embolization. Catheter-based myoblast transfer seems to have been equally uneventful. Indeed, the only adverse event that could possibly be ascribed to cell transplantation is ventricular arrhythmia. Thus, non-fatal episodes of sustained ventricular tachycardia occurred in four of our patients,[2] all during the first three postoperative weeks, and required implantation of an automatic internal cardioverter defibrillator (AICD). This early post-procedural timing has important implications for patient monitoring, as close follow-up is mandatory during the initial weeks following transplantation. In contrast, the rate of late recurrences seems to be extremely low, as demonstrated by the observation that only one of these four implanted patients (followed up from 8 to 14 months) has experienced two appropriate shocks, while the Holter tracings of the remaining non-implanted patients have failed to detect new arrhythmic events. Two episodes of early postoperative ventricular tachycardia were also reported by the Polish group,[3] and two sudden deaths most likely attributable to arrhythmias have led to the stopping of the catheter-based trial. Thus, although data derived from phase I studies, which, by definition, lack a control group, do not allow us to conclusively establish a causal relationship between cell transplantation and arrhythmias, in particular in a patient population prone to this complication by virtue of the underlying disease, it currently appears sound to consider this relationship as likely until it has eventually been ruled out by randomized trials involving comparison with a placebo group receiving intramyocardial injections of suspension medium alone (as planned in our ongoing phase II trial).

The mechanisms of these potentially cell grafting-related arrhythmias are still elusive. One possibility is that they may be caused by the inflammatory response triggered by needle punctures and cell injections. Although such a hypothesis would fit the early post-transplantation time-frame of these arrhythmias, we rather favor an alternative hypothesis based on the differences in membrane properties between engrafted myotubes and host cardiomyocytes. To further test this hypothesis, we designed an experimental protocol entailing transfection of rat myoblasts with the gene encoding green fluorescent protein followed by transplantation of these cells into post-infarction myocardial scars. One month later, hearts were removed, and

213

while the left ventricular explant was kept beating in an organ chamber, fluorescence microscopy was used to track the grafted fluorescent cells and guide their puncture by microelectrodes, allowing us to record membrane properties. The major result is that the action potential of these intramyocardially engrafted myotubes featured a quite typical skeletal muscle pattern and was thus significantly shorter than that of a cardiomyocyte.[5] In addition, these engrafted myotubes demonstrated depolarizing rebounds from which bursts of action potentials were fired. Thus, although grafted cells do not seem to be coupled with host cardiomyocytes, a finding consistent with the previous observation that connexin 43 and N-cadherin are downregulated following myoblast engraftment,[6] it is conceivable that firing of these repetitive action potentials may initiate a re-entry circuit leading to ventricular tachycardia, particularly if the excitable myotube is in close physical contact with a native cardiac cell (which is not unlikely, given the patchy pattern of human infarcts). This hypothesis could account for the efficacy, in our experience, of amiodarone in blunting these arrhythmias, since one of the mechanisms of action of this drug is to reduce repolarization dispersion,[7] and thus to 'homogenize' intracardiac conduction of electrical impulses.

Thus, regardless of the mechanism(s), our data suggest that the incidence and/or severity of these arrhythmias can be reduced by appropriate prophylaxis with amiodarone started at the time of the biopsy and continued thereafter for 2–3 months (although it is possible that this period could be shortened). Others are strong believers that these patients should be systematically implanted with an internal cardioverter defibrillator. We currently disagree with this risk management policy but recognize that this debate may be somewhat academic, since, independently of the cell transplant, many of these high-risk heart failure patients meet the implantation criteria of the MADIT II trial[8] and, as such, are likely to receive a defibrillator at some point during the postoperative course.

It should finally be mentioned that, so far, oncogenicity has not been a concern. This is not unexpected, since, as long as primary cultures are used, cells remain strictly committed to a skeletal muscular phenotype. Indeed, no tumor development was seen in any of the immunodeficient mice which were injected with the myoblasts of our phase I patients.

Efficacy

By virtue of their design (small sample size, lack of control groups, concomitant revascularization), no definite conclusions can yet be drawn from the phase I trials which have been undertaken. In our study, approximately

60% of the initially akinetic (as assessed by low-dose dobutamine echocardiography) and metabolically non-viable (as demonstrated by fluorodeoxyglucose positron emission tomography) cell-grafted scarred areas featured new postoperative systolic thickening, and this result was sustained over time (there was no deterioration of the benefit during the 1–2.5-year follow-up). These data are encouraging if one considers that at most 10% of myocardial segments meeting these inclusion criteria (lack of contractile reserve and of metabolic viability) are expected to improve following bypass surgery alone.[2] The results of Siminiak et al[3] are also good but they focus on the assessment of global left ventricular function, which could obviously be influenced by the associated revascularization. Overoptimistic results have been reported in the US dose-escalating adjunct-to-bypass trial, which is somewhat surprising, given the relatively small number of injected cells, which peaked at 300 million. Finally, improved function of the grafted areas has been reported by the investigators of the percutaneous trial. Put together, these data are encouraging but definitely need to be validated by randomized phase II trials designed and powered so as to demonstrate efficacy, if any. It is in this context that we have implemented a multicenter dose-ranging study planned to include 300 patients with severe post-infarction left ventricular dysfunction (ejection fraction $\leq 35\%$), a residual akinetic scar not amenable to revascularization and an indication for bypass in remote ischemic areas. The primary endpoint is the change in the contractility of cell-grafted non-revascularized myocardial segments, as assessed after 6 months by echocardiography in a core laboratory by blinded observers, and the comparison of data gathered in the placebo group (injections of culture medium alone) and the two transplanted cohorts (which differ by the number of injected cells) should allow more meaningful conclusions about the efficacy of the procedure.

The mechanism of this putative efficacy still remains elusive. While early post-infarct cell injections could limit scar expansion, those implemented at a later stage, i.e. when the remodeling process is completed, are unlikely to reverse it,[9] and, in fact, postoperative end-diastolic dimensions of our phase I patients, whose infarcts were on average 6 years old, have not changed compared with preoperative values. The alternative mechanism of the improvement consistently observed in experimental studies involving both small[10–12] and large[13] animal models of myocardial infarction is an increase in contractility. This, in turn, could occur through two distinct pathways. The first pathway entails a *direct* effect of the engrafted myotubes which, by virtue of their intrinsic contractile properties, would contribute to improvement of the kinetics of the area they are implanted in and, subsequently, overall pump function. In support of this hypothesis are the pathologic observations

215

made in explanted hearts of assist device-supported patients[14] as well as in the heart of one of our patients who died late (17.5 months after transplantation) of an unrelated cause (stroke). These observations demonstrate in-scar engraftment of myotubes with preservation of the contractile apparatus (which is expected to disappear in non-functional muscle cells) and an increased proportion of fibers expressing a slow-type myosin,[15] which could account for resistance of these cells to fatigue and their subsequent ability to withstand a cardiac workload and thus to provide sustained functional benefits, as actually supported by our follow-up data. However, a direct contribution of engrafted myotubes to increased inotropism requires that they directly couple with host cardiomyocytes. As indicated previously, our electrophysiologic studies[5] have not been able to demonstrate such a coupling, in that stimulation of cardiomyocytes only elicits passive displacement of the neighboring myotubes (scar tissue most likely providing the physical link between the two cell populations). This finding does not preclude the possibilities that some coupling may occasionally occur, particularly in border zones, due to electrotonic phenomena distinct from connexin-mediated gap junctions, and thus account for the above-mentioned arrhythmic events. Furthermore, our electrophysiologic studies have also shown that engrafted myotubes retained their excitable properties in that a strong depolarizing current could elicit firing of action potentials by engrafted myotubes (as recorded directly by intracellular microelectrodes) followed by active contractions. This observation suggests that at least some transplanted cells remain alive, which has led us to consider a second possible pathway of improved function. This pathway is *indirect*, in that it could entail paracrine mechanisms whereby secretion of pleiotrophic factors by engrafted myotubes would benefit the damaged heart. These factors could, for example, promote angiogenesis (although we have failed to document increased neovascularization in transplanted hearts compared with controls) or, more likely, recruit the purported population of cardiac resident stem cells[16] and thus trigger endogenous regeneration leading to an increased number of contractile elements. Whereas this hypothesis is still unproven, it is noteworthy that recent data from our laboratory have documented that human myoblasts and myotubes produced substantial amounts of insulin growth factor-1, a factor implicated in muscle cell regeneration[17] and whose cardioprotective effects have been demonstrated by several experimental studies.[18] Two lines of experimental evidence provide additional support for the paracrine paradigm. First, in the rat model, the functional benefits of myoblast transplantation remain sustained over time, despite a decreasing number of detectable cells.[19] A similar temporal dissociation was recently reported with gene transfection of hepatocyte growth factor (HGF) in a canine model of pacing-induced heart failure,[20] as perfusion and function were found to be improved 4 weeks after treatment, while neither HGF nor its messenger ribonucleic acid were still detectable in left ventricular myocardium. By analogy, one can thus speculate that if myotubes trigger some form of endogenous repair, the process, once initiated, proceeds on its own even if the factor-delivering platforms are no longer present. Second, in the sheep model, myoblast transplantation was associated with a significant reduction of fibrosis,[13] which could reflect a paracrine effect of myoblasts on the extracellular matrix.[21] While each of the previously mentioned hypotheses (limitation of remodeling, direct increase in contractility, paracrine mobilization of new cardiac cells) requires further testing, it is also important to note that none of them is mutually exclusive.

Regardless of the mechanism(s) whereby myoblast transplantation exerts beneficial effects of post-infarction function, it is critically important to emphasize that these effects are likely to be dramatically hindered by the early rate of cell death occurring shortly after cell injections. In fact, up to 90% of transplanted cardiomyocytes have been shown to die within the first 24 h,[22] and we have made quantitatively similar observations with myoblasts. The mechanisms of this high attrition rate are multiple and include, in particular, physical strain during injections, ischemia due to the poor vascularity of the target scar and apoptosis. Thus, the development of cell survival-enhancing strategies appears to be critical for optimizing the functional benefits of the procedure. Two of these strategies deserve special attention. The first is targeted at enhancing angiogenesis to limit the ischemic component of cell death. The rationale of this approach is supported by the observation that cell survival is significantly improved when injections are made in a richly vascularized granulation tissue, as compared with an acute cryoinjury-induced scar.[22] In practice, increased angiogenesis can be achieved by genetically engineering cells so as to make them overexpress vascular growth factors[23] or, perhaps more realistically in a clinical perspective, by co-injecting these factors directly.[24] Furthermore, although it appears important that *current* clinical trials do not involve concomitant revascularization of cell-grafted areas to avoid confounding factors in the interpretation of efficacy data, it sounds equally reasonable to consider that in the *future*, once efficacy is demonstrated and transplantation really enters clinical practice, the benefits of cell implantation could be enhanced by simultaneous surgical or catheter-based restoration of flow in the grafted areas. The second strategy aimed at increasing the survival rate of transplanted cells relies on limitation of apoptosis. In practice, the simplest approach might consist of heat-shocking cells during the late stages of the expansion process, a process which has been shown to markedly increase survival of both cardiomyocytes[22] and skeletal myoblasts[25] following implantation into infarcted myocardium. Furthermore, it is also possible that cell survival could be improved by the initial selection of a behaviorally more resistant subpopulation of myoblasts.[26] This hypothesis is conceptually attractive but its clinical applicability requires additional investigations. Finally, it is also likely that cells can be killed by the inflammatory response triggered by needle punctures. This mechanism is expected to be still more significant if it is superimposed on a pre-existing inflammatory state resulting from a fresh infarct. As previously mentioned, late injections may equally be less than optimal because of their inability to reverse a fully completed remodeling process. These observations suggest that there is probably an optimal time window for cell transplantation following myocardial infarction and that bracketing this time-frame is another means of optimizing the benefits of the procedure.

Clinical myoblast transplantation in perspective

It will still take several years before we can reach meaningful conclusions regarding the ability of myoblast transplantation to improve ischemic left ventricular dysfunction and the extent to which this purported improvement affects clinical outcome in a relevant manner. In the meantime, one can reasonably expect parallel advances in the management of heart failure, whether they rely on new drugs, multisite stimulation, surgical constraint and shape-change devices or even genetic manipulations. It is thus realistic to view cell therapy, if its efficacy is definitely proven, as one option within a multifaceted armamentarium; it will therefore be complementary, not competitive, with other validated therapeutic approaches.

In the restricted field of cell therapy, it is also important to better define the place of myoblasts by comparison with autologous bone marrow-derived stem cells (we currently consider the use of embryonic cells much more problematic from a clinical standpoint and more relevant to basic research than to patient care). As the use of bone marrow cells is addressed in another chapter of this book, this paragraph will be limited to three general comments. (1) Whether bone marrow-derived stem cells can *fully* convert into *true* cardiomyocytes (i.e. expressing at least the cardiospecific markers most critical for function) is still a matter of debate. Assuming, however, that such conversion really does occur, there is good agreement that it involves only a small number of cells, which raises the question of the functional relevance of this transdifferentiation. (2) The optimal type of bone marrow cells to be grafted remains unsettled. Whole unfractionated bone marrow is clinically appealing (hence its use in early trials) because immediate transplantation of the bone marrow aspirate looks simple and straightforward in that it avoids the problems associated with expansion procedures. However, analysis of the literature data and of our laboratory findings suggests that *in-scar* injection of whole bone marrow is functionally ineffective.[27] Only injections in the *border zone*[28] have been reported to provide some local benefits, which fail, however, to translate into an improvement in global heart function. The other setting in which this approach has been efficacious entailed early post-infarct transplantation.[29] This raises the problem of the optimal timing of cell delivery, which is discussed below. Another option is to use selected populations of well-defined progenitors (in humans, the CD34[+] or CD133[+] cells, which can be phenotypically characterized by specific antibodies). This approach has two major theoretical advantages: the immaturity of these cells, which should make them particularly sensitive to local signals, and their ability to give rise to endothelial cells, probably deriving from putative hemangioblasts. In practice, however, the percentage of these progenitors is very low, and they most likely require scale-up if functional benefits are to be expected. This, in turn, could be achieved by in vitro expansion, which is technically challenging, or in vivo cytokine-induced mobilization, which can raise tolerance concerns in patients with severe left ventricular dysfunction or acute myocardial infarcts. In parallel with observations made with whole unpurified bone marrow, positive experimental results with progenitors have so far been reported when injections were made in border zones[30] or in the early post-infarct period.[31] Conversely, clinical transplantation of CD133[+] cells into post-infarct scars is less than convincing and has only demonstrated the safety of this procedure.[32] Finally, the greatest promise is possibly held by mesenchymal (or stromal) cells, which are easier to expand in culture. However, apart from preimplantation processing with agents like 5-azacytidine, which would raise clinically relevant safety concerns, their cardiomyogenic differentiation seems to require direct cell-to-cell contact with cardiomyocytes, which probably accounts for the improvement in function recently reported in pig models of myocardial infarction when injections were targeted at the border zones[33] or when cells had been co-cultured with fetal cardiomyocytes.[34] Whether these results could be optimized by the more specific use of the multipotent adult mesenchymal cells (MAPCs) isolated by the group of Verfaillie[35] remains to be demonstrated, but it should be kept in mind that, so far, the results of this group have been difficult to reproduce and that, although MAPCs have been shown to give rise to cells of mesodermal, ectodermal and endodermal lineages, their cardiomyogenic

219

differentiation is yet to be more conclusively established.[3] The optimal timing of bone marrow cell delivery also remains to be defined. It makes sense that if grafted early after the infarct, bone marrow stem cells may find appropriate cues for transdifferentiation; conversely, it is likely that, at the later stage of the fibrous scar, these signals are lost and, at worst, could convey transdifferentiation of grafted cells into fibroblasts. Thus, in this setting, efficacy of bone marrow stem cells can only be expected if their implantation is targeted to the border zones which may still harbor living cells that could potentially emit the appropriate differentiation cues. These considerations highlight the number of still unknown factors in this area, which makes surprising the speed with which some groups have embarked on clinical trials. It is equally important to stress that assessment of bone marrow cells transplanted at the late stage of fibrous scars should be made comparatively not only with 'controls' receiving injection medium but also with myoblasts, which now represent a legitimate benchmark.

Regardless of the type of cells to be transplanted, improvements in delivery techniques appear mandatory both for reducing injury to the graft at the time of implantation and for making the procedure less invasive than the current surgical transepicardial approach. The latter entails multiple punctures across the scar with a 27-gauge pre-bent needle so as to make injections parallel to the epicardium and avoid the inadvertent delivery of cells into the left ventricular cavity. Although the procedure is by itself technically simple, the patchy pattern of human infarcts and their frequent thinness require it to be performed with meticulous care. It is thus important to ensure that catheter-based cell transfer techniques are at least equivalent to the 'open vision' approach in terms of accuracy of cell shooting, material retention, cell viability and cell functionality (i.e. their ability to differentiate into myotubes). So far, these percutaneous techniques, whether endoventricular or transvenous, have been shown to be technically feasible, but data conclusively establishing their functional efficacy are still scarce. The same caveat applies to the intracoronary route, which sounds logical in the setting of early post-infarct cell injections concomitant with revascularization, and has actually been already used for delivering bone marrow stem cells in this context,[36] but the validation of this strategy still awaits the experimental demonstration that these cells can effectively cross the endothelium to gain access to the myocardial tissue.

In conclusion, the early results of autologous myoblast transplantation have established the technical feasibility of the procedure as well as its safety, with the caveat of an arrhythmogenic potential which now requires to be further characterized but can be controlled by drugs and/or devices. The initial efficacy data look encouraging, but the small number of patients and the

220

multiplicity of confounding factors should lead to a very careful interpretation of these functional data, which need to be validated by large prospective randomized trials complying with the stringent methodological rules commonly applied to drug trials. Only such an approach will allow us to draw meaningful conclusions and conclusively establish whether myoblast transplantation can really 'rejuvenate' areas of scar tissue and to what extent this regeneration process affects patient function and clinical outcome.

References

1. Menasché P, Hagège AA, Scorsin M et al. Myoblast transplantation for heart failure. Lancet 2001; 357: 279–80.

2. Menasché Ph, Hagège AA, Vilquin JT et al. Autologous skeletal myoblast transplantation for severe postinfarction left ventricular dysfunction. J Am Coll Cardiol 2003; 41: 1078–83.

3. Siminiak T, Kalawski R, Fiszer D et al. Transplantation of autologous skeletal myoblasts in the treatment of patients with postinfarction heart failure. Early results of phase I clinical trial. Circulation 2002; 106(suppl II): II-626 (abstract).

4. Dib N, McCarthy P, Dinsmore J et al. Safety and feasibility of autologous myoblast transplantation in patients with ischemic cardiomyopathy: interim analysis from the United States experience. Circulation 2002; 106(suppl II): II-463 (abstract).

5. Léobon B, Garcin I, Menasche P, et al. Myoblasts transplanted into rat infarcted myocardium are functionally isolated from their host. Natl Acad Sci USA 2003; 100: 7808–11.

6. Reinecke H, MacDonald GH, Hauschka SD, Murry CE. Electromechanical coupling between skeletal and cardiac muscle: implications for infarct repair. J Cell Biol 2000; 149: 731–40.

7. Drouin E, Lande G, Charpentier F. Amiodarone reduces transmural heterogeneity of repolarization in the human heart. J Am Coll Cardiol 1998; 32: 1063–7.

8. Moss AJ, Zareba W, Hall J et al. Prophylactic implantation of a defibrillator in patients with myocardial infarction and reduced ejection fraction. New Engl J Med 2002; 346: 877–83.

9. Li RK, Mickle DAG, Weisel RD et al. Optimal time for cardiomyocyte transplantation to maximize myocardial function after left ventricular injury. Ann Thorac Surg 2001; 72: 1957–63.

10. Taylor DA, Atkins BZ, Hungspreugs P et al. Regenerating functional myocardium: improved performance after skeletal myoblast transplantation. Nat Med 1998; 4: 929–33.

11. Jain M, DerSimonian H, Brenner DA et al. Cell therapy attenuates deleterious ventricular remodeling and improves cardiac performance after myocardial infarction. Circulation 2001; 103: 1920–7.

12. Pouzet B, Ghostine S, Vilquin JT et al. Is skeletal myoblast transplantation clinically relevant in the era of angiotensin-converting enzyme inhibitors? Circulation 2001; 104(suppl I): I-223–8.

13. Ghostine S, Carrion C, Guarita Sousa LC et al. Long-term efficacy of myoblast transplantation on regional structure and function after myocardial infarction. Circulation 2002; 106(suppl I): I-131–6.

14. Pagani F, DerSimonian R, Zawadska A et al. Autologous skeletal myoblasts transplanted in ischemia damaged myocardium in humans: histological analysis of cell survival and differentiation. Circulation 2002; 106(suppl II): II–463 (abstract).

15. Hagege AA, Carrion C, Menasché Ph et al. Autologous skeletal myoblast grafting in ischemic cardiomyopathy. Clinical validation of long-term cell viability and differentiation. Lancet 2003; 361: 491–2.

16. Anversa P, Nadal-Ginard B. Myocyte renewal and ventricular remodelling. Nature 2002; 415: 240–3.

17. Wang PH. Roads to survival. Insulin-like growth factor-1 signaling pathways in cardiac muscle. Circ Res 2001; 88: 552–4.

18. Welch S, Plank D, Witt S et al. Cardiac-specific IGF-1 expression attenuates dilated cardiomyopathy in tropomodulin-expressing transgenic mice. Circ Res 2002; 90: 641–8.

19. Al Attar N, Carrion C, Ghostine S et al. Long-term (1 year) functional and histological results of autologous skeletal muscle cells transplantation in rat. Cardiovasc Res 2003; 58: 142–8.

20. Ahmet I, Sawa Y, Iwata K, Matsuda H. Gene transfection of hepatocyte growth factor attenuates cardiac remodeling in the canine heart: a novel gene therapy for cardiomyopathy. J Thorac Cardiovasc Surg 2002; 124: 957–73.

21. Zhao LR, Duan WM, Reyes M et al. Human bone marrow stem cells exhibit neural phenotypes and ameliorate neurological deficits after grafting into the ischemic brain of rats. Exp Neurol 2002; 174: 11–20.

22. Zhang M, Methot D, Poppa V et al. Cardiomyocyte grafting for cardiac repair: graft cell death and anti-death strategies. J Mol Cell Cardiol 2001; 33: 907–21.

23. Suzuki K, Murtuza B, Smolenski RT et al. Cell transplantation for the treatment of acute myocardial infarction using vascular endothelial growth factor-expressing skeletal myoblasts. Circulation 2001; 104(suppl I): I-207–12.

24. Sakakibara Y, Nishimura K, Tambara K et al. Prevascularization with gelatin microspheres containing basic fibroblast growth factor enhances the benefits of cardiomyocyte transplantation. J Thorac Cardiovasc Surg 2002; 124: 50–6.

25. Suzuki K, Smolenski RT, Jayakumar J et al. Heat shock treatment enhances graft cell survival in skeletal myoblast transplantation to the heart. Circulation 2000; 102(suppl III): III-216–21.

26. Beauchamp JR, Morgan JE, Pagel CN, Partridge TA. Dynamics of myoblast transplantation reveal a discrete minority of precursors with stem cell-like properties as the myogenic source. J Cell Biol 1999; 144: 1113–21.

27. Bel A, Messas E, Agbulut O et al. Transplantation of autologous fresh bone marrow into infarcted myocardium: a word of caution. Circulation 2002; 106(suppl II): II-463 (abstract).

28. Hamano K, Li TS, Kobayashi T et al. Therapeutic angiogenesis induced by local autologous bone marrow cell implantation. Ann Thorac Surg 2002; 73: 1210–15.

29. Kamihata H, Matsubara H, Nishiue T et al. Implantation of bone marrow mononuclear cells into ischemic myocardium enhances collateral perfusion and regional function via side supply of angioblasts, angiogenic ligands, and cytokines. Circulation 2001; 104: 1046–52.

30. Barlucchi L, Chimenti S, Jakoniuk I et al. The injection of c-kit-derived cardiac lineages in vitro repairs infarcted scarred myocardium in vivo. Circulation 2002; 106(suppl II): II-131 (abstract).

31. Kocher AA, Schuster MD, Szabolcs MJ et al. Neovascularization of ischemic myocardium by human bone-marrow-derived angioblasts prevents cardiomyocyte apoptosis, reduces remodeling and improves cardiac function. Nat Med 2001; 4: 430–6.

32. Stamm C, Westphal B, Kleine HD et al. Bone marrow stem cell transplantation for myocardial regeneration in post-infarction CABG patients. Circulation 2002; 106(suppl II): II-375 (abstract).

33. Makkar RR, Price M, Lill M et al. Multilineage differentiation of transplanted allogenic mesenchymal stem cells injected in a porcine model of recent myocardial infarction improves left ventricular function. Circulation 2002; 106(suppl II): II-34 (abstract).

34. Min JY, Sullivan MF, Yang Y et al. Delayed co-transplantation of human mesenchymal stem cells and fetal cardiomyocytes in infarcted porcine hearts. Circulation 2002; 106(suppl II): II-419 (abstract).

35.   Jiang Y, Jahagirdar BN, Reinhardt RE et al. Pluripotency of mesenchymal stem cells derived from adult marrow. Nature 2002; 418: 41–9.

36.   Strauer BE, Brehm M, Zeus T et al. Repair of infarcted myocardium by autologous intracoronary mononuclear bone marrow cell transplantation in humans. Circulation 2002; 106: 1913–18.

16. Challenges of Myogenesis and Repair of the Heart

Patrick W Serruys, Pieter C Smits, Wim van der Giessen, Howard B Haimes, John M Harvey and James L Green

A damaged myocardium cannot effectively regenerate and repair itself subsequent to either acute or chronic pathologic insult. The emerging field of cell transplantation has attempted to address some of the issues and has progressed from preclinical studies to proof-of-concept clinical studies conducted in humans. Different cell types are being researched, including autologous skeletal muscle-derived myoblasts, bone marrow-derived mesenchymal stem cells and autologous bone marrow-derived stem cells. Other ongoing efforts are seeking to promote homing of bone marrow-derived cells to convert to cardiomyocytes in the myocardium, enhancement of the ability of cardiomyocytes to replicate and efforts to derive pluripotent stem cells from human blastocysts. While a variety of other cell types such as embryonic cardiomyocytes and embryonic stem cells have been investigated through preclinical studies, they have not progressed to clinical applications, for logistic and ethical reasons. The goal of any such therapy is to restore both an angiogenic and a muscular component to the myocardium by replacing damaged, fibrous scar tissue with compliant, elastic muscle tissue that would convert an akinetic or dyskinetic scar into tissue that augments systolic and diastolic function. The unique ability of skeletal muscle-derived stem cells (myoblasts) to form myotubes within the infarcted zones of the heart has led to the promotion of early pilot studies in humans.[1-5] A secondary benefit would be that the compliance of the scar would be modified such that the pathologic remodeling process would be altered and would progress towards the baseline normal state.[6-8] The challenge of replacing a large amount of dysfunctional and necrotic tissue is immense, and the ability to deliver, retain and engraft cells into a mechanically disadvantaged and neurohormonally altered environment has yet to be adequately addressed.

Autologous skeletal muscle-derived myoblasts are stem cells that are capable of being expanded in culture. These cells appear to be advantageous, in that they are resistant to ischemia, form skeletal muscle and provide angiogenic and mitogenic stimuli that are beneficial to cell engraftment. An additional factor that may limit the use of autologous myoblasts is their lack of ability to couple with host cardiomyocytes, since their differentiated form

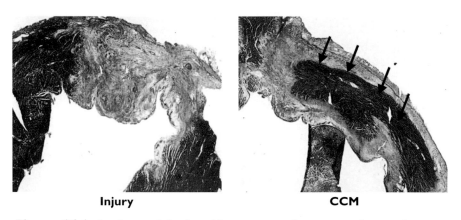

Injury **CCM**

Figure 16.1 *Autologous skeletal myoblasts can engraft into injured myocardium. The pink stained area on the figure labeled CCM depicts the presence of engrafted myoblasts circumscribed within the fibrous scar resulting from cryoablation of the left ventricle of a rabbit. (Reprinted from Taylor et al,[6] with permission).*

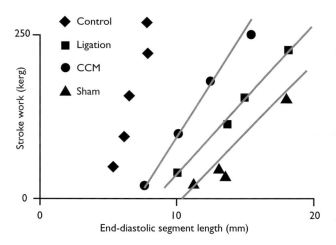

Figure 16.2 *Skeletal myoblast CCM effect on systolic performance. The injection of autologous skeletal muscle derived myoblast results in an increase in stroke work of the infarcted LV. Controls continue to degrade systolic function over time.(Reprinted from Taylor et al,[6] with permission).*

downregulates both N-cadherin and Connexin 43 necessary for electromechanical coupling.[9] Several preclinical studies have determined that autologous myoblasts appear to provide some benefit to the hemodynamic status of the heart. The induction of myocardial insult through ischemia–reperfusion, coronary artery ligation, microembolization of the coronary vasculature and cryoablation in a variety of animal species points towards the ability of autologous myoblasts to restore systolic function[1,6–8] (Figures 16.1 and 16.2). The goal of such therapy is to translate these hemodynamic changes into enhanced quality of life for the patients.[10–12]

Autologous myoblast implantation for repair of damaged cardiac muscle begins with a skeletal muscle biopsy. Approximately 2–10 g of muscle are

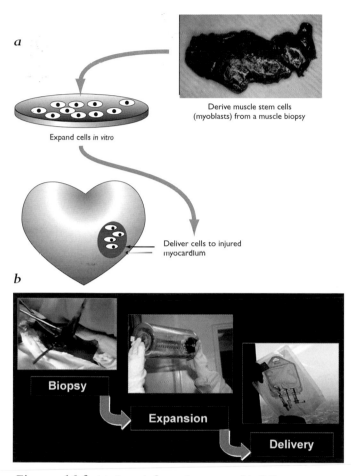

Figure 16.3 (a) Straightforward concept. (b) Cell expansion process.

obtained from the vastus lateralis in an outpatient procedure using local anesthetics (Figure 16.3). Once acquired, the biopsy is transported to a cell culture facility for further processing. Early clinical studies included manipulation of the biopsy (mincing) at the clinical site and rapid transport to a local culture facility. As clinical studies increase in their scope and the therapy comes closer to commercialization, manipulation at the clinical site will need to be minimized, and the times required to transport to centralized culture facilities will increase significantly. Bioheart, Inc. has developed systems and procedures that allow for shipment of biopsy material to distant locations within 48 h while retaining the integrity of the biopsy (Figure 16.4).

The process of culturing cells for therapeutic use requires strict adherence

227

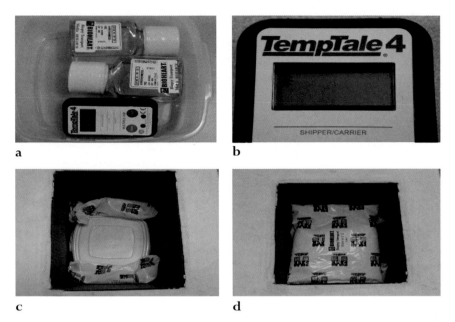

Figure 16.4 (a) Biopsy packaged with temperature control. (b) Sun symbol indicates monitor is activated. (c,d) Biopsy packaged for shipment in a thermo-controlled container.

to high quality standards. Cell culture facilities should operate in accordance with cGMPs (current Good Manufacturing Practices). Once a biopsy arrives at the culture facility, it is entered into that facility's quality assurance and documentation system. Batch record documentation should capture all of the biopsy and cell culture processing activities. Operations should be done within controlled areas by trained and gowned personnel. Typically, these areas are composed of Class 100 bio-safety cabinets for open processing contained within Class 10 000 suites. Equipment should be calibrated and maintained, and programs and processes should be validated. Cells for therapeutic use cannot be sterilized after culture completion. Therefore, rigorous adherence to aseptic processing guidelines is required. Processing suites and bio-safety cabinets must be cleaned and monitored for possible contaminants. Personnel must be appropriately gowned and trained to prevent introduction of a contaminant into the culture. Multiple quality control (QC) tests for sterility and purity of the culture must be performed for the duration of the processing.

Myoblast cell culture is initiated by processing the skeletal muscle biopsy. Excess tissue is trimmed away and the biopsy is washed several times to remove excess blood (Figure 16.5). The biopsy is then minced into small

228

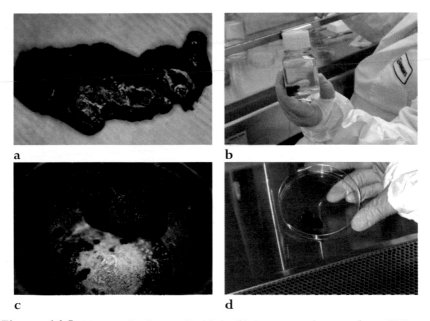

Figure 16.5 *(a) Muscular biopsy (5–10 g). (b) Biopsy sample received in cGMP cell culture facility. (c) Minced muscle. (d) Enzymatic dissociation.*

pieces (<1 mm) and treated with a digestive enzyme. Typically, collagenase is utilized, although blends of collagenase, trypsin and other enzymes are not uncommon. The enzymes break down the minced tissue further into a nearly single-cell suspension. This slurry is then washed several times to remove the enzymes and eventually placed into culture.

Myoblasts and other muscle-derived cells stick to the surface of the culture vessel, creating what is referred to as an adherent culture. The cells liberated from the initial processing will proliferate and proceed to coat the culture surface. Myoblast cultures need to be monitored closely, as they will differentiate into myotubes as the confluence of the culture increases. Typically, myoblast cultures are harvested enzymatically as they reach higher confluences. The harvested cells are washed, quantified and returned to culture, using either more vessels or larger vessels to reduce confluence. Typically, a biopsy of skeletal muscle results in a mixed population of myoblasts and fibroblasts (Figure 16.6). The derivation of sufficient numbers of myoblasts from such biopsies may be challenging, since their numbers in skeletal muscle appear to decrease with age.

QC testing of myoblasts and other cells for therapeutic use needs to establish that the cells are suitable for implantation. Freedom from

229

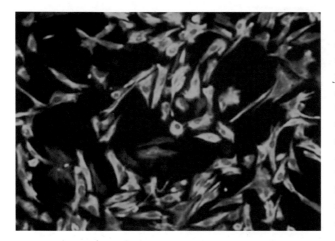

Figure 16.6 *A culture of 94% myoblasts; the other cells are presumably fibroblasts. Myoblast cultures are characterized using an antibody against desmin, a muscle specific marker (green). All nuclei are stained with a nucleus marker (red). Skeletal myoblast characterization by Desmond stain.*

adventitious contaminants is established by performing USP/EP sterility tests, assaying endotoxin levels and testing for the presence of mycoplasma. Cell viability and the identity of the desired cell type need to be established. Typically, this is accomplished with immunohistochemistry techniques. Unique antibodies can be used to identify specific cell types. For myoblasts, the markers most commonly used are CD56 (NCAM) and desmin. CD56 is a cell surface marker but it should be noted that CD 56 is not specific to myoblasts and can be found on a variety of cell types including T cells and renal tubular epithelium. Desmin is a cytoskeletal protein expressed by myoblasts. Finally, the potency (activity) of the cells needs to be established. The potency of myoblast cultures can be established by performing a bioassay where the cells are placed in conditions where they are guided to differentiate and form myotubes. The major challenge to the QC paradigm is the short shelf-life of therapeutic cells. The shelf-life for these types of therapies is typically between 72 h and 96 h. Parametric QC protocols need to be established, as testing of the final cell product cannot be completed prior to the expiration of the shelf-life.

Perhaps the final consideration with regard to the cell culture process for myoblast implantation is the delivery of the cells to the clinical site. Early studies (as previously stated) have been conducted with the culture facility in close proximity to the clinical site, which minimizes delivery issues. As studies expand and therapies progress towards commercialization, delivery issues increase in significance. Product shelf-life must be determined and maximized to allow for transport flexibility. Packaging and shipping systems must be developed that allow for extended transport of cells. Quality systems need to be able to monitor shipments and ensure that the product is suitable for use upon arrival. An important consideration is the extent to which the

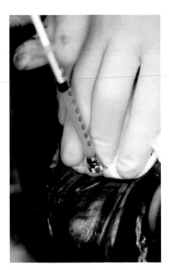

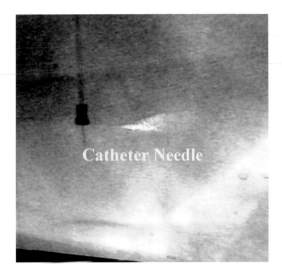

Figure 16.7 *Surgical injections of cells. Cells are injected into the scarred region of the LV by direct injection tangential to the surface.*

Figure 16.8 *Cell transplantation via endocardial delivery. Cells are injected via a percutaneous catheter to the endocardial surface of dysfunctional left ventricle.*

clinical site must manipulate the product upon arrival prior to administration. The more extensive the manipulation at the clinical sites, the greater the quality challenges become.

The delivery of cells epicardially, endocardially or intramyocardially through transvenous access and by intracoronary infusion have all met with some modest success (Figures 16.7 and 16.8). Several percutaneous catheters, including the Myocath (Bioheart), Myostar (Cordis-Webster), Stiletto (Boston Scientific) and Transvenous Access Catheter (Transvascular), as well as the ability to inject cells under direct observation with a tangentially directed hypodermic needle using direct pericardial access, are under formal evaluation. The retention of large numbers of cells is challenging, since several studies have indicated that the percutaneous endovascular route retains only approximately 15% of delivered cells. Similar estimates have been given for epicardial injections. Additional concerns include the concern that many of the implanted cells are unable to engraft into the ischemic cardiac environment. Estimates that less than 1% of delivered cells are actually able to survive and adapt to the cardiac environment. Biodistribution using radiolabeled cells has indicated that the majority of injected cells are distributed through the venous vasculature to sites of the reticuloendothelial system, notably in the heart, lung, liver and spleen (Figure 16.9).

231

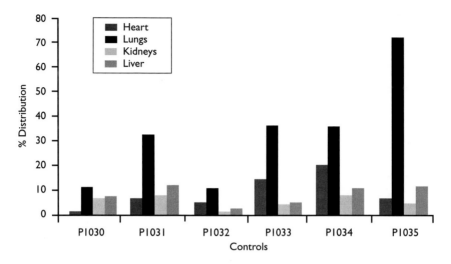

Figure 16.9 *Biodistribution of injected myoblasts. Technitium-99 labelled cells were injected into the infarcted zones of the LV and their ultimate deposition shortly after injection was studied and quantified by scintography.*

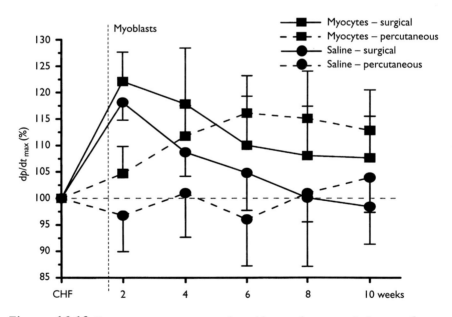

Figure 16.10 *Percutaneous versus surgical myoblast implantation. Induction of a chronic stable state of heart failure was accomplished by repetitive microembolization of the coronary vasculature. Autologous canine myoblasts were injected into the dysfunctional myocardium via direct epicardial access or percutaneous routes. Animals were assessed for LV hemodynamic parameters. (Courtesy of Dr Daniel Burkhoff, Columbia University, New York.)*

Conventional wisdom suggests that implantation of skeletal muscle-derived myoblasts is able to modify the remodeling process of the heart, resulting in more favorable mechanical attributes of the left ventricle.

Cellular cardiomyoplasty using autologous derived skeletal muscle-derived myoblasts has resulted in advantageous changes in left ventricular (LV) function as assessed by changes in dp/dt, sonomicrometry and echocardiography[1,6–8] (Figure 16.10). Although the long-term fate of such implanted cells is unclear, pioneering studies have suggested that myotube formation does occur along with a change in skeletal muscle phenotype from the fast-twitch to the slow-twitch form of heavy chain myosin, indicating that the cells can adapt to the cardiac workload[2] (Figure 16.11). The evidence for active contraction and coupling of myoblasts with native cardiomyocytes is lacking, but early safety studies have pointed towards modest improvements in hemodynamic parameters. It is clear that myoblasts, once injected into the myocardium, form myotubes and lose the ability to form gap junctions and intercalated disks by the downregulation of connexin 43 and N-cadherin proteins[9] (Figure 16.12). Preclinical studies have been conducted in mouse,

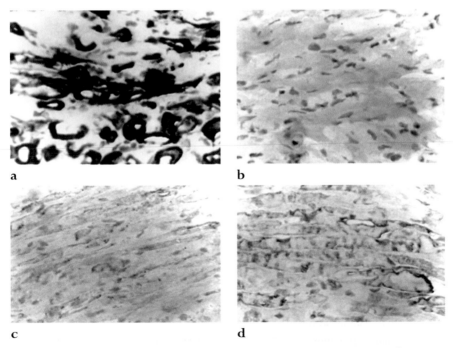

a   b

c   d

Figure 16.11 Phenotype conversion in skeletal muscle grafts. (a) 1 week, fast skeletal MHC. (b) 1 week, slow β-MHC. (c) 7 weeks, fast skeletal MHC. (d) 7 weeks, slow β-MHC. (Courtesy of Dr Charles Murry, University of Washington, Seattle.)

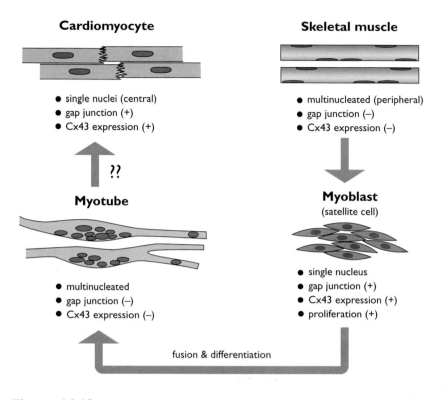

Figure 16.12 *Cardiomyocytes versus skeletal muscle.*

rat, rabbit, dog, pig and sheep, and have in general indicated that therapy is safe, well tolerated and results in advantageous functional changes.[10,11]

Over 10 years of preclinical data in both small and large animal models have demonstrated that skeletal myoblasts implanted into damaged myocardium can engraft, exhibit cell proliferation and myotube formation and ultimately augment ventricular function.[1,10,11] Based on these data, a single-center (Erasmus Medical Center) pilot clinical study evaluating safety and feasibility in five patients was initiated. For reasons stated previously, autologous skeletal myoblasts (ASMs) were chosen for endocardial injection into non-viable scar tissue via a percutaneous needle injection catheter. Only patients with symptomatic NYHA functional Class II under optimal medical therapy were selected. All patients had a previous anterior wall myocardial infarction (MI) 4 weeks old at the time of implantation and depressed LV function (left ventricular ejection fraction (LVEF)) of 20–45% by radionuclide ventriculography. The presence of myocardial scar was defined by akinesia or

234

dyskinesia at rest during echocardiography, LV angiography, magnetic resonance imaging (MRI), no contractile reserve during dobutamine stress echocardiography (DSE) and hyper-enhancement by gadolinium on MRI scan (Figure 16.13). Patients with target region wall thickness <5 mm by echocardiography or MRI, history of syncope or sustained ventricular tachycardia or fibrillation or an ICD implanted were excluded from trial enrollment. Written informed patient consent and a negative serology panel were required prior to skeletal muscle biopsy. Patients enrolled were on average 59 years old (49–78 years), were in NYHA Class III heart failure and had an average age of infarct of 6 years (2–11 years). All five patient biopsies were uneventful, with an average of 8.4 g of tissue being excised and shipped in a temperature-controlled container to a cGMP cell culture facility (Cambrex Corporation, Walkersville, MD, USA) for isolation and expansion using a proprietary process (Bioheart, Inc., Weston, FL, USA). With an approximate culture time of 17 days, an average of 269×10^6 cells was taken at harvest. An average of 55% of the cells stained positive for the immunohistochemical marker desmin, confirming their commitment to myogenic differentiation. Harvested cells were formulated into a ready-to-use injectate medium and were returned to the cardiac catheterization laboratory in a temperature-controlled container for implantation. Cell viability remained high, at 97%, throughout transportation. The transplantation procedure was

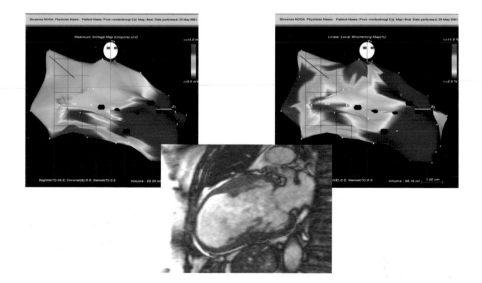

Figure 16.13 MRI and NOGA map at baseline. (Courtesy of the Interventional Cardiology Department, Thoraxcenter.)

235

performed in the cardiac catheterization laboratory. Access was obtained via the femoral artery. After a coronary biplane LV angiogram (LAO 60° and RAO 30°) was made, an outline of the LV chamber was drawn on transparent tabloids that were taped to the fluoroscopy monitors. An electromechanical NOGA map of the left ventricle was then obtained by use of a 7F NOGASTAR catheter connected to the NOGA console (Biosense-Webster, Waterloo, Belgium). Areas exhibiting low voltages and linear shortening on the NOGA map were considered as target areas if they were geographically concordant with scar areas assessed by pre-procedural DSE, MRI and LV angiogram (Figure 16.13). Using an 8F Myostar (Biosense-Webster, Waterloo, Belgium) injection catheter, an average of 200×10^6 cells was delivered into the endocardial wall (Figure 16.14). The number of injections made was based on the size of the infarct, with an average spacing of 1 cm between injection sites. In a follow-on multicenter clinical trial, injections were guided solely by biplane fluoroscopy with the 8F Myocath (Bioheart, Inc., Weston, FL, USA) injection catheter system (Figure 16.15). Additionally, clinical work is ongoing using an injection system to deliver intramyocardial injections via the transvenous approach to improve cell retention post-injection. Each patient's arrythmogenic profile was assessed at baseline and follow-up at 3 and 6 months with 24h ECG monitoring. Ventricular remodeling (wall motion and wall thickening changes) was assessed at baseline and at 3 and 6 months via DSE with pulse-wave Doppler

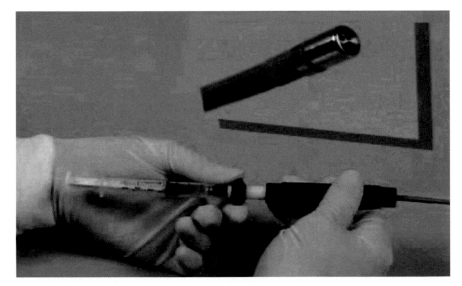

Figure 16.14 Biosense-Webster Myostar injection catheter.

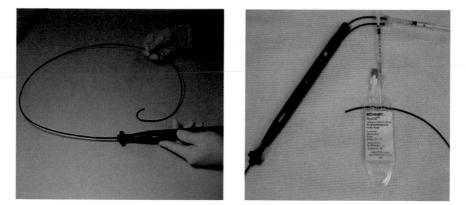

Figure 16.15 *Myocath™ injection catheter system by Bioheart, Inc.*

tissue sampling (TDI) and MRI (Figure 16.16). Furthermore, at baseline and at 3 and 6 months of follow-up, LV volume and ejection fractions were assessed with LV angiography and radionuclide scintigraphy. The results from this phase I, single-center, pilot study are in the process of publication and as such will not be reviewed in this chapter.

In terms of patient safety, all procedures have been completed without any acute complications. Echocardiography is performed post-transplantation to ensure there is no pericardial effusion caused through injection perforation. All patients are monitored in hospital immediately following procedures and generally are released within 48 h based on normal ECG monitoring or adverse events. One area of concern, which has been reported in the literature, is the presence of arrhythmias and non-sustained tachycardia post-transplantation. It is well known that congestive heart failure patients are prone to having rhythm abnormalities, and recent studies (MADIT II) have shown the benefits of ICD implantation in patients with LV function depressed between 20% and 30% in reducing sudden cardiac death due to arrhythmia.[13] In response to this question, we have adjusted patient inclusion criteria to require patients to either be ICD patients or have an ICD implanted a minimum of 30 days prior to cell transplantation. Continuous Holter monitoring with review of saved event information from the ICD both before and after cell transplantation has been increased to improve our understanding of the arrythmogenic profile of patients treated before cell transplantation and the window of vulnerability for arrhythmias post-transplantation. Our conclusions are that cell transplantation via a percutaneous injection catheter is feasible, the procedure is safe, and improvements in LV function and reduction NYHA class are encouraging, warranting additional safety and efficacy clinical trials.

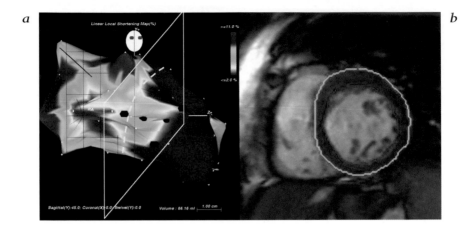

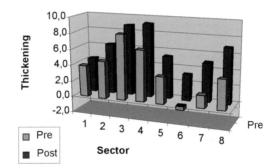

Figure 16.16 MRI – *Quantitative LV function (a,b) First patient: treatment effect. (c) Wall thickness changes by MRI.*

Issues still to be addressed through preclinical as well as clinical studies are: how to improve the method of delivery for accurate placement and enhance cell retention to improve our ability to replace large masses of dysfunctional tissue; reduction of adverse events related to therapy, such as the potential for arrhythmogenesis; and exploring what zones of the infarcted tissue should be targeted and what is the ideal patient population that would benefit from cell transplantation, resulting in enhanced quality of life.

References

1. Taylor DA. Cellular cardiomyoplasty with autologous skeletal myoblasts for ischemic heart disease and heart failure. Curr Controlled Trials Cardiovasc Med 2001; 2: 208–10.

2. Murry CE, Wiseman RW, Schwartz SM, Hauschka SD. Skeletal myoblast transplantation for repair of myocardial necrosis. J Clin Invest 1996; 98: 2512–23.

3. Chiu RC-J, Zibaitis A, Kao RL. Cellular cardiomyoplasty: myocardial regeneration with satellite cell implantation. Ann Thorac Surg 1995; 60: 12–18.

4. Pagani FD, DerSimonian H, Zawadzka A et al. Autologous skeletal myoblasts transplanted to ischemia-damaged myocardium in humans: histological analysis of cell survival and differentiation. J Am Coll Cardiol 2003; 41: 879–88.

5. Hagège AA, Carrion C, Menasché P et al. Viability and differentiation of autologous skeletal myoblast grafts in ischaemic cardiomyopathy. Lancet 2003; 361: 491–2.

6. Taylor DA, Atkins BZ, Hungspreugs P et al. Regenerating functional myocardium: improved performance after skeletal myoblast transplantation. Nat Med 1998; 4: 929–33.

7. Atkins BZ, Hueman MT, Meuchel JM et al. Myogenic cell transplantation improves in vivo regional performance in infarcted rabbit myocardium. J Heart Lung Transplant 1999; 18: 1173–80.

8. Chachques J, Rajnoch C, Berrebi A et al. Cellular therapy reverses myocardial dysfunction. In: Proceedings of the American Association for Thoracic Surgery. 80th Annual Meeting, 2000.

9. Reinecke H et al. Electromechanical coupling between skeletal and cardiac muscle: implications for infarct repair. J Cell Biol 2000; 149: 731–40.

10. Penn MS, Francis GS, Ellis SG et al. Autologous cell transplantation for the treatment of damaged myocardium. Prog Cardiovasc Dis 2002; 45: 21–32.

11. Oakley RME, Ooi OC, Bongso A, Yacoub MH. Myocyte transplantation for myocardial repair: a few good cells can mend a broken heart. Ann Thorac Surg 2001; 71: 1724–33.

12. Murry CE, Wiseman RW, Schwartz SM, Hauschka SD. Skeletal myoblast transplantation for repair of myocardial necrosis. J Clin Invest 1996; 98: 2512–23.

239

13. Moss AJ, Zareba W, Hall WJ et al. Prophylactic implantation of a defibrillator in patients with myocardial infarction and reduced ejection fraction. N Engl J Med 2002; 346: 877–83.

17. Myoblast Genome Therapy and the Regenerative Heart

Peter K Law, Eugene KW Sim, Husnian Kh Haider, Gwendolyn Fang, Florence Chua, Tea Kakuchaya, Vadim S Repin and Leo A Bockeria

Introduction

Heart muscle degeneration is the leading cause of debilitation and death in humans. It is the common pathway underlying congenital and infectious cardiomyopathies, myocardial infarction, congestive heart failure, angina, coronary artery disease and peripheral vascular disease, all of which constitute the cardiovascular diseases. Global healthcare spending on the latter topped $280 billion in 2001. In the USA alone, approximately $186 billion is spent every year in treating some 60 million cardiovascular disease patients. About 50% of the patients suffering congestive heart failure will die within 5 years of diagnosis.

Bioengineering the regenerative heart may provide a novel treatment for cardiovascular diseases. Through endomyocardial injections of cultured skeletal myoblasts, the latter spontaneously transfer their nuclei into cardiomyocytes to impart myogenic regeneration. Donor myoblasts also fuse among themselves to form new myofibers, depositing contractile filaments to improve heart contractility. These myofibers contain satellite cells with regenerative vigor to combat heart muscle degeneration.

Three myogenesis mechanisms were elucidated as proof of concept with 17 human/porcine xenografts using cyclosporine as immunosuppressant. Some myoblasts transdifferentiated to become cardiomyocytes. Others transferred their nuclei into host cardiomyocytes through natural cell fusion. Yet others formed skeletal myofibers with satellite cells. De novo production of contractile filaments augmented heart contractility. Human myoblasts transduced with the $VEGF_{165}$ gene produced six times more capillaries in porcine myocardium than placebo. Xenograft rejection was not observed for up to 30 weeks despite cyclosporine discontinuation at 6 weeks.

First in man (FIM) studies using cGMP-produced pure myoblasts of autogenic and allogenic origins are documented. The advantages and disadvantages of autografts vs. allografts are compared to guide the future development of heart cell therapy.

241

Heart muscle degeneration

Heart muscle degeneration cascades with cardiomyocyte membrane leakage, uncontrolled Ca^{2+} influx, mitochondrial ATP shutdown, inability to exude Ca^{2+} through the cell surface and to reabsorb Ca^{2+} into the sarcoplasmic reticulum, myofibrillar hypercontracture and disarrangement. Apoptosis ensues. Fibroblasts proliferate and infiltrate. The heart muscle, which was once populated by live cardiomyocytes with proteinaceous contractile filaments such as myosin, actin, troponin and tropomyosin, is now partially occupied by fibrous scars that are incapable of electrical conduction, mechanical contraction and revascularization. These scars continue to exert negative effects on the heart and the circulation despite the remodeling that occurs after a myocardial infarction.

Natural heart muscle repair

Ultimately, heart muscle degeneration results in loss of live cardiomyocytes, contractile filaments, contractility, heart function and healthy circulation. The damaged heart responds by cell division of cardiomyocytes. However, such regenerative capacity is hardly significant. Cardiomyocytes in culture will undergo no more than three to five divisions, yielding an insufficient number of cells to repopulate any myocardial infarct.

Cardiomyocytes do not multiply significantly, because the human telomeric DNA repeats[1] in these terminally differentiated cells are minimal. Telomerasing cardiomyocytes in vivo remains a technical challenge. Without significant mitotic activity, surviving cardiomyocytes cannot provide enough new cells to deposit the contractile filaments necessary to maintain normal heart function.

The degenerative heart also transmits biochemical signals to recruit stem cells from the stroma and the bone marrow in an attempt to repair the muscle damage. Being pluripotent, embryonic or adult stem cells exhibit uncontrolled differentiation into various lineages to produce bone, cartilage, fat, connective tissue, skeletal and heart muscles (Figure 17.1). Because fibroblast growth factor level is elevated in the degenerative heart, many of the recruited stem cells differentiate to become fibroblasts instead of cardiomyocytes, thus depositing fibrous scars and not contractile filaments.

Despite the claimed success of transmyocardial revascularization using lasers, angiogenic factors and genes, the damaged myocardium really needs additional live myogenic cells to deposit contractile filaments to regain heart function, preferably before fibroblast infiltration, which leads to scar formation.

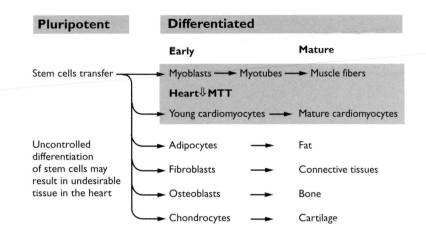

Figure 17.1 *Advantages of using myoblasts over stem cells in treating heart failure. MTT, myoblast transfer therapy.*

Myoblasts regenerate muscles

Myoblasts are differentiated cells destined to become muscles. Unlike cardiomyocytes, myoblasts have long telomeric DNA subunits and are capable of extensive mitosis. Myoblasts obtained from young adults can undergo 50 divisions without any loss of myogenicity or development of tumorigenicity. Myoblasts survive and proliferate in intercellular fluid. Their survival does not depend on vascularization or nerve innervation.

During ontogeny, human myoblasts migrate and fuse spontaneously, beginning at day 53 of gestation, sharing their nuclei in a common gene pool, and forming multinucleated myotubes within the somites. The abilities to undergo mitosis, to migrate and to fuse are conserved in mononucleated satellite cells, which are essentially myoblast reserves in adult muscles.

Satellite cells are found between the basement membrane and the plasma membrane of every skeletal muscle fiber. Approximately 11% of all skeletal myonuclei belong to satellite cells in young rats, declining to about 6% in the aged. In human beings over the age of 26 years, there are fewer satellite cells, with shorter telomeres. Their muscle biopsies thus yield less satellite cells, which also exhibit less proliferative vigor in cell culture.

Upon single myofiber injury, the satellite cells are activated to divide and migrate from beneath the basement membrane. They divide extensively, forming hundreds of myoblasts that fuse spontaneously at the site of injury to repair the host myofiber. They also fuse among themselves to form new myofibers to substitute for lost function. The signals to stop myoblast division and to initiate myotube formation appear to be cell confluence and low serum level.

Newly formed myotubes have to be vascularized and innervated within 10 days, or they will perish. When successfully innervated and vascularized, they deposit actin, myosin, troponin and tropomyosin, which eventually organize into sarcomeres, the structural units of muscle contraction. This maturation process takes approximately 3 months.

Myoblasts strengthen dystrophic muscles

Progressive skeletal muscle degeneration is the hallmark of the 12 forms of human hereditary muscular dystrophy. An enabling technology called myoblast transfer therapy (MTT) has been developed in the past 27 years to treat these degenerative genetic diseases, with success.[2] MTT is a platform technology of cell transplantation, nuclear transfer and tissue engineering.[3] It is the only human genome therapy in existence.[4]

MTT involves taking a 2-g muscle biopsy from the quadriceps of a young normal male aged between 13 and 26 years, culturing some 10 000 released satellite cells to become 50 billion pure myoblasts in 45 days and injecting the myoblasts into 82 large muscle groups of the dystrophic patient under general anesthesia.

The patient takes oral cyclosporine as immunosuppressant for 2 months to suppress rejection of the allografts. Since myoblast fusion is completed within 3 weeks after MTT, and since myotubes and mature myofibers do not express MHC-1 surface antigens, it is not necessary to administer life-long immunosuppression, as in heart transplants.

As a cell therapy, MTT provides normal myoblasts that fuse with each other, forming new myofibers to *replenish* myofiber loss. As a genome therapy, MTT provides normal myoblasts that spontaneously insert their nuclei (carrying the software[5] and the hardware[6] of the complete genome) into the dystrophic myofiber to effect genetic complementation *repair*. Whereas the dystrophic myofiber degenerates because of the deletion of an essential gene product, the donor myonuclei within the syncytial heterokaryon are now activated to regenerate and produce the therapeutic mRNAs. The dystrophin gene which is deleted in Duchenne muscular dystrophy (DMD) is stably integrated, regulated and expressed at least 6 years after MTT.[7,8]

The results of over 240 MTT procedures (on muscular dystrophy) in the past 12 years have demonstrated an absolute safety record, with no death or coma or failure in heart, lung, kidney or liver function in 2 years of follow-up studies. Myoblast-injected DMD muscles showed dystrophin and improved histology as compared to placebo-injected muscles, which showed no dystrophin but fat and connective tissue.[2] Their average isometric force increase at 18 months after MTT was 123% ±18% (mean ±SD) compared to the natural controls.

The regenerative heart

The goal of bioengineering the regenerative heart seems to be within reach with MTT. Five grams of muscle biopsies would be taken from both quadriceps of a heart patient aged 40–90 years, and approximately one billion myoblasts would be cultured for 4 weeks and then injected or surgically implanted between the vascularized and the non-vascularized infarcted myocardium.

Heart cell therapy (HCT),[4] as this is called, is administered with the idea that the myoblasts will survive, develop and function as aliens in the heart, and their nuclei as aliens within cardiomyocytes and myofibers. The myocardial aliens are newly formed skeletal myofibers that contribute to cardiac output through production of contractile filaments. They are donor in origin and, as skeletal myofibers, will have satellite cells and regenerative capability. The cardiomyocyte aliens are donor myoblast nuclei carrying chromosomes with long telomeric DNA subunits that are essential for mitosis. Upon injury of the transdifferentiated or heterokaryotic cardiomyocyte, the myoblast regenerative genome will be activated to produce foreign contractile filaments such as myosin.

Proof of concept

The human myoblast transfer into the heart revealed that it was safe to administer one billion myoblasts at 100×10^6/ml through the Myostar catheter of the NOGA system (Biosense Webster, Inc.) using 20 injections at different locations inside the left ventricle of a pig.[9] It was determined that 0.3–0.5 ml would be the optimal volume per injection. ECG was normal throughout the study without arrhythymia.

Human myoblasts were manufactured according to our in-house SOPs and trade secrets with a license of the US Patent No. 5,130,141[10]. This method of culture yielded a purity of 99% by human desmin immunostaining (Figure 17.2).

In the myogenesis study, cultured myoblasts derived from satellite cells of human rectus femoris biopsies were transduced with retroviral vector carrying the LacZ reporter gene, and about 75% of the myonuclei were successfully transduced. Trypan blue stain revealed >95% cell viability immediately before injection.

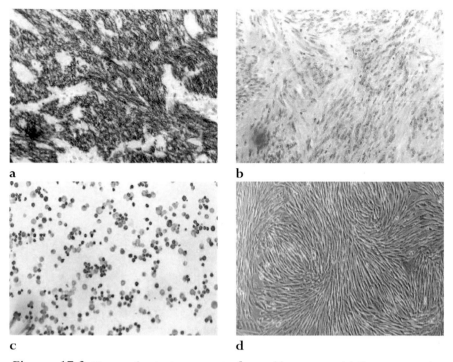

Figure 17.2 *Human desmin immunostain for myoblast purity. (a) Positive control of leiomyosarcoma, staining brown. (b) Negative control. (c) Pure human myoblasts immunostained with desmin. (d) Pure human myoblasts in culture.*

A porcine heart model of chronic ischemia (control = 3; myoblast implanted = 6) was produced by clamping an ameroid ring around the left circumflex artery. Four weeks later, the heart was exposed by left thoracotomy.

Twenty injections (0.25 ml each) containing 300 million myoblasts, or 5 ml total volume of basal Dulbecco's modified Eagle's medium (DMEM) as control, were given into the left ventricle intramyocardially. Left ventricular function was assessed using MIBI-^{99m}Tc SPECT scanning 1 week before injection to confirm myocardial infarction and at 6 weeks after injection.

Animals were maintained on cyclosporine at 5 mg/kg body weight from 5 days before until 6 weeks after cell transplantation. The animals were euthanized at 6 weeks to 7 months postoperatively, and the hearts were processed for histologic, immunocytochemical and ultrastructural studies.

Laser nuclear capture, together with single-nucleus RT-PCR, was performed to delineate host and donor nuclei. In situ hybridization using fluorescent DNA probes specific for human Y-chromosome and chromosomes 1 and 10 of the pig were used.

246

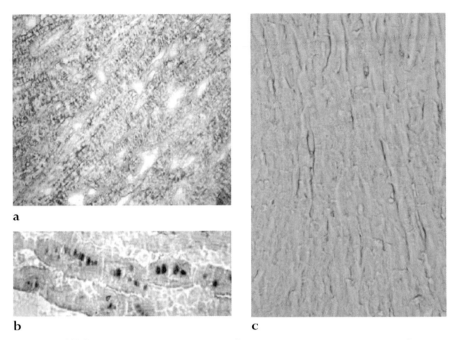

a

b   c

Figure 17.3 *(a) Brownish immunostain of human myosin in porcine myocardium 12 weeks after human myoblast injection. (b) Cardiomyocytes with LacZ-positive nuclei and human myosin stain, indicative of their being donor or myoblastic in origin. (c) Negative immunostain (gray) of human myosin in porcine myocardium sham-injected without myoblasts.*

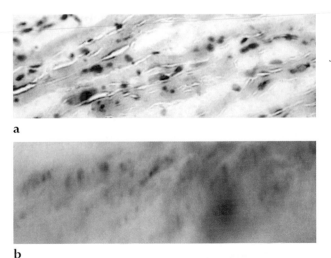

a

b

Figure 17.4 *(a) Heterokaryons derived from fusion of porcine cardiomyocytes and human myoblasts showing LacZ-positive human myoblast nuclei (bluish green) and porcine cardiomyocyte nuclei (purple) in the heterokaryotic syncytium. (b) These heterokaryons expressed human myosin heavy chain.*

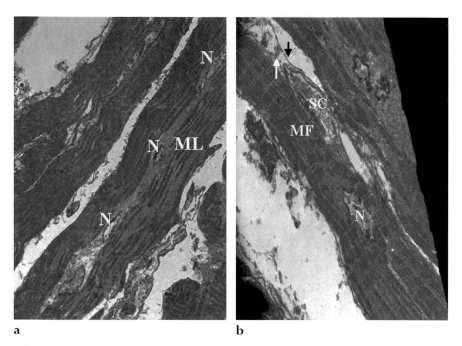

a   b

Figure 17.5 *Electron microscopy of the myoblast-injected porcine myocardium showing (a) myotubes with central nuclei and myfibril (ML) deposits, and (b) skeletal myofiber with satellite cell (SC) and nucleus (N). The satellite cell is located between the basement membrane (black arrow) and the plasma membrane (white arrow). Sarcomeres show proper alignment of newly formed contractile filaments.*

Histologic examination of myoblast-injected myocardium showed cardiomyocytes containing LacZ-positive nuclei (of donor origin) after 12 weeks (Figure 17.3b). More than 80% of the LacZ-positive cardiomyocytes immunostained positively for human myosin heavy chain (Figure 17.3a). The human genome was integrated (LacZ-labeled nuclei) and expressed (myosin immunostain) in the porcine myocardium. Donor myoblasts transdifferentiated to become cardiomyocytes containing four to five nuclei each. The control heart without myoblast injection did not show LacZ-positive myonuclei or human myosin (Figure 17.3c). Triple stain of myoblast-injected myocardia demonstrated multinucleated heterokaryons containing human and porcine nuclei with expression of human myosin (Figure 17.4). Electron microscopy demonstrated human myotubes and skeletal myofibers with satellite cells in the porcine myocardium (Figure 17.5).

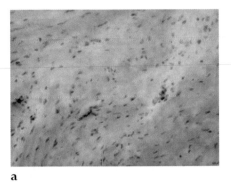

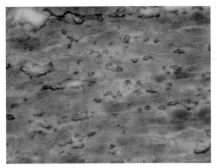

a

b

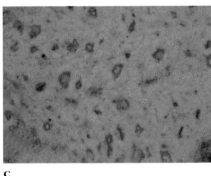

Figure 17.6 *(a) Control myocardium immunostained for von Willebrand factor (vWF) VIII and counterstained with eosin to show capillaries. (b) VEGF₁₆₅- transduced myoblasts produced increased vascular density. (c) As (b), but without eosin counterstain.*

c

Angiomyogenesis

In the angiomyogenesis study, the human myoblasts were transduced with retroviral and adenoviral vectors carrying the LacZ and human $VEGF_{165}$ genes, respectively. The cells were characterized for $VEGF_{165}$ transduction and expression efficiency by immunostaining, ELISA, immunoblotting and RT-PCR. A porcine heart model of infarction was created in eight female pigs by left circumflex artery ligation. The animals were placed into control $(n = 3)$ and myoblast-implanted $(n = 5)$ groups. Angiography was performed to ensure complete occlusion of the blood vessel. Infarction was confirmed with MIBI-^{99m}Tc SPECT scanning. Four weeks later, 5 ml basal DMEM without or with 3×10^8 human myoblasts carrying the $VEGF_{165}$ and LacZ genes was injected into the left ventricle intramyocardially. The animals were maintained on cyclosporine (5 mg/kg body weight) for 6 weeks postoperatively. Hearts were then explanted and processed for immunocytochemical studies.

249

Table 17.1 Autograft versus allograft for the regenerative heart

Autograft	Allograft
Advantages	
No immunosuppression	HCT within 12 h ↛ scar
	Good cells readily available
	Patients with infections and genetic disease can be treated
Disadvantages	
HCT in 1 month → scar	2-month immunosuppression
Cell limitations: age, contamination	
Infected/mutated tissues not usable	

The transduction efficiencies for the LacZ and $VEGF_{165}$ genes were 75–80% and >95%, respectively. The transduced myoblasts continued to secrete $VEGF_{165}$ for longer than 18 days, at a significantly higher level $(37 \pm 3\,ng/ml)$ than the non-transduced ones $(200 \pm 30\,pg/ml)$. Dye exclusion test revealed >95% cell viability at the time of injection. Histologic examination showed extensive survival of the grafted myoblasts expressing the LacZ gene in and around the infarct. The vascular density (mean $\pm$SEM) counted in an average of 12 low-power fields ($\times200$) in control animal hearts was 4.18 ± 0.42, as compared to 28.31 ± 1.84 in the $VEGF_{165}$ myoblast-transplanted group (Figure 17.6). The SPECT scans showed improved perfusion in the infarcted region.

Discontinuation of cyclosporine after 6 weeks prompted no xenograft rejection for up to 30 weeks. There are many advantages of developing allografts, as shown in Table 17.1.

Future perspective

Menasché et al reported feasibility and safety data for five patients using 650 million to 1.2 billion cells during coronary artery bypass surgery.[12,13] The myoblast purity was determined using $CD56^+$, an antibody that reacts with stem cells, neurons and fibroblasts rather than with myoblasts. $CD56^+$ antibody yields false data on myoblast purity.

The great demand for normal myoblasts, the labor-intensiveness and high cost of cell culturing, harvesting and packaging, and human imprecision, will soon necessitate the production of automated cell processors[14,15] capable of

250

manufacturing huge quantities of viable, sterile, genetically well-defined and functionally demonstrated biologicals, examples of which are the myoblasts and myoblast-derived heterokaryons.

This development will be one of the most important offspring of modern-day computer science, mechanical engineering and cytogenetics. The material used will be biopsics of various human tissues. The computer will be programmed to process tissue(s), with precise control of time, space, proportions of culture ingredients and apparatus maneuvers. Cell conditions can be monitored at any time during the process, and flexibility is built in to allow changes. Different protocols can be programmed into the software for culture,[10] controlled cell fusion,[11] harvest and package. The outputs of the system will be injectable cells ready for cell therapy or shipment. The cell processor will be self-contained in a sterile enclosure large enough to house the hardware in which cells are cultured and manipulated.

The automated cell processor will replace the current bulky inefficient culture equipment, and eliminate the high manpower demands and human error. It will decentralize cell production, allowing the latter to be conducted in hospitals where transport of patients' muscle biopsies and the autologous myoblasts is cut to a minimum.

The development of CardioChip[16] allows the early diagnosis of cardiovascular diseases using 10 368 expressed sequence tags (ESTs). Subjects so identified can have a muscle biopsy taken before any symptom occurs. Myoblasts can be processed and deposited in a cell bank for future HCT or be injected into the subject to prevent sudden heart attack.

First in man (FIM) studies

Myoblast autograft

On 14 May, 2002, a 55-year-old man suffering acute ischemic myocardial infarction received cGMP-produced pure myoblasts into his beating myocardium as an adjunct to off-pump coronary artery bypass grafting (CABG). Professor Eugene Sim of the National University Hospital of Singapore led his team in the operation.

Coronary angiography previously demonstrated a right dominant system, 80% occlusion of the mid-left anterior descending artery, 70% occlusion of the proximal first diagonal branch and 50% stenosis of the circumflex artery. The mid-right coronary artery was occluded with good collateral supply from the left coronary artery. Echocardiography 5 days later revealed akinetic apex, anterior wall and septum of the left ventricle, with a left ventricular ejection fraction of 31%. Tomographic Tc^{99m} tetrofosmin scan 25 days after the acute

251

myocardial infarction revealed a large partially reversible defect on the anterior wall and a moderately-sized reversible defect on the inferior wall. After qualifying for the inclusion/exclusion criteria, signing patients' informed consent, and obtaining approval from the hospital ethics committee, the patient was included as a volunteer for myocardial cell transplantation adjunct to CABG at 2 months after the initial presentation

Approximately 2.5 g of rectus femoris muscle biopsy was taken under local anesthesia from the patient and cultured under cGMP for 32 days to produce one billion cells. Myoblast purity of >99% was ascertained by positive immunostain for human desmin.

Under direct vision and stabilization with the Octopus III tissue stabilizer, 4.65×10^8 autologous myoblasts in 3 ml serum were injected into the myocardium within 15 minutes using a 27-gauge needle. Twenty-five injections were made on the anterior wall, near the apex, on the posterior wall, in and around the infarcted areas. These injections of 0.1 ml to 0.2 ml each were performed at 0.5–1 min intervals to observe for dysrhythmias.

The patient recovered well from the operation. Serum creatine kinase was 222 µg/l and the MB fraction was 6 µg/l at 3 h postoperatively, and 385 µg/l and 6 µg/l, respectively, at 12 h. Postoperative 24-h Holter monitoring revealed no arrhythmia. The patient was discharged on the eighth postoperative day.

His ECG has shown no arrhythmia in 10 months. He has shown good effort tolerance, no dyspnea or angina, and a significant increase in ejection fraction at 3 weeks post-operatively. This case study suggests that beating-heart cellular cardiomyoplasty can be a safe and viable option. Additional results will be reported.

Myoblast allograft

Myoblast allograft is being developed to prevent and to alleviate heart muscle degeneration.[17] We report its first application in man.

The feasibility and safety of myoblast allograft was assessed by injecting the infarcted myocardia of two men, aged 63 and 49, with 1.1 and 1.2 billion myoblasts respectively, using 2-month cyclosporine immunosuppression.

Donor myoblasts were manufactured in compliance with current Good Manufacture Practice (cGMP) and ISO 9001 conditions. About 2.18 g of muscle biopsy was taken under local anesthesia from the *rectus femoris* of a 20 year-old pathogen-free male volunteer, after he had met muscle donor criteria and had signed informed consent. At harvest, the culture yielded 3.64×10^9 myoblasts that were 98.3% pure by positive desmin immunostain. It was 91.5% viable according to vital dye exclusion tests. The cells were potent in myogenecity in that myotubes comprised more than 99% of the culture in fusion medium. Throughout the culture and for the final injectates, the myoblasts were free of endotoxin, mycoplasma, and negative for sterility (14 day test) and gram stain (absence of gram positive or negative bacteria) according to certified laboratory analyses.

Both patients enrolled as clinical trial subjects after qualifying for inclusion/exclusion criteria, signing patients' informed consents, and obtaining institutional and academy approval. They had atherosclerosis, coronary artery disease, history of acute myocardial infarction, stable angina Functional Class IV (CCS), and arterial hypertension II (risk 4). Positron emission tomography (PET) with [18]FDG revealed scarred myocardium in LV septal, apical, and anterior/posterior wall regions. Echocardiography showed regional akinesis/hypokinesis, LVEF being 41% and 38% for the subjects respectively. Single-photon emission computed tomography (SPECT) with 30 mCi ^{99m}Tc-tetrofosmin was performed during exercise with bicycle and during rest. Ischaemic changes and scars were confirmed, with significant perfusion defective areas (Figure 17.7). Total LVEF were 39% and 38% for the two subjects respectively. Coronarography revealed calcination, stenosis, and occlusion of the left and right coronary arteries. Left ventriculography demonstrated hypokinesis in segments II, III, IV, and V in the older subject.

Before	After

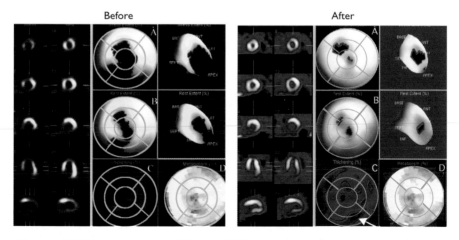

Figure 17.7 *Polar views on PET and SPECT tomograms of the left ventricular myocardium before and at 3 months after myoblast allograph for the 63 y.o. patient. Before surgery — (A) 35% perfusion detect during exercise and (B) 20% at rest, (C) significant decrease of systolic thickening and (D) preserved metabolism are indicative of scarred and hibernated myocardium.*
After surgery — (A) 14% perfusion defect during exercise and (B) 5% at rest. (C) Decrease in systolic thickening is less, and perfusion in the posterior wall (arrow) has been retrieved. (D) Metabolism is preserved and shows no change.

Our 12 years of experience of injecting allogenic myoblasts into 240 muscular dystrophy patients and 28 years of animal allograft/xenograft studies suggested that 8 weeks of cyclosporine immunosuppression are sufficient to allow foreign myoblast engraftment in heart patients. The subjects took two oral doses of cyclosporine totaling 5 to 7 mg/kg body weight per day, beginning at five days before grafting, weaning at half-doses in the last two weeks, and off cyclosporine at eight weeks after grafting. Whole blood trough level of cyclosporine was monitored every three days at 23 hours after the morning dose. Doses were adjusted to maintain the level at about 250 ng/mL.

Professor Leo A. Bockeria of the Russian Academy of Medical Sciences injected the hearts of patients with allogenic myoblasts. The patients underwent bypass grafting immediately prior to myoblast implantation. They received 18/19 injections totaling 1.1/1.2 billion myoblasts respectively. The 10-min procedure was performed open-chest on an ice-chilled, non-beating heart with the subject under general anesthesia and on a respirator. Cells were injected at 100×10^6/ml. The 0.5 ml injections were made under direct vision between the infarcted and viable myocardium, and into scarred tissue.

The patients recovered from the general anesthesia with no rash or fever. Holter EKG monitor registered sporadic ventricular arrhythmias and ventricular extrasystoles that were eventually eliminated with Amiodarone treatment. Both patients were discharged after careful observation for 3 weeks. There was no evidence of overt blood pressure changes or renal failure.

Despite cyclosporine discontinuation at 2 months postoperatively, no sign of rejection was observed. At 3-month follow-up, both subjects were in stable condition at Class I-II (CCS). They no longer suffered angina or shortness of breath. Echocardiography showed 14.6% and 10.5% increases in LVEF respectively with no local akinetic/hypokinetic regions. SPECT with 30 mCi ^{99m}Tc-tetrofosmin confirmed similar LVEF increases and demonstrated reduction on perfusion defective areas during exercise and rest (Figure 17.7). [18]FDG accumulation was equable throughout LV myocardium, and glucose metabolism changes were not revealed.

Human myoblast allografts may provide an alternative therapy for heart muscle degeneration and prevention of heart attack, with virtually unlimited cell availability and only 2-month immunosuppression. Cell potency from young donors is much higher than that of autografts from older heart patients. The regenerative heart is also a rejuvenated heart. Whereas good cells are readily available from cell banks in allografts, autograft patients have to be biopsied and wait approximately one month for their own myoblasts to grow to reach one billion in number. In acute myocardial infarction, the immediate allografts may prevent fibroblast infiltration and eventual scar formation. Patients with infectious diseases such as AIDS can be treated with allografts without fear of contamination of the cell culture system.[17] Furthermore, heart patients with genetic diseases such as the muscular dystrophies can be treated with genetically normal allografts.

The survival of the two patients without any sign of rejection after cyclosporine withdrawal confirmed our report on safety in the human/porcine cardiac xenografts.[17] Cyclosporine immunosuppression for 3 months allowed allogeneic myoblasts to survive, develop, and function in a muscle of a Duchenne muscular dystrophy patient, expressing the therapeutic protein dystrophin at 3 months[7] unto 6 years[8] after myoblast transfer. Myoblast autograft has been demonstrated to have survived and developed up to 17.5 months after implantation[18] in an ischaemic heart patient. Patients who received autografts following CABG had shown improvement that might have been the result of myoblasts in addition to CABG.[12,13]

More than 70 patients have received myoblasts worldwide since the initial procedure in June 2000. Mortality has been less than 10%. If future myoblast allografts prove to be safe and efficacious in treating heart dysfunction, the 2-month immunosuppression, when compared to life-long immunosuppression in heart transplant patients, will greatly improve life expectancy and quality of life for heart patients. Moreover, myoblast allografts can significantly reduce medical cost considering quality control and analysis tests as one lot of 50 billion myoblasts are much less costly than the same tests on 50 lots of one billion myoblasts. Future allograft studies are warranted.

It will be of major interest to determine if the subjects will continue to survive after cyclosporine weaning. Nine more subjects are to be included in this study. The cessation of akinesis/hypokinesis, reduction in perfusion defects, and increase in LVEF suggest that future myoblast allograft studies are warranted.

The future of HCT lies with myoblast allograft, 90% delivered endovascularly and 10% epicardially in adjunct to CABG. Myoblasts will likely be transduced with VEGF, TGF-ß, or similar factors to allow concomitant angiomyogenesis (Figure 17.7).

Conclusion

Our ongoing clinical trial is based on unequivocal evidence of cGMP-produced pure human myoblasts and proof of concept for heart cell therapy.

Human myoblasts survive and integrate into porcine ischemic myocardium, allowing concomitant cell therapy and gene therapy to produce angiomyogenesis. Whereas the newly formed myofibers harbor satellite cells and impart regenerative capacity to the heart muscle, the genetic transformation of cardiomyocytes in vivo to become regenerative heterokaryons through myoblast genome transfer[4] constitutes the ultimate heart repair. The regenerative heart[19] also contains transdifferentiated cardiomyocytes of myoblastic origin. In all three scenarios, new contractile filaments are deposited to improve heart contractility. This can be translated into improvement in the quality of life of heart patients and in the prevention of heart attacks.

It can be concluded that pure $VEGF_{165}$ myoblasts, when injected intramyocardially, are potential therapeutic transgene vehicles for concurrent angiogenesis and myogenesis to treat heart failure.[19,20] Immunosuppression using cyclosporine for 6 weeks is effective for long-term survival of xenografts or allografts. The feasibility and preliminary safety/efficacy observed in the world's first human myoblast allografts lead the way in developing a low-cost, easy-to-use treatment for heart failure and prevention of heart attacks, with virtually unlimited cell availability and short-term immunosuppression.

References

1. Ishikawa F, Matunis MJ, Dreyfuss G, Cech TR. Nuclear proteins that bind the pre-mRNA 3' splice site sequence r(UUAG/G) and the human telomeric DNA sequence d(TTAGGG)$_n$. Mol Cell Biol 1993; 13: 4301–10.

2. Law PK et al. Myoblast transfer as a platform technology of gene therapy. Gene Ther Mol Biol 1998; 1: 345–63.

3. Law, PK. Myoblast transfer as a platform technology of gene therapy. Regul Affairs Focus (Technol) 1999; 4: 25–7.

4. Law PK. Nuclear transfer and human genome therapy. Business Briefing – Future Drug Discovery (Genomics) 2001; 38–42.

5. Venter JC, Adams MD, Myers EW et al. The sequence of the human genome. Science 2001; 291: 1304–51.

6. Bird RC, Stein GS, Lian JB, Stein JL, eds. Nuclear structure and gene expression. New York: Academic Press, 1997: 1–296.

7. Law PK et al. Dystrophin production induced by myoblast transfer therapy in Duchenne muscular dystrophy. Lancet 1990; 336: 114–15.

8. Law PK et al. First human myoblast transfer therapy continues to show dystrophin after 6 years. Cell Transplant 1997; 6: 95–100.

9. Law PK et al. World's first human myoblast transfer into the heart. Frontier Physiol 2000: A85.

10. Law PK. Compositions for and methods of treating muscle degeneration and weakness. US Patent No. 5,130,141, issued 14 July 1992.

11. Law PK. Myoblast therapy for mammalian diseases. Singapore Patent No. 34490 (WO 96/18303), issued 22 August 2000.

12. Menasché P, Hagege AA, Scorsin M et al. Myoblast transplantation for heart failure. Lancet 2001; 357: 279–80.

13. Menasché P et al. Early results of autologous skeletal myoblast transplantation in patients with severe ischemic heart failure. Circulation 2001; 104: II-598.

14. Law PK. Automated cell processor. US Patent No. 6,261,832, issued 17 July 2001.

15. Law PK. Instrument for cell culture. Singapore Patent No. 74036, issued 14 December 2001.

16. Barnes JD, Stamatiou D, Liew CC. Construction of a human cardiovascular cDNA microarray: portrait of the failing heart. Biochem Biophys Res Commun 2001; 280: 964–9.

17. Law PK. Mechanisms of myoblast transfer in treating heart failure. Adv Heart Failure 2002: 43–48.

18. Hagege A, Carrion C, Menasche P et al. Viability and differentiation of autologous skeletal myoblast grafts in ischaemic cardiomyopathy. Lancet 2003; 361: 491–492.

19. Law PK. The regenerative heart. Business Briefing: PharmaTech 2002. 2002: 65–70.

20. Law PK. Concomitant angiogenesis/myogenesis in the regenerative heart. Business Briefing: Future Drug Discovery 2002: 64–7.

18. Transplantation of Autologous Mononuclear Bone Marrow Cells: Clinical Results and Perspectives

Michael Brehm, Tobias Zeus and Bodo E Strauer

Introduction

Ischemic heart disease accounts for approximately 50% of all cardiovascular deaths and is the leading cause of congestive heart failure.[1] With 1.1 million myocardial infarctions and more than 400 000 new cases of congestive heart failure each year in the USA, cardiovascular disease severely impacts on men and women. For patients diagnosed with congestive heart failure, a consequence of chronic heart failure, the 1-year mortality rate is 20%. Myocardial necrosis is due to myocardial infarction and is, by nature, an irreversible injury.[2] After coronary artery occlusion the cardiomyocytes are destroyed irreversibly.[2,3] The extent of the infarction, with respect to the loss of cardiomyocytes, depends on the duration and severity of the perfusion defect.[4] However, the extent of infarction is also modulated by a number of factors, including collateral blood supply, medications and ischemic preconditioning.[5] Beyond contraction and fibrosis of myocardial scar, progressive ventricular remodeling of non-ischemic myocardium can further reduce cardiac function in the weeks to months after the initial event.[6] Many of the therapies available to clinicians today can significantly improve the prognosis of patients with acute myocardial infarction.[7] Although angioplasty and thrombolytic agents can relieve the cause of the infarction by prompt reperfusion of the occluded artery, the time from onset of occlusion to reperfusion determines the degree of irreversible myocardial injury.[8] However, post-infarction heart failure remains a major challenge, resulting from ventricular remodeling processes, characterized by progressive expansion of the infarct area and dilatation of the left ventricular (LV) cavity.[9]

The major goal of reversing LV remodeling would be the enhancement of regeneration of cardiac myocytes as well as the stimulation of neovascularization within the infarct area, by repopulation of the damaged myocardium with healthy autologous cells or by induced proliferation of endogenous resident cardiac stem cells.[10–14] Experimental studies have suggested that bone marrow-

259

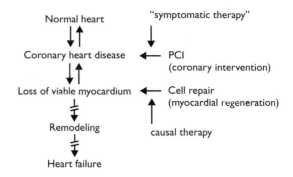

Figure 18.1 *Development of heart failure in coronary artery and therapeutic interventions for prevention. PCI, percutaneous coronary intervention.*

derived or blood-derived progenitor cells may contribute to the regeneration of the infarcted myocardium[15] and enhance neovascularization of ischemic myocardium.[16–18] Indeed, either intravenous infusion or intramyocardial injection of adult progenitor cells resulted in sustained improvement of cardiac function after experimentally induced myocardial infarction.[19,20] Therefore, clinical studies were performed to investigate the feasibility, safety and initial clinical outcome of transplantation of autologous progenitor cells in patients with acute myocardial infarction or ischemic LV impairment (Figure 18.1).

Physiologic cell regeneration after myocardial infarction

Until very recently, there was widespread consensus that the proliferation of cardiac myocytes ceases permanently soon after birth and that there is no replacement with new cardiomyocytes either physiologically or after damage. Although binucleated cardiomyocytes do arise by nuclear division, cytokinesis appears to be blocked in humans. This block of cellular proliferation occurs as a specific event in human cardiac muscle, as human skeletal myocytes and cardiac cells in other species seem to be endowed with considerably greater mitotic potential.[21,22] New data suggest, however, that there is a low level of myocyte proliferation also in the human postnatal heart, amounting to approximately 14 cells per million in normal heart, which is increased 10-fold in heart disease. Since there is also a progressive loss of cardiomyocytes, calculated at 6×10^6 cardiomyocytes per year, it now appears that there may indeed be a slow turnover of cardiac myocytes throughout life.[23,24] Understanding cell cycle control of human cardiomyocytes has since become an area of intensive scientific research, but the master regulators of postnatal cardiomyocyte mitosis are currently still largely unclear.[25]

The traditional understanding has been that, following myocardial infarction, cardiomyocytes were unable to undergo mitosis and proliferated, but were limited to – albeit considerable – hypertrophy in order to compensate the loss of functional tissue.[26–28] Proliferative repair mechanisms were thought to be restricted to vascular cells in the form of angiogenesis and arteriogenesis for the formation of collateral vessels and also fibroblasts, replacing cardiac muscle with connective tissue (scar formation). A notable study has recently extended the findings on myocardial cell proliferation described above to the immediate post-infarction period.[29] Analyzing cardiac tissue samples from the border of the infarct zone and from areas distant from the infarct for the expression of a nuclear proliferation marker, the authors demonstrated re-entry into the cell cycle in about 0.08% of myocytes in the infarct zone and in 0.03% in the distant area, both significant elevations over the levels found in control hearts. In addition, events characteristic for cell division – the formation of mitotic spindles, karyokinesis and cytokinesis – were identified. Overall, these results raise the possibility that the regeneration of myocytes may, indeed, contribute to a true increase in muscle mass following myocardial infarction. Despite the enormous impact of this report, the actual origin of the dividing cells found in the infarcted hearts remains unclear, i.e. whether these were locally resident heart muscle cells re-entering a cell division program or whether circulating cells endowed with a preserved higher mitotic potential had infiltrated the infarct area and other parts of the functionally impaired heart. This question becomes even more intriguing when viewed in the context of another seminal study, investigating the contribution of bone marrow-derived stem cells to the repair of mechanisms operative in ischemically damaged heart muscle in an animal model.[30] A certain subpopulation of highly enriched hematopoietic stem cells from the bone marrow cells, the so-called side-population cells, were transplanted into lethally irradiated mice. The side-population cells were taken from a transgenic mouse strain, expressing a marker antigen in all cells of the body. Ten weeks after the bone marrow transplantation, the recipient mice were rendered ischemic by coronary artery occlusion for 60 min followed by reperfusion. Subsequent histologic examination showed that the engrafted side-population cells or their progeny had migrated into ischemic cardiac muscle and blood vessels, differentiated to cardiomyocytes and endothelial cells, and contributed to the formation of functional tissue. Donor-derived cardiomyocytes were found primarily in the peri-infarct region at a prevalence of around 0.02%. Endothelial engraftment was found at a prevalence of around 3.3%,

261

primarily in small vessels adjacent to the infarct. These results demonstrate the cardiomyogenic potential of hematopoietic stem cells and suggest a possible alternative explanation for the presence of dividing cells in the infarct area as described above,[29] especially as in the study performed in human hearts the presence of stem cell markers had not specifically been investigated. In this regard, it is interesting to note that similar infiltration of bone marrow-derived or circulating stem cells or progenitor cells has now been reported by several authors as a (patho)physiological event after cardiac transplantation,[31,32] a situation in which the presence of non-resident cells in the heart can be demonstrated very easily, because of their different tissue type and gender.

Overall, in contrast to long-standing dogma, there is now evidence to support some proliferation of postnatal cardiomyocytes in humans, especially after heart damage. The origin of such proliferating cardiomyocytes currently remains enigmatic, but contributions by bone marrow-derived stem cells or circulation progenitor cells appear highly likely. Nonetheless, these human data should be interpreted as nothing more than a proof of principle for physiologic repair mechanisms after myocardial infarction, because the functional relevance of these findings is still entirely unproven. In contrast to some animal investigations, the issues of true myocardial differentiation and the development of intercellular contacts for force transmission and electrical conductance have not been rigorously addressed in these studies. Furthermore, it should not be overlooked that these autoreparative processes, either through local proliferation or the invasion of stem/progenitor cells, are exceedingly infrequent and cannot significantly mitigate the adverse functional consequences of myocardial infarction in animals or humans.[33] The realization that self-healing processes are clearly insufficient to counter the loss of functional tissue after ischemic injury to the heart is of course very much in line with our clinical experience of myocardial infarction under current standard medical care. On the other hand, the increasing understanding of mechanisms of repair and regeneration of the damaged heart forms the indispensable foundation for exciting novel approaches to the treatment of myocardial infarction.

Cell replacement therapy of the infarcted heart

When we are confronted with the problem of therapy of heart damage after infarction, replacement of myocytes is the only causal and therefore ideal treatment, as only full regeneration of functional cardiac tissue lost through necrosis can avoid the unwanted consequences of cardiac remodeling. Because of the recent data on cardiac autoregeneration and the increasing amount of stimulating animal data, there is increasing interest in cell transplantation as potential therapy for cardiovascular disease. Independent of the type of cell or tissue used for cellular regeneration therapy, there are some basic principles to be borne in mind when assessing the relative usefulness of such treatment strategies. To be clinically effective, the enhancement of cardiomyocyte proliferation after damage must be rapid if the organism is to survive any acute insult that disrupts heart function through damage to the individual cardiac myocytes. In cases in which there is chronic damage to the heart muscle, the proliferation might need to be sustained to slowly but continually replace myocytes as necessary during the course of disease. Whatever the source of the cells and the use to which they are put, concurrent revascularization must also keep pace with repopulation of the infarct to ensure viability and survival of the repaired region and prevent further scar tissue formation. Finally, the newly formed myocardium must integrate into the existing myocardial wall if it is to assume the function of the tissue it replaces. All of this must occur while the heart continues to beat and perform the essential work of supplying blood throughout the organism. Furthermore, even small areas of imperfectly integrated tissues are likely to severely alter electrical conduction and syncytial concentration of the heart, with long-term life-threatening consequences.

The ideal cellular source for transplantation and regeneration is currently an issue of intensive scientific debate;[25,34] for both theoretical and practical purposes, the following cell types seem to hold some promise for an eventual clinical application in the treatment of acute myocardial infarction: (1) adult stem cells; (2) embryonic stem cells; (3) umbilical cord stem cells; and (4) endothelial progenitor cells (Table 18.1).

Table 18.1 Different types of cells with therapeutic potential in cellular cardiomyoplasty after myocardial infarction

Clinical trials:
    Adult stem cells
    Endothelial progenitor cells
    Angioblasts (AC133+ cells)
    Skeletal myoblasts

Animal models:
    Embryonic stem cells
    Umbilical cord stem cells
    Neonatal cardiomyocytes
    Adult cardiomyocytes

263

Route of cell administration

The appropriate route of cell administration to the damaged organ is an essential prerequisite for the success of organ repair (Figure 18.2). Large cell concentrations within the area of interest and prevention of homing of transplanted cells into other organs are desirable. Different routes of application may be important for different kinds of heart disease. Therefore, targeted and regional administration and transplantation of cells should be preferred.

In regional heart muscle disease, as in myocardial infarction, selective cell delivery by intracoronary catheterization techniques leads to effective accumulation and concentration of cells within the infarcted zone, a

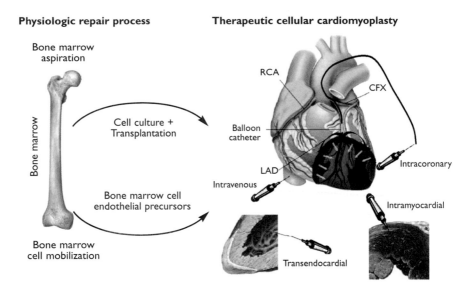

Figure 18.2 *Cellular mobilization routes of endogenous cells for physiologic regeneration processes and various therapeutic administration routes of exogenous autologous cells for cellular repair after myocardial infarction. Bone marrow-derived cells become mobilized from their niches after myocardial infarction and engraft in the infarct zone. Stem cells and precursor cells were readministered by the intracoronary, intramyocardial or transendocardial routes: the red area represents an apical lesion of the left ventricle by myocardial infarction. The balloon catheter is localized in the infarct-related artery and is placed above the border zone of the infarction area. The blue and green arrows suggest the possible route of cell infusion and migration in the infarct. The other two pictures depict the transendocardial and intramyocardial administration route. RCA, right coronary artery; LAD, left anterior descending coronary artery; CFX, circumflex artery.*

mechanism which offers the stem cells the best chance of finding their niche within the myocardium. This can be realized in humans with bone marrow-derived cells. With intracoronary administration, all cells must pass the infarct and peri-infarct tissue during the immediate first passage. Accordingly, with the intracoronary procedure, the infarct tissue can be enriched with and infiltrated by the maximum available number of cells at all times.[35]

The second way, the transendocardial and transpericardial administration method, has been used in large animal experiments,[36] and was also tested recently in patients.[37,38] Current clinical experience is limited to one injection system, using electromechanical mapping to generate three-dimensional LV reconstruction prior to the injection. Intraventricular catheter manipulation, however, can injure the myocardium, inducing ventricular premature beats and short runs of ventricular tachycardia.[18,39] Future developments with steerable transendocardial injection and delivery systems with mapping of the injured zone are needed.

The third application route, intravenous administration, is easiest. However, it has the disadvantage that only approximately 3% of normal cardiac output will flow per minute through the left ventricle, and it is also limited due to the transpulmonary first-pass attenuation effect on the cells. Therefore, this administration technique will require many circulation passages to enable infused cells to come into contact with the infarct-related artery. During that time, homing of infused cells to other organs will considerably reduce the number of cells that will populate the infarcted area. This homing effect has been evaluated, and large amounts of injected stem cells in various extracardiac organs such as liver, spleen and lungs, but only a minor proportion in the heart, have been demonstrated.[40] Thus, direct application of cells into the target organ is desirable, e.g. by selective catheterization techniques to avoid homing to non-desired organs.

Another approach, especially in animal experiments, is the fourth possibility, direct intramuscular cell injection, which has also been used in open heart surgery[41] for coronary artery bypass grafting (CABG), showing improvement in myocardial perfusion in three of five treated patients. These changes were determined by pre- and postoperative thallium scintigraphy.[42] It is conceivable that different and individual cell application routes are necessary for specific heart muscle diseases for coronary as well as for valve disease.

Detection of transplanted stem cells

Another experimental and clinical problem concerns the identification and localization of transplanted autologous stem cells within the injured area of the heart. The transplanted cell or cell population is a single unit in a complex biological network of other cells. Therefore, for both localization and gate mapping of stem cells within the target organ, specific cell markers are desirable. However, a hallmark of most stem cells is the lack of expression of a specific stem cell marker. Therefore, analysis of stem cell behavior will require in situ labeling of a single cell or a transplanted population or transplantation of already in vitro-labeled cells or cell populations. For labeling in animal experiments, retroviral transduction with a marker gene or labeling with thymidine or bromodeoxyuridine (BrdU) have been used. For clinical detection of stem cells, magnetic labeling and in vivo tracking of bone marrow cells by the use of magnetodendrimers or radioactive detection methods may be useful. Single-photon emission computed tomography (SPECT) and positron emission tomography (PET) imaging can determine myocardial perfusion and viability. Magnetic resonance imaging (MRI) evaluates cardiac anatomy and volumes.[43] Furthermore, after stem cells have been labeled with iron particles,[44,45] their distribution can be detected non-invasively with MRI in the healthy and infarcted myocardium. These methods, however, have not yet been established in humans. Myocardial biopsies will hardly be justifiable under these circumstances.

Stem cells for cardiac repair — clinical data

Endogenous bone marrow cells infiltrate non-hematopoietic organs

Therapeutic transplants of sex-mismatched bone marrow and orthotopic organ transplants in male recipients have been used to study human bone marrow stem cell plasticity. Archival samples of liver and heart obtained from female recipients of male bone marrow transplants and male patients who had received liver or heart transplants from female donors were positive for the Y-chromosome.[46,47] Although there were wide differences in the percentage of Y-positive myocytes detected, several reports[31,32] conclude that recipient cells repopulate the myocardium in transplanted heart.[48] Taken together, these data provide evidence that circulating human bone marrow stem cells traffic to non-hematopoietic organs, where they give rise to cells of completely different origin and phenotype.[49]

Exogenous bone marrow cells for cardiac regeneration

A clinical study with direct intracoronary autologous transplantation of adult stem cells was performed in 2001 in patients following acute myocardial infarction.[40] Twenty patients participated in this trial. Ten patients were treated by intracoronary transplantation of autologous, mononuclear bone marrow cells in addition to standard therapy of infarction. The other 10 patients received standard therapy solely, consisting of balloon angioplasty and subsequent stent implantation, in parallel with medication consisting of a beta-blocker, an angiotensin-converting enzyme inhibitor and a statin.

Cells were directly transplanted into the infarcted zone. This was accomplished by the use of a balloon catheter, which was placed within the infarcted-related artery. After exact positioning of the balloon at the site of the former infarct vessel occlusion, percutaneous coronary intervention (PCI) was performed six or seven times for 2–4 min each. During this time, intracoronary cell transplantation via the balloon catheter was performed, using six or seven fractional high-pressure infusions of 2–3 ml of cell suspension, each of which contained 1.5 million to 4 million mononuclear cells. PCI (balloon inflation) thoroughly prevented the backflow of cells and at the same time produced a stop-flow beyond the site of the balloon inflation to facilitate high-pressure infusion of cells into the infarcted zone. Thus, prolonged contact time for cellular migration was allowed.

At 3 months after intracoronary transplantation, the infarct area decreased significantly compared with 10 patients not given cell therapy. The treated patients showed improved LV end-systolic volume and contractility. The therapeutic effect can be attributed to bone marrow cell-associated myocardial regeneration and neovascularization. This is the first report[50] to demonstrate the feasibility and safety of intracoronary administration of bone marrow cells for myocardial repair.

Seiler et al recently reported the effects of intracoronary and systemic administration of granulocyte–macrophage colony-stimulating factor (GM-CSF) in patients with coronary artery disease. GM-CSF is a cytokine with effects on bone marrow similar to those of the more commonly utilized G-CSF, albeit with less potency for bone marrow stem cell mobilization. Twenty-one patients who were not amenable to or refused CABG participated in this randomized, double-blind, placebo-controlled study. The individuals received GM-CSF via intracoronary infusion into the vessel believed to subserve ischemic myocardium, and this was followed by systemic administration of GM-CSF daily for 2 weeks. Analysis of mobilization of bone marrow stem cells was not performed in this study, but because the leukocyte counts were only twice the baseline values, it was suggested that only modest bone marrow stem cell mobilization was achieved.

An invasive measure of collateral artery bloodflow (estimated by coronary artery pressure distal to balloon occlusion) before and after administration of GM-CSF or placebo indicated improved collateral flow in the GM-CSF group at 2 weeks, but not in the placebo group, with reduced ECG signs of myocardial ischemia during coronary balloon occlusion.[51] Because the quantity of bone marrow stem cells mobilized with GM-CSF was probably low, the coronary vascular benefit determined in this study may have resulted from direct effects of this cytokine on angiogenesis or on collateral vascular dilator tone with improved regional bloodflow. No clinically relevant endpoints (e.g. exercise-induced myocardial ischemia or LV contractile response to stress) were assessed in this study.

Patients with severe ischemic heart disease also profit from intramyocardial implantation of bone marrow cells. Eight patients with stable angina refractory to maximum medical therapy and with LV ejection fraction above 30% participated in this phase I trial.[38] The individuals received isolated autologous mononuclear bone marrow cells obtained by bone marrow puncture of the iliac crest and administered after non-fluoroscopic LV electromechanical mapping to guide the later injections of bone marrow cells to areas of ischemic myocardium, which were documented by stress SPECT-sestamibi investigations. There were no ECG changes or sustained ventricular or atrial arrhythmias, and no increase in concentrations of creatine kinase-MB, echocardiographic evidence of pericardial effusion and bleeding or excessive pain at the site of harvesting of bone marrow cells after the procedure.

Clinically, the number of angina episodes per week among the patients declined and the consumed number of nitroglycerin tablets per week decreased during the 3 months of follow-up. MRI showed that the radial motion and thickening of the target wall were significantly less than those of the normal wall at baseline during pharmacologic stress. Three months after implantation of bone marrow cells, MRI showed an improvement in target wall thickening and in target wall motion. Furthermore, the percentage of hypoperfused myocardium was reduced at 3 months, in comparison with baseline. Although an improvement in symptoms and myocardial perfusion and function was noted, the study involved only a few patients and the benefits of the procedure may have been due to the placebo effect or attributable to the variability of MRI.

Stamm et al. recently reported the effects of implantation of bone marrow stem cells in patients with transmural myocardial infarction who had undergone CABG. Six patients with a transmural myocardial infarction greater than 10 days but less than 3 months participated in this clinical phase 1 trial to assess the safety and feasibility of stem cell transplantation in coronary artery bypass patients.[52] The individuals received isolated autologous bone marrow stem cells obtained by bone marrow puncture of the iliac crest. Purified AC133+ cells were injected into the circumference of the infarct border after all bypasses to coronary artery anastomoses had been completed. Within the AC133+ population, the non-hematopoietic (CD34−) subpopulation is included, this has a high potential for multiplication and angiogenic differentiation. After the procedure, some patients developed atrial arrhythmia, pneumonia, bleeding from the left internal mammary artery and relevant pericardial effusion. Up to now, no malignant neoplasia, ventricular arrhythmia or ventricular tachycardia has occurred.

Echocardiography showed that the LV ejection fraction and diastolic LV dimension (LVEDD) definitely improved during follow-up, compared with baseline. Furthermore, myocardial perfusion improved strikingly in the non-perfused or hypoperfused infarct zone. However, the effectiveness of stem cell transplantation cannot be readily assessed alone, because the cell implantation was done in association with surgical revascularization.

Conclusions and perspectives

Stem cell therapy represents a fascinating new approach for the management of heart disease. Recent clinical results have shown the feasibility of adult autologous cell therapy in acute myocardial infarction in humans. However, many unresolved questions for experimental and clinical cardiology are still open for future research, especially many basic problems concerning, among others, the following issues: (1) the long-term fate of transplanted stem cells in the recipient tissue; (2) the ability of transplanted stem cells to find their optimum myocardial 'niche'; (3) the variable potency of stem cells to transdifferentiate into heart muscle cells; (4) the optimal angiogenic milieu needed for transplanted cells in hypoperfused tissue; (5) the ability of the recipient tissue to enable an enhanced environment to offer optimum, milieu-dependent differentiation of engrafted cells; (6) the specific detection of engrafted cells or cell populations by labeling techniques; (7) the optimal time course of availability and application for stem cell replacement therapy in cardiovascular disease; (8) the arrhythmogenic potential of implanted cells; (9) the specific characterization of the progenitor cells that should be measured to predict the therapeutic effect of transplanted cells; (10) the development of safe and reproducible catheter-based delivery systems for depositing stem cells in recipient heart muscle; and (11) the adequate assessment of myocardial function and viability after cell transplantation.

With regard to the clinical practicability, to ethical problems and to hazards of immunogenity, actual and future research will focus preferably on adult stem cells, whereas research on embryonic stem cells may lead to clinical applications many years in the future. According to our present experience, autologous transplantation of adult human stem cells represents a very effective and safe therapeutic procedure for the restoration of damaged myocardium.

References

1. American Heart Association. Heart and stroke statistical update. Dallas, TX: American Heart Association, 2001.

2. Ho KK, Anderson KM, Kannel WB et al. Survival after the onset of congestive heart failure in Framingham Heart Study subjects. Circulation 1993; 88: 107–15.

3. Heyndrickx GR, Baig H, Nellens P et al. Depression of regional blood flow and wall thickening after brief coronary occlusions. Am J Physiol 1978; 234: H653–9.

4. Reimer KA, Lowe JE, Rasmussen MM, Jennings RB. The wavefront phenomenon of ischemic cell death. 1. Myocardial infarct size vs duration of coronary occlusion in dogs. Circulation 1977; 56: 786–94.

5. Murry CE, Jennings RB, Reimer KA. Preconditioning with ischemia: a delay of lethal cell injury in ischemic myocardium. Circulation 1986; 74: 1124–36.

6. Pfeffer MA. Left ventricular remodeling after acute myocardial infarction. Annu Rev Med 1995; 46: 455–66.

7. Ryan TJ, Antman EM, Brooks NH et al. 1999 update: ACC/AHA guidelines for the management of patients with acute myocardial infarction. A report of the American College of Cardiology/American Heart Association Task Force on Practice Guidelines (Committee on Management of Acute Myocardial Infarction). J Am Coll Cardiol 1999; 34: 890–911.

8. Schwarz F, Schuler G, Katus H et al. Intracoronary thrombolysis in acute myocardial infarction: duration of ischemia as a major determinant of late results after recanalization. Am J Cardiol 1982; 50: 933–7.

9. Pfeffer MA, Braunwald E. Ventricular remodeling after myocardial infarction. Experimental observations and clinical implications. Circulation 1990; 81: 1161–72.

10. Blau HM, Brazelton TR, Weimann JM. The evolving concept of a stem cell: entity or function? Cell 2001; 105: 829–41.

11. Pittenger MF, Mackay AM, Beck SC et al. Multilineage potential of adult human mesenchymal stem cells. Science 1999; 284: 143–7.

12. Graf T. Differentiation plasticity of hematopoietic cells. Blood 2002; 99: 3089–101.

13. Reyes M, Lund T, Lenvik T et al. Purification and ex vivo expansion of postnatal human marrow mesodermal progenitor cells. Blood 2001; 98: 2615–25.

14. Strauer BE, Kornowski R. Stem cell therapy in perspective. Circulation 2003; 107: 929–34.

15. Orlic D, Kajstura J, Chimenti S et al. Bone marrow cells regenerate infarcted myocardium. Nature 2001; 410: 701–5.

16. Kocher AA, Schuster MD, Szabolcs MJ et al. Neovascularization of ischemic myocardium by human bone-marrow-derived angioblasts prevents cardiomyocyte apoptosis, reduces remodeling and improves cardiac function. Nat Med 2001; 7: 430–6.

17. Kawamoto A, Gwon HC, Iwaguro H et al. Therapeutic potential of ex vivo expanded endothelial progenitor cells for myocardial ischemia. Circulation 2001; 103: 634–7.

18. Fuchs S, Baffour R, Zhou YF et al. Transendocardial delivery of autologous bone marrow enhances collateral perfusion and regional function in pigs with chronic experimental myocardial ischemia. J Am Coll Cardiol 2001; 37: 1726–32.

19. Asahara T, Masuda H, Takahashi T et al. Bone marrow origin of endothelial progenitor cells responsible for postnatal vasculogenesis in physiological and pathological neovascularization. Circ Res 1999; 85: 221–8.

20. Orlic D, Kajstura J, Chimenti S et al. Mobilized bone marrow cells repair the infarcted heart, improving function and survival. Proc Natl Acad Sci USA 2001; 98: 10344–9.

21. Olivetti G, Quaini F, Sala R et al. Acute myocardial infarction in humans is associated with activation of programmed myocyte cell death in the surviving portion of the heart. J Mol Cell Cardiol 1996; 28: 2005–16.

22. Li F, Wang X, Bunger PC, Gerdes AM. Formation of binucleated cardiac myocytes in rat heart: I. Role of actin–myosin contractile ring. J Mol Cell Cardiol 1997; 29: 1541–51.

23. Kajstura J, Leri A, Finato N et al. Myocyte proliferation in end-stage cardiac failure in humans. Proc Natl Acad Sci USA 1998; 95: 8801–5.

24. Soonpaa MH, Field LJ. Survey of studies examining mammalian cardiomyocyte DNA synthesis. Circ Res 1998; 83: 15–26.

25. Grounds MD, White JD, Rosenthal N, Bogoyevitch MA. The role of stem cells in skeletal and cardiac muscle repair. J Histochem Cytochem 2002; 50: 589–610.

26. Adler CP, Friedburg H, Herget GW et al. Variability of cardiomyocyte DNA content, ploidy level and nuclear number in mammalian hearts. Virchows Arch 1996; 429: 159–64.

27. Sun Y, Weber KT. Infarct scar: a dynamic tissue. Cardiovasc Res 2000; 46: 250–6.

28. Buschmann I, Schaper W. The pathophysiology of the collateral circulation (arteriogenesis). J Pathol 2000; 190: 338–42.

29. Beltrami AP, Urbanek K, Kajstura J et al. Evidence that human cardiac myocytes divide after myocardial infarction. N Engl J Med 2001; 344: 1750–7.

30. Jackson KA, Majka SM, Wang H et al. Regeneration of ischemic cardiac muscle and vascular endothelium by adult stem cells. J Clin Invest 2001; 107: 1395–402.

31. Quaini F, Urbanek K, Beltrami AP et al. Chimerism of the transplanted heart. N Engl J Med 2002; 346: 5–15.

32. Laflamme MA, Myerson D, Saffitz JE, Murry CE. Evidence for cardiomyocyte repopulation by extracardiac progenitors in transplanted human hearts. Circ Res 2002; 90: 634–40.

33. Rosenthal N. High hopes for the heart. N Engl J Med 2001; 344: 1785–7.

34. Goodell MA, Jackson KA, Majka SM et al. Stem cell plasticity in muscle and bone marrow. Ann NY Acad Sci 2001; 938: 208–18.

35. Strauer BE, Brehm M, Zeus T et al. Intrakoronare, humane autologe Stammzelltransplantation zur Myokardregeneration nach Herzinfarkt. Dtsch Med Wochenschr 2001; 126: 932–8.

36. Kornowski R, Fuchs S, Leon MB, Epstein SE. Delivery strategies to achieve therapeutic myocardial angiogenesis. Circulation 2000; 101: 454–8.

37. Fuchs S, Weisz G, Kornowski R. Catheter-based autologous bone marrow myocardial injection in no-option patients with advanced coronary artery disease: a feasibility and safety study. Circulation 2002; 106(suppl II): I-I655–6.

38. Tse HF, Kwong YL, Chan JK et al. Angiogenesis in ischaemic myocardium by intramyocardial autologous bone marrow mononuclear cell implantation. Lancet 2003; 361: 47–9.

39. Losordo DW, Vale PR, Hendel RC et al. Phase 1/2 placebo-controlled, double-blind, dose-escalating trial of myocardial vascular endothelial growth factor 2 gene transfer by catheter delivery in patients with chronic myocardial ischemia. Circulation 2002; 105: 2012–18.

40. Toma C, Pittenger MF, Cahill KS et al. Human mesenchymal stem cells differentiate to a cardiomyocyte phenotype in the adult murine heart. Circulation 2002; 105: 93–8.

41. Menasche P, Hagege AA, Scorsin M et al. Myoblast transplantation for heart failure. Lancet 2001; 357: 279–80.

42. Hamano K, Nishida M, Hirata K et al. Local implantation of autologous bone marrow cells for therapeutic angiogenesis in patients with ischemic heart disease: clinical trial and preliminary results. Jpn Circ J 2001; 65: 845–7.

43. Orlic D, Hill JM, Arai AE. Stem cells for myocardial regeneration. Circ Res 2002; 91: 1092–102.

44. Lederman RJ, Guttman MA, Peters DC et al. Catheter-based endomyocardial injection with real-time magnetic resonance imaging. Circulation 2002; 105: 1282 4.

45. Zhao M, Beauregard DA, Loizou L et al. Non-invasive detection of apoptosis using magnetic resonance imaging and a targeted contrast agent. Nat Med 2001; 7: 1241–4.

46. Theise ND, Nimmakayalu M, Gardner R et al. Liver from bone marrow in humans. Hepatology 2000; 32: 11–16.

47. Korbling M, Katz RL, Khanna A et al. Hepatocytes and epithelial cells of donor origin in recipients of peripheral-blood stem cells. N Engl J Med 2002; 346: 738–46.

48. Muller P, Pfeiffer P, Koglin J et al. Cardiomyocytes of noncardiac origin in myocardial biopsies of human transplanted hearts. Circulation 2002; 106: 31–5.

49 Thiele J, Varus E, Wickenhauser C et al. Chimerism of cardiomyocytes and endothelial cells after allogeneic bone marrow transplantation in chronic myeloid leukemia: an autopsy study. Pathologe 2002; 23: 405–10.

50. Strauer BE, Brehm M, Zeus T et al. Repair of infarcted myocardium by autologous intracoronary mononuclear bone marrow cell transplantation in humans. Circulation 2002; 106: 1913–18.

51. Seiler C, Pohl T, Wustmann K et al. Promotion of collateral growth by granulocyte–macrophage colony-stimulating factor in patients with coronary artery disease: a randomized, double-blind, placebo-controlled study. Circulation 2001; 104: 2012–17.

52. Stamm C, Westphal B, Kleine HD et al. Autologous bone-marrow stem-cell transplantation for myocardial regeneration. Lancet 2003; 361: 45–6.

19. Therapeutic Angiogenesis for Cardiac and Peripheral Vascular Diseases by Autologous Bone Marrow Cell Transplantation

Hiroaki Matsubara

Introduction

Blood vessels are primarily composed of two cell types: endothelial cells, lining the inside, and smooth muscle cells, covering the outside. While angiogenesis research has generally been focused on these two vascular cell types, recent evidence indicates that the bone marrow may also contribute to this process, both in the embryo and in the adult. Following commitment to the endothelial lineage, marrow-derived angioblasts assemble into a primitive vascular plexus of veins and arteries, a process called vasculogenesis. This primitive vasculature is subsequently refined into a functional network by angiogenesis (vascular sprouting from pre-existing vessels, vascular fusion and intussusception) and by remodeling and muscularization (arteriogenesis) of newly formed vessels.[1]

Preclinical studies have indicated that angiogenic growth factors promote the development of collateral arteries, a concept called 'therapeutic angiogenesis'.[2] Angiogenesis can be achieved by the use of either growth factor proteins or genes encoding these proteins. Limited clinical data from protein and gene delivery trials suggest that both approaches are safe. However, much more clinical experience will be necessary to resolve the safety concerns, such as potentiation of pathologic angiogenesis (e.g. malignancy) and 'bystander' effects of the delivered factors (e.g. effects on kidney or atheroma).[3] Given the investment of the formed mature vessels with periendothelial matrix and pericyte/smooth muscle cells, combination with various angiogenic growth factors may be preferable in future therapies.[4]

We discovered that endothelial progenitor cells (EPCs) in the CD34$^+$ stem cell fraction of adult human peripheral blood participate in postnatal neovascularization after mobilization from the bone marrow.[5–7] We[7] and Kalka et al[8] reported that mononuclear cells from adult human peripheral

275

or cord blood improved capillary density in hindlimb ischemia. Marrow stromal cells have many of the characteristics of stem cells for mesenchymal tissues, and also secrete a broad spectrum of angiogenic cytokines,[9] raising the possibility that marrow implantation into ischemic limbs effectively enhances angiogenesis by supplying EPCs as well as angiogenic cytokines or factors. We have demonstrated in animal studies that bone marrow mononuclear cell (BM-MNC) implantation into ischemic limbs[7] or myocardium[10,11] promotes collateral vessel formation with incorporation of EPCs into new capillaries, and that local concentrations of angiogenic factors (basic fibroblast growth factor (bFGF), vascular endothelial growth factor (VEGF) and angiopoietin-1) or angiogenic cytokines (interleukin-1ß (IL-1ß and tumor necrosis factor-alpha (TNF-α) are increased in implanted tissues. Neither tissue injury caused by inflammatory cytokines released from injected cells nor differentiation into other lineage cells such as osteoblasts or fibroblasts was observed in implanted ischemic tissues. Side-effects, such as an increase in cardiac enzymes, malignant arrhythmia or differentiation into other lineage cells, were not observed in the BM-MNC-implanted myocardium. On the basis of these animal studies, we have started a clinical trial to test the therapeutic availability by cell therapy using autologous BM-MNCs in patients with ischemic limbs or ischemic myocardium. In this review, I summarize the results of clinical trials of angiogenic cell therapy by implantation of bone marrow cells or peripheral blood-derived cells.

Therapeutic angiogenesis for ischemic limbs by autologous transplantation of bone marrow cells

CD34[+] hematopoietic stem cells include EPCs and play a key role in neocapillary formation.[4,5] Although CD34[-] cells enhance CD34[+] cell-mediated angiogenesis,[4] the underlying mechanism remains undefined. As BM-MNCs include both CD34[+] and CD34[-] cells, we hypothesized that these cell fractions may release angiogenic factors to enhance angiogenesis in addition to the supply of EPCs. Interestingly, we found that CD34[-] rather than CD34[+] cells mainly expressed bFGF >> VEGF > angiopoietin-1 mRNAs but not angiopoietin-2, while CD34[+] cells predominantly expressed their receptors (Figure 19.1), suggesting that BM-MNCs have the natural ability of the marrow cells to supply EPCs as well as to secrete various angiogenic factors or cytokines. We have reported that autologous marrow implantation in rabbit or rat ischemic limbs augmented collateral vessel formation, and the implanted cells were incorporated into neocapillaries.[7,12] Neither tissue injury by inflammatory cytokines released from injected cells nor differentiation into other lineage cells such as osteoblasts or fibroblasts was observed in implanted ischemic tissues.[7,10] On the basis of these animal studies, we have started a clinical trial to test therapeutic availability by cell therapy using autologous BM-MNCs in patients with ischemic limbs.[13]

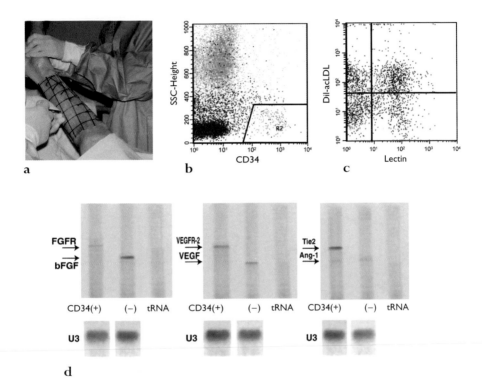

Figure 19.1 Identification of endothelial lineage cells and expression of angiogenic factors in BM-MNCs (a) Concentrated BM-MNCs (~30 ml) were intramuscularly injected into the ischemic lower limb using a 3 cm × 3 cm grid and 26-gauge needle (×40 sites, 1.5 cm deep). (b,c) The CD34⁺ fraction of BM-MNCs (R2 area in (b)) was analyzed by fluorescence-activated cell sorting (FACS) using dialkylcarbocyanine (DiI)–acLDL uptake and Ulex lectin-binding (c). The upper right area in (c) indicates endothelial lineage cells. (d) The CD34⁺ and CD34⁻ fractions were separated from BM-MNCs with the use of CD34 magnetic microbeads. The mRNAs for bFGF and its receptor FGFR-1, VEGF and its receptor VEGFR-2 and angiopoietin-1 (Ang-1) and its receptor Tie2 were analyzed by RNase protection assay. The same amounts of RNA were analyzed by Northern blotting using a U3 rRNA probe as an internal standard. Representative pictures from eight different patients in group A are shown.

Patients qualified for marrow implantation if they had chronic critical limb ischemia including rest pain and/or non-healing ischemic ulcers and were not candidates for non-surgical or surgical revascularization. Requisite hemodynamic deficits included a resting ankle–brachial pressure index (ABI) <0.6 in the affected limb on two consecutive examinations performed at least 1 week apart. Patients with poorly controlled diabetes mellitus (HbA1c >6.5 and proliferative retinopathy) or with evidence of malignant neoplasm (during the last 5 years) were excluded. The patients ($n = 45$) were included in a multicenter, randomized, double-blind trial; BM-MNCs (active treatment) or peripheral blood mononuclear cells (PB-MNCs) (control cells) were randomly, double blindly implanted into right or left ischemic limbs. We used PB-MNCs as a more appropriate cell control than saline, since peripheral blood was partially contaminated during the marrow aspiration procedure ($\sim$10% of marrow cells) and the number of CD34$^+$ cells including EPCs was $\sim$500-fold less in PB-MNCs than that in BM-MNCs.

We obtained $\sim$500 ml of marrow cells from each patient and isolated 2.8×10^9 to 0.7×10^9 MNCs (1.6×10^9 cells (SD 0.6)), which included 9.6×10^7 to 0.84×10^7 CD34$^+$ cells (3.7×10^7 (SD 1.8)). The BM-MNCs were implanted by intramuscular injection into gastrocnemius of ischemic lower limbs ($\times$40 sites) using a 26-gauge needle. ABI values in BM-MNC-implanted limbs were increased by 0.1 (95% CI 0.07–0.12) from 0.37 (0.31–0.42) at baseline to 0.46 (0.40–0.52) at week 4 ($P < 0.0001$). In contrast, PB-MNC-injected limbs showed much smaller increases in ABI (0.02 increase, 95% CI 0.01–0.024). In the follow-up study, improvement of ischemic status (ABI, tissue oxygen concentration, rest pain scale, pain-free walking time, improvement of ischemic ulcers) was maintained over 24 weeks of observation (Figure 19.2).[13] Angiography revealed a marked increase in visible collateral vessel numbers in 60% of patients (Figure 19.3). Vessel numbers assessed by capillary/muscle fiber ratio (2.3 (SD 0.6)) were markedly increased compared with the contralateral saline-injected muscle (0.74 (0.31)) (Figure 19.4a). CD31-positive endothelial cells express Ki-67 in the marrow-implanted limb (Figure 19.4b). Ki-67 is a nuclear protein that is expressed in proliferating cells and nearly absent in normal vessels. No Ki-67 expression was detected in the saline-injected limb, suggesting the presence of proliferating endothelial cells in newly formed vessels.

In considering the clinical potential of therapeutic angiogenesis, it is important to determine whether growth of new capillaries (vasculogenesis) or of pre-existing collaterals (angiogenesis) is the therapeutic goal. For newly formed vessels to survive, they must be remodeled and acquire a smooth muscle coat.[14] Given the complexity of vessel formation, therapies using a single angiogenic factor may produce incompletely functioning endothelial

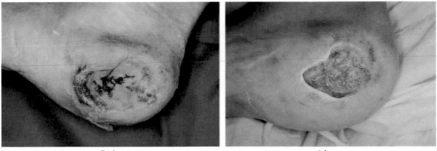

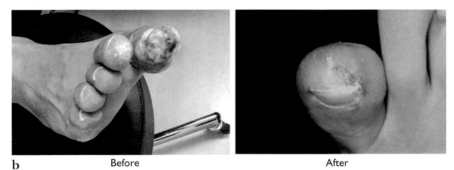

Figure 19.2 *Limb salvage after marrow implantation. A non-healing ulcer on the heel (a) and ischemic necrosis involving the big toe (b) were markedly improved 8 weeks after BM-MNC implantation.*

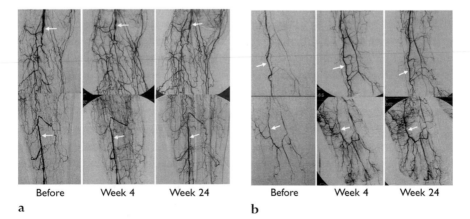

Figure 19.3 *Angiographic analysis of collateral vessel formation. Angiographically visible collateral branches were markedly increased at the knee and upper tibia levels (a) and lower tibia, ankle and foot levels (b) 4 and 24 weeks after BM-MNC implantation. Note that contrast densities in the suprafemoral, posterior–tibial and dorsal pedal arteries (indicated by arrows) are similar in the 'before' and 'after' figures.*

279

channels.[3] We found that the CD34⁻ fraction in BM-MNCs synthesized not only angiogenic growth factors (VEGF and bFGF) but also angiopoietin-1, which is known to have important functions in the maturation and maintenance of the vascular system. Recently, infusion of EPCs or CD34⁺ cells was shown to induce angiogenesis in ischemic limbs.[6,7] Thus, it is concluded that the efficacy of BM-MNC implantation therapy is due to the supply of EPCs (included in the CD34⁺ fraction) as well as multiple angiogenic factors (released from the CD34⁻ fraction). These combined

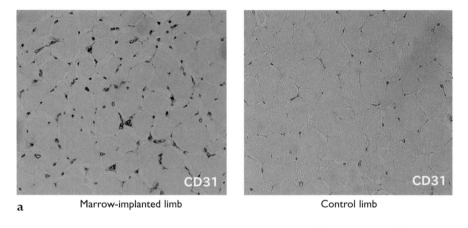

a   Marrow-implanted limb   Control limb

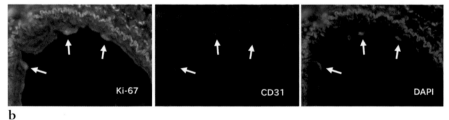

b

Figure 19.4 *Immunohistochemical analysis of new proliferating vessel formation. (a) Vessel formation in specimens of BM-MNC-implanted limb (gastrocnemius) was analyzed with anti-CD31 antibody (DAKO) specific to vascular endothelial cells. Staining was viewed by the immunoperoxidase reaction with diaminobenzidine. CD31-positive vessels (brown staining) were markedly increased in the BM-MNC-implanted limb compared with those in the saline-injected control limb (×200). (b) Sections from BM-MNC-implanted limb were double-immunostained with mouse monoclonal anti-CD31 antibody (DAKO) and rabbit polyclonal anti-Ki-67 antibody (DAKO), and counterstained with DNA binding dye diamidino-phenylindole (DAPI) (Molecular Probe), followed by incubation with fluorescein isothiocyonate (FITC)-conjugated anti-rabbit antibody or TRITC-conjugated anti-mouse secondary antibody (×400). Arrows indicate Ki-67- and CD31-positive endothelial cells.*

280

therapies may lead to the formation of stable capillary vessels, as suggested by
the findings that improvement of limb ischemia was sustained during 1 year
of follow-up.

Therapeutic angiogenesis for ischemic limbs by peripheral blood-derived mononuclear cells

PB-MNCs,[15] polymorphonuclear leukocytes (PMNs)[16] and platelets[17] synthesize
and release high levels of VEGF as well as platelet-derived growth factor
(PDGF) and TGF-β, which are known to be prerequisites for investment of
stable vessels with pericytes.[18] We have used PB-MNCs as control injection
cells and compared their angiogenic activity with that of BM-MNCs in patients
with ischemic limbs.[13] Although the increase in limb blood pressure was
significantly lower than with BM-MNCs, we found a moderate improvement in
ischemic status, implying a potential angiogenic effect of PB-MNC implantation.
Our study using immunodeficient nude rats demonstrated that intramuscular
implantation of human PB-MNCs enhanced neocapillary formation in a PB-
MNC-derived VEGF-dependent mechanism, while PMNs reduced PB-MNC-
mediated angiogenesis by PMN-derived neutrophil elastase.[7] In contrast,
Minamino et al[19] reported that intramuscular implantation of PB-MNCs induces
a greater increase in limb blood pressure and a greater improvement of
ischemic status compared with our previous observation,[13] suggesting that the
efficacy of angiogenic therapy with PB-MNCs may depend on the degree of
limb ischemia of patients. Inaba et al[20] showed that intramuscular implantation
of CD34+ cells isolated from G-CSF-mobilized PB-MNCs also enhanced blood
perfusion in ischemic limbs; however, the angiogenic action appeared to be
weaker than that of PB-MNCs. Taken together with our data,[13] these clinical
studies suggest the feasibility of angiogenic cell therapy using peripheral blood-
derived cells for the treatment of ischemic tissues. As the ischemic status of
limbs or numbers of injected cells are different between patients in these pilot
studies, further controlled studies using large numbers of patients will be
needed to define the efficacy of PB-MNCs and CD34+ cells.

Therapeutic angiogenesis for ischemic myocardium by bone marrow cells

Myogenic cell grafting in a damaged myocardium is a promising approach to
the treatment of heart failure. We and others have previously shown the

efficacy of intramyocardial transplantation of BM-MNCs in animal models of ischemic heart failure.[10,11] Side-effects, such as an increase in cardiac enzymes, malignant arrhythmia or differentiation into other lineage cells, were not observed in the BM-MNC-implanted myocardium,[10,11] A marked increase in cardiac function may be due to not only neovascularization but also partly cardiomyogenesis by marrow-derived hematopoietic cells[21] and/or marrow-derived mesenchymal cells.[22] On the basis of the results of these preclinical experiments using porcine models,[10,11] we performed the first clinical trial of sole cell therapy using BM-MNC implantation targeted into an ischemic hibernating myocardium.

A 65-year-old man suffered from refractory angina (CCS class IV) due to posterolateral ischemia in spite of repeated bypass surgery (two times) and angioplasty (five times). Echocardiography showed severe posterolateral hypokinesia, and viability in the posterolateral wall was confirmed by a biphasic response with low-dose and high-dose dobutamine. The hibernating myocardium focus was identified on NOGA electromechanical mapping (Biosense-Webster) by preserved viability (voltage mapping) associated with an impairment in linear local shortening (mechanical mapping)[5] (Figure 19.5). The average number of NTG sprays was 10–15 per day. Based on the severity of refractory angina as well as the presence of hibernating myocardium, we decided to perform BM-MNC implantation to improve regional blood perfusion. After aspiration of the marrow cells, an intercostal space was opened to visualize the left ventricular lateral wall. BM-MNCs (0.1 ml) were injected into 30 different sites (total 3×10^8 cells) on the left ventricular posterolateral wall with a 27G needle.

Angina occurrence decreased dramatically as early as 7 days after BM-MNC implantation, and at 1-year follow-up the patient's clinical status was markedly improved and he had stable CCS class 1 disease (no NTG spray use). There was no substantial arrhythmia on 24 h Holter recordings performed monthly for 1 year. NOGA electromechanical analysis (Figure 19.5) indicated that the reduced motion of the posterolateral hibernating area (shown in red in mechanical mapping), identified by preserved viability associated with impaired linear local shortening, markedly improved towards the normal wall motion level (shown in purple) 4 months after BM-MNC implantation. The area of ischemic myocardium decreased from 36% before BM-MNC implantation to 11% after implantation. The result of SPECT-sestamibi myocardial perfusion scans corresponded to improved perfusion in the posterolateral myocardium observed in NOGA electromechanical analysis (Figure 19.6), and reduced blood perfusion in the posterolateral region after pharmacologic stress was not observed 3 months after BM-MNC implantation. Echocardiography showed systolic function improvement in the

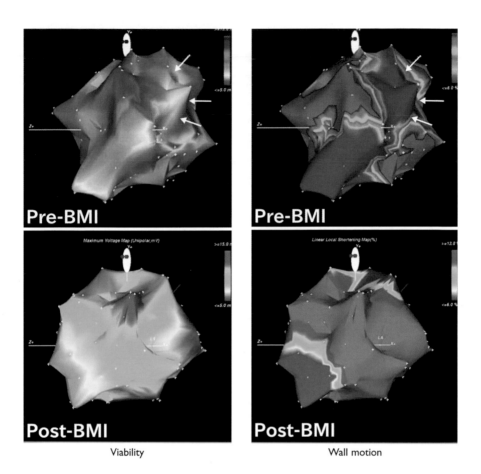

Viability Wall motion

Figure 19.5 NOGA *electromechanical mapping performed in a 65-year-old man.*
NOGA *images in left lateral projection before BM-MNC implantation (pre-BMI) show
myocardial viability and wall motion; the red zone (which depicts abnormal wall
motion) on the linear local shortening map (wall motion, top right), together with
observed viability (green–yellow in viability, top left) on the unipolar voltage map
constitute the focus of electromechanical uncoupling that suggests ischemic hibernating
myocardium of the posterolateral region. BM-MNCs were injected into the hibernating
area, indicated by arrows. The same projection 4 months after BMI (post-BMI) shows
almost complete resolution of wall motion in the hibernating region (shift from red
zone to purple zone), corresponding to changes observed on the SPECT scan (Figure
19.2a). The vertical and horizontal axes are represented by red and white lines,
respectively.*

283

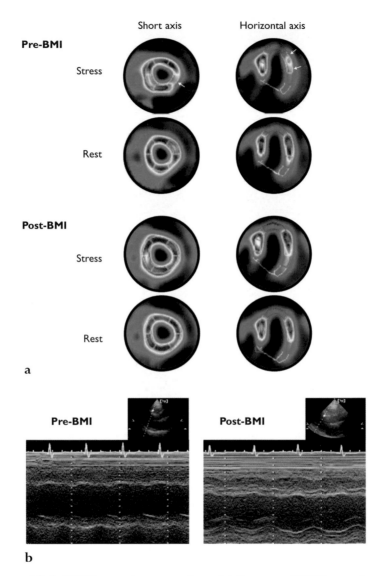

Figure 19.6 *SPECT-sestamibi scan analysis. (a) Persantine SPECT-sestamibi scans recorded before and after cell implantation. White color depicts maximal uptake of radionuclide. Scans before cell implantation (pre-BMI) show a reversible posterolateral wall defect (indicated by arrows). Scans 4 months after cell implantation (post-BMI) show complete normalization of posterolateral wall perfusion after pharmacologic stress. (b) M-mode echocardiograms before (pre-BMI) and after (post-BMI) BM-MNC implantation. An increase in left ventricular posterior wall contractility occurred after cell implantation. Echocardiography showed the improvement of systolic function in the posterior wall (fractional shortening: 19–33%) and a decrease in left ventricular end-diastolic dimension (from 61 to 43 mm).*

posterior wall (fractional shortening: 19–33%) and a decrease in the left ventricular end-diastolic dimensions (from 61 to 43 mm). On angiographic analysis, the numbers of detectable collateral vessels did not appear to change, while ejection fraction (EF) calculated by left ventriography increased from 42% to 53%.

Together, these results suggest that improved systolic function of the hibernating myocardium is related to the implanted BM-MNCs. We[10,11] demonstrated revascularization of an ischemic myocardium by BM-MNC-derived neocapillary formation, while BM-MNCs were also shown to include cardiomyocyte-committed hematopoietic stem cells[21] as well as cardiomyocyte-committed mesenchymal stem cells.[22]. Thus, our findings show the feasibility of autologous BM-MNC implantation in a patient with an ischemic myocardium. Very recently, two research teams have reported catheter-mediated implantation of BM-MNCs as sole therapy in eight patients with stable angina[23] and injection of AC133+ hematopoietic cells in six patients with recent myocardial infarction at the time of coronary artery bypass.[24] Although the number of patients is too small to derive any meaningful efficacy and definitive safety data, most patients had significant improvement in symptoms and many had improvement in physiologic variables such as regional wall motion and target area perfusion, consistent with our present observation. Thus, cell-based investigational therapies for ischemic heart diseases were shown to be safe and feasible. Additional larger randomized placebo-controlled double-blind studies with mechanistic and clinical endpoints are in progress.

References

1. Carmeli P, Luttun A. The emerging role of the bone marrow-derived stem cells in (therapeutic) angiogenesis. Thromb Haemost 2001; 86: 289–97.

2. Isner M, Asahara T. Angiogenesis and vasculogenesis as therapeutic strategies for postnatal neovascularization. J Clin Invest 1999; 103: 1231–6.

3. Simons M, Bonow RO, Chronos NA et al. Clinical trial in coronary angiogenesis: issues, problems, consensus. Circulation 2000; 102: e73–89.

4. Ferrara N, Alitalo K. Clinical application of angiogenic growth factors and their inhibitors. Nat Med 1999; 5: 1359–64.

5. Asahara T, Murohara T, Sullivan A et al. Isolation of putative progenitor endothelial cells for angiogenesis. Science 1997; 275: 964–7.

6.   Asahara T, Masuda H, Takahashi T et al. Bone marrow origin of endothelial progenitor cells responsible for postnatal vasculogenesis in physiological and pathological neovascularization. Circ Res 1999; 85: 221–8.

7.   Iba O, Matsubara H, Nozawa Y et al. Angiogenesis by implantation of peripheral blood mononuclear cells and platelets into ischemic limbs. Circulation 2002; 106: 2019–25.

8.   Kalka C, Masuda H, Takahashi T et al. Transplantation of ex vivo expanded endothelial progenitor cells for therapeutic neovascularization. Proc Natl Acad Sci USA 2000; 97: 3422–7.

9.   Prockop DJ. Marrow stromal cells as stem cells for nonhematopoietic tissues. Science 1997; 276: 71–4.

10. Kamihata H, Matsubara H, Nishiue T et al. Implantation of autologous bone marrow cells into ischemic myocardium enhances collateral perfusion and regional function via side-supply of angioblasts, angiogenic ligands and cytokines. Circulation 2001; 104: 1046–52.

11. Kamihata H, Matsubara H, Nishiue N et al. Improvement of collateral perfusion and regional function by catheter-based implantation of peripheral blood mononuclear cells into ischemic hibernating myocardium. Arterioscler Thromb Vasc Biol 2002; 22: 1804–10.

12. Shintani S, Murohara T, Ikeda H et al. Augmentation of postnatal neovascularization with autologous bone marrow transplantation. Circulation 2001; 103: 897–903.

13. Tateishi-Yuyama E, Matsubara H, Murohara T et al. Therapeutic angiogenesis for patients with limb ischemia by autologous transplantation of bone marrow cells: a pilot study and a randomised controlled trial. Lancet 2002; 360: 427–35.

14. Carmeliet P. VEGF gene therapy: stimulating angiogenesis or angioma – genes? Nat Med 2000; 6: 1102–3.

15. Salven P, Orpana A, Joensuu H. Leukocytes and platelets of patients with cancer contain high levels of vascular endothelial growth factor. Clin Cancer Res 1999; 5: 487–91.

16. Gaudry M, Bregerie O, Andrieu V et al. Intracellular pool of vascular endothelial growth factor in human neutrophils. Blood 1997; 90: 4153–61.

17. Wartiovaara U, Salven P, Mikkola H et al. Peripheral blood platelets express VEGF-C and VEGF which are released during platelet activation. Thromb Haemost 1998; 80: 171–5.

18. Folkman J, D'Amore PA. Blood vessel formation: what is its molecular basis? Cell 1996; 87: 1153–5.

19. Minamino T, Toko H, Tateno K et al. Peripheral-blood or bone-marrow mononuclear cells for therapeutic angiogenesis. Lancet 2002; 360: 2083–4.

20. Inaba S, Egashira K, Komori K. Peripheral-blood or bone-marrow mononuclear cells for therapeutic angiogenesis. Lancet 2002; 360: 2083–4.

21. Anversa P, Nadal-Ginard B. Myocyte renewal and ventricular remodeling. Nature 2002; 415: 240–3.

22. Makino S, Fukuda K, Miyoshi S et al. Cardiomyoctes can be generated from marrow stromal cells in vitro. J Clin Invest 1999; 103: 697–705.

23. Tse HF, Kwong YL, Chan JKF et al. Angiogenesis in ischaemic myocardium by intramyocardial autologous bone marrow mononuclear cell implantation. Lancet 2003; 361: 47–9.

24. Stamm C, Westphal B, Kleine HD et al. Autologous bone-marrow stem-cell transplantation of myocardial regeneration. Lancet 2003; 361: 45–6.

20. BONE MARROW AND BONE MARROW-DERIVED MONONUCLEAR STEM CELL THERAPY FOR THE CHRONICALLY ISCHEMIC MYOCARDIUM

Ron Waksman and Richard Baffour

Despite recent advances in revascularization interventions (endovascular therapy or surgery), advanced arterial obstructive disease that causes chronic ischemia or acute myocardial infarction is associated with high rates of morbidity and mortality. Cardiac muscle does not have an inherent mechanism for repair and renewal, which according to current paradigms reflects the lack of an organ-specific stem cell able to proliferate along a cardiomyogenic lineage. Scar formation with subsequent congestive heart failure and vulnerability to arrhythmia remain major causes of morbidity and mortality. Myocardial infarction causes irreversible cardiomyocyte injury, which initiates myocardial remodeling that may produce ventricular dilatation and loss of cardiac function. By some means that remain unclear, myocardial infarction causes increased release of bone marrow stem cells into the circulation, and these cells home in on areas of injured tissue. These localized stem cells may then set off repair of the myocardium, but in some patients the number of cells in the injured tissue may not be adequate to prevent cardiovascular events. Clinical evidence suggests that the number of circulating endothelial progenitor cells, presumably from bone marrow, is negatively correlated with combined cardiovascular risk, and also positively correlated with vascular function as measured by flow-mediated brachial artery reactivity in healthy men.[1] The ability to initiate and augment the repair process starting immediately after acute myocardial infarction by in vivo administration of an adequate number of stem cells would be a significant therapeutic advance, since bone marrow and bone marrow-derived stem cells have been shown to differentiate into various phenotypes, including endothelial cells and cardiomyocytes.[2–5]

Optimal angiogenesis and arteriogenesis require expression of multiple growth factors in appropriate sequence and concentration. Such complexity would be impossible to achieve therapeutically by administration of arbitrarily selected individual growth factors. Therefore, it appears unlikely that a single growth factor (either the gene or peptide) given to the patient with myocardial or leg ischemia will optimally increase collateral flow.[6–8] Cultured bone marrow cells or bone marrow-derived stem cells secrete growth factors, including vascular endothelial growth factor (VEGF) and MCP1, and conditioned medium from the cultured cells can cause changes in vitro (endothelial cell proliferation and migration, and tube formation by both endothelial and smooth muscle cells) that, in vivo, would be associated with angiogenesis and arteriogenesis.[9,10] These findings lend mechanistic support to the concept that bone marrow stem cells may offer a unique strategy for therapeutic angiogenesis and arteriogenesis.

Bone marrow and mononuclear bone marrow stem cells

Bone marrow or bone marrow-derived mononuclear stem cells contain hematopoietic and non-hematopoietic cells, which have the potential for self-renewal and differentiation. Hematopoietic stem cells include hemangioblasts and endothelial progenitor cells, and have been shown to play a part in angiogenesis and differentiate into other cell types, including endothelial cells, smooth muscle cells and cardiomyocytes.[3,11–15] The number of hematopoietic stem cells in bone marrow is relatively very low, and for that reason cell culture expansion is required for cell therapy that may be associated with a greater potential for contamination. Non-hematopoietic cells can also differentiate into several cell types such as skeletal and smooth muscle cells, fibroblasts, myoblasts and cardiomyocytes. Because mononuclear bone marrow stem cells contain both hematopoietic and non-hematopoietic cells, it has been suggested that perhaps unfractionated mononuclear bone marrow cells may be more appropriate for cell therapy.[16]

Timing and delivery routes of stem cells in transplantation

Because of inflammatory processes in the myocardial tissues immediately after infarction, early cell therapy may be ineffective. Conversely, late transplantation of cells after scar formation may be similarly ineffective. Therefore, the microenvironment into which cells are injected plays a key role in the subsequent differentiation of the injected cells. For example, bone marrow stromal cells injected into the border area of an infarct differentiate into cardiomyocytes, but similar cells in the scar of an infarct become fibroblasts.[17] The optimal therapeutic window for cell transplantation after myocardial infarction is suggested to be between 3 and 6 days in the clinical situation.[18] There is no evidence that the timing of cell therapy has any influence on the ensuing differentiation of the injected cells in the setting of chronically ischemic and non-infarcted myocardium.

Several delivery routes including intravenous, intracoronary, intrapericardial, intramyocardial and transepicardial have been suggested as methods of cell transplantation delivery. Each one of these routes has potential problems however. For example, intravenous delivery may cause most cells to locate in non-targeted tissues, with much fewer cells in the targeted area. Intracoronary delivery may lead to a substantial number of cells in the targeted tissue, but if it is not done appropriately, most of the injected cells will end up in the systemic circulation. In addition, intracoronary delivery has the potential to cause blockage of capillaries that may exacerbate the ischemic insult if clumps of cells are infused. The problem with intramyocardial delivery is that it remains unclear how the injected cells can gain access to the vasculature of the targeted tissue for dispersion. Transepicardial delivery requires an open heart surgical procedure, which is associated with some risks. Which of these delivery routes for cell transplantation is most safe and effective remains to be determined. It seems that local stem cell delivery using direct intramuscular or intracoronary injection may be more effective than the other routes since stem cells can be targeted to specific areas of damaged myocardium.

Animal studies

Several studies in various animal models suggest that implantation of different types of stem cells including bone marrow, bone marrow-derived mononuclear cells and mesenchymal stem cells, into ischemic or infarcted tissue beds is helpful.[2-5,9,19,20] Unfractionated bone marrow cells injected into damaged muscle differentiate into myocytes, which then form part of the regenerated cardiac fibers.[2] Autologous bone marrow cells, when injected transendocardially into ischemic porcine myocardium, increase collateral flow and myocardial function.[9] Similarly, transplantation of mononuclear bone marrow cells in a porcine model of acute myocardial infarction has been shown to enhance collateral perfusion and regional function.[19] Mesenchymal stem cells, when injected into myocardium, express muscle protein and may attenuate contractile dysfunction.[20] Side-population cells (a subset of

291

hematopoietic stem cells), when injected into lethally irradiated mice and followed by acute coronary artery occlusion and reperfusion, have been shown to be incorporated into both regenerating endothelial cells and cardiomyocytes.[21] This implies that circulating stem cells may play a part in the repair of damaged tissues.

Clinical experiences

In a pilot study at the Washington Hospital Center, Fuchs et al evaluated the feasibility of transendocardial delivery of autologous bone marrow in patients with severe symptomatic chronic myocardial ischemia not amenable to conventional revascularization.[22] Ten patients received transendocardial injections of freshly aspirated and filtered unfractionated autologous bone marrow (Figure 20.1). These injections were delivered into ischemic, non-infarcted myocardium pre-identified by SPECT perfusion imaging. In these patients, there were no serious adverse effects including arrhythmia, infection, myocardial inflammation or increased scar. At 3-month follow-up, the patients showed significant improvement as measured by Canadian Cardiovascular Society angina score. There was a trend towards increased treadmill exercise duration in nine patients whose data were available. This investigation was limited to a small cohort of patients and lacked a control group. Nevertheless, the study demonstrated the feasibility of transendocardial delivery of autologous bone marrow to ischemic myocardium. Other studies have also shown that bone marrow-derived stem cells can improve function and perfusion in cardiac injury.[18,23–25] Strauer et al treated patients with myocardial infarction by intracoronary transplantation of autologous mononuclear bone marrow as an adjunct to standard endovascular therapy.[23] Five to 9 days after standard therapy, 10 patients received these cells in their infarcted area during brief periods (3 min) of intermittent balloon dilatation to facilitate adhesion and subsequent migration of the injected cells. A control group ($n = 10$) had undergone prior standard therapy as well, but no subsequent cell treatment. At 3-month follow-up, the autologous mononuclear bone marrow cell-treated group showed significant improvement as measured by infarct size, infarction wall movement, stroke volume index and myocardial perfusion compared with the control group.

These clinical studies showed the safety and feasibility of various cell therapies. None of the studies conclusively shows the efficacious nature of such a treatment, let alone suggesting the mechanisms by which this therapy improves healing. Then again, gaining mechanistic insights into such therapy

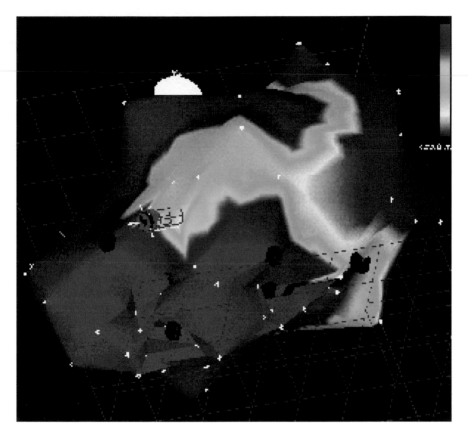

Figure 20.1 *Injections of bone marrow via NOGA mapping labeled as black dots.*

may be impossible to accomplish in the clinical setting.

Other cells used in stem cell therapy are myoblasts, which have been shown in both animal and human studies to improve heart function following cardiac injury.[26–29] However, myoblast transplantation has been shown to cause arrhythmias in some patients.[29]

Conclusion

Although stem cell therapy has been shown to be safe and feasible in both animal and human studies, the efficacy and the mechanisms by which this therapy improves healing after ischemic injury remain unexplored. Other unanswered questions are as follows. Which stem cells (e.g. unfractionated bone marrow, bone marrow-derived mononuclear or any of the multiple subpopulations of the latter) will produce an optimal therapeutic effect in damaged myocardium? What is the optimal delivery approach (e.g. intravenous, intracoronary, intramyocardial or transepicardial)? What is the optimal dosage and timing of the administration of cell therapy? What is the durability of any observed functional improvements as well as the long-term effects of cell therapy? Answers to these questions may require additional animal studies.

It has been suggested that stem cell therapy after myocardial infarction may be more appropriate since stem cells have the potential to secrete growth factors, which can enhance tissue perfusion and myocardial remodeling. On the other hand, myoblast therapy may be better in the setting of chronic ischemia. A combination of stem cell and myoblast therapy, sequentially or in concert to achieve more effective therapy, may be needed depending on the stage and the associated symptoms of myocardial disease.

Carefully planned randomized, double-blind, placebo-controlled clinical trials with appropriate endpoints must be completed to determine the effectiveness of stem cell or myoblast therapy. Much still needs to be learned before cell transplantation in damaged myocardium becomes successful in patients.

References

1. Hill JM, Zalos G, Halcox JPJ et al. Circulating endothelial progenitor cells, vascular function, and cardiovascular risk. N Engl J Med 2003; 348: 593–600.

2. Ferrari G, Cusella-De Angelis G, Coletta M et al. Muscle regeneration by bone marrow-derived myogenic progenitors. Science 1998; 279: 1528–30.

3. Orlic D, Kajstura J, Chimenti S et al. Bone marrow cells regenerate infarcted myocardium. Nature 2001; 410: 701–5.

4. Orlic D, Kajstura J, Chimenti S et al. Mobilized bone marrow cells repair the infarcted heart, improving function and survival. Proc Natl Acad Sci USA 2001; 98: 10344–9.

5. Kamihata H, Matsubara H, Nishiue T et al. Implantation of bone marrow mononuclear cells into ischemic myocardium enhances collateral perfusion and regional function via side supply of angioblasts, angiogenic ligands, and cytokines. Circulation 2001; 104: 1046–52.

6. Helisch A, Schaper W. Angiogenesis and arteriogenesis – not yet for prescription. Z Kardiol 2000; 89: 239–44.

7. Epstein SE, Fuchs S, Zhou YF et al. Therapeutic interventions for enhancing collateral development by administration of growth factors: basic principles, early results and potential hazards. Cardiovasc Res 2001; 49: 532–42.

8. Folkman J. Angiogenic therapy of the human heart. Circulation 1998; 97: 628–9.

9. Fuchs S, Baffour R, Zhou YF et al. Transendocardial delivery of autologous bone marrow enhances collateral perfusion and regional function in pigs with chronic experimental myocardial ischemia. J Am Coll Cardiol 2001; 37: 1726–32.

10. Baffour R, Zhou YF, Fuchs S et al. Bone marrow-induced stimulation of endothelial and smooth muscle cell proliferation, migration, tube formation, and production of growth factors. J Am Coll Cardiol 2001; 37(suppl A): 232A (abstract).

11. Kocher AA, Schuster MD, Szabolcs MJ et al. Neovascularization of ischemic myocardium by human bone-marrow-derived angioblasts prevents cardiomyocyte apoptosis, reduces remodeling and improves cardiac function. Nat Med 2001; 7(4): 430–6.

12. Goodell MA, Jackson KA, Majka SM et al. Stem cell plasticity in muscle and bone marrow. Ann NY Acad Sci 2001; 938: 208–18.

13. Krause DS, Theise ND, Collector MI et al. Multi-organ, multi-lineage engraftment by a single bone marrow-derived stem cell. Cell 2001; 105: 369–77.

14. Orlic D, Kajstura J, Chimenti S et al. Transplanted adult bone marrow cells repair myocardial infarcts in mice. Ann NY Acad Sci 2001; 938: 221–9; discussion 229–30.

15. Reyes M, Lund T, Lenvik T et al. Purification and ex vivo expansion of postnatal human marrow mesodermal progenitor cells. Blood 2001; 98: 2615–25.

16. Brehm M, Zeus T, Strauer BE. Stem cells – clinical application and perspectives. Herz 2002; 27(7): 611–20.

17. Wang JS, Shum-Tim D, Chedrawy E, Chiu RC. The coronary delivery of marrow stromal cells for myocardial regeneration: pathophysiologic and therapeutic implications. J Thorac Cardiovasc Surg 2001; 122: 699–705.

18. Assmus B, Schachinger V, Teupe C et al. Transplantation of progenitor cells and regeneration enhancement in acute myocardial infarction (TOPCARE-AMI). Circulation 2002; 106: 3009–17.

19. Kamihata H, Matsubara H, Nishiue T et al. Implantation of bone marrow mononuclear cells into ischemic myocardium enhances collateral perfusion and regional function via side supply of angioblasts, angiogenic ligands, and cytokines. Circulation 2001; 104(9): 1046–52.

20. Shake JG, Gruber PJ, Baumgartner WA et al. Mesenchymal stem cell implantation in a swine myocardial infarct model: engraftment and functional effects. Ann Thorac Surg 2002; 73: 1919–25.

21. Jackson KA, Majka SM, Wang H et al. Regeneration of ischemic cardiac muscle and vascular endothelium by adult stem cells. J Clin Invest 2001; 107: 1395–402.

22. Fuchs S, Satler L, Kornowski R et al. Catheter-based autologous bone marrow myocardial injection in no-option patients with advanced coronary artery disease – a feasibility study. J Am Coll Cardiol 2003; 41: 1721–4.

23. Strauer BE, Brehm M, Zeus T et al. Repair of infarcted myocardium by autologous intracoronary mononuclear bone marrow cell transplantation in humans. Circulation 2002; 106: 1913–18.

24. Stamm C, Westphal B, Kleine HD et al. Autologous bone-marrow stem-cell transplantation for myocardial regeneration. Lancet 2003; 361: 45–6.

25. Tse HF, Kwong YL, Chan KF et al. Angiogenesis in ischaemic myocardium by intramyocardial autologous bone marrow mononuclear cell transplantation. Lancet 2003; 361: 47–9.

26. Taylor DA, Atkins BZ, Hungspreugs P et al. Regenerating functional myocardium: improved performance after skeletal myoblast transplantation. Nat Med 1998; 4: 929–33.

27. Murry CE, Wiseman RW, Schwartz SM, Hauschka SD. Skeletal myoblast transplantation for repair of myocardial necrosis. J Clin Invest 1996; 98: 2512–23.

28. Menasche P, Hagege AA, Scorsin M et al. Myoblast transplantation for heart failure. Lancet 2001; 27(357): 279–80.

29. Menasche P. Myoblast transplantation: feasibility, safety and efficacy. Ann Med 2002; 34: 314–15.

21. CELL TRANSPLANTATION: FIRST US CLINICAL EXPERIENCE

Marc S Penn and Patrick M McCarthy

Differentiated cell-based therapy

Acute myocardial infarction (MI) remains a leading cause of morbidity and mortality in Western countries, and over 10% of the US population over 65 years of age has been diagnosed with congestive heart failure. In an attempt to develop novel therapeutic strategies to improve outcomes in patients with ischemic heart disease, investigators have assessed the role of autologous cell transplantation using differentiated cells,[1] including smooth muscle cells, skeletal myoblasts, cardiac fibroblasts and other cell types.[2-6] The goal of this approach is to replace dead scarred tissue with living cells. The majority of work to date has focused on the use of skeletal myoblasts. While the majority of this preclinical work was done prior to complete remodeling of the left ventricle following MI (mostly within 4 weeks of MI), there is also hope that skeletal myoblast transplantation will benefit clinical populations, even at times remote from MI.[7,8] This approach has demonstrated efficacy and safety in animal models and is now under investigation in clinical populations.[8]

The mechanism of functional left ventricular (LV) improvement with skeletal myoblast transplantation is not clear and is still under investigation. Transplanted skeletal myoblasts do not result in the development of new cardiac myocytes, and the transplanted cells do not integrate into the electrical syncytium of the myocardium.[9] Increases in LV ejection fraction with the introduction of skeletal myoblasts into the infarct zone are modest.[2,10-12] However, the improvement in systolic function combined with the improvements in diastolic function that have been demonstrated ultimately appear to lead to overall improved cardiac performance.[13,14]

Cell transplantation: first in man trial in the USA

The first in man US trial of skeletal myoblast transplantation was sponsored by and performed in collaboration with Diacrin Inc. This study was a phase 1 trial designed to study intracardiac injection of autologous skeletal myoblasts into transmural scar in patients undergoing coronary artery bypass grafting (CABG). The goals of the trial were to establish safety and feasibility data.

The trial was designed with escalating doses of skeletal myoblasts, starting with 10 million cells, with a maximum dose of 300 million cells. While efficacy with respect to recovery of myocardial function and perfusion was measured, it was not a predefined primary endpoint of the study.

Study design

This study was an open-label, non-randomized, multicenter pilot study. The centers in the USA include the Cleveland Clinic Foundation, University of California, Los Angeles, Arizona Heart Institute and Ohio State University. All the patients had MI at some time, often years, prior to surgery that resulted in transmyocardial scar and LV dysfunction. The patients screened for this study included those requiring elective CABG surgery, and who could wait the required time for myoblast expansion prior to open heart surgery. Initially, those requiring other surgical procedures, such as ventricle reduction/remodeling surgery, AICD placement or valvular surgery, were excluded (Table 21.1).

Study protocol

Baseline evaluations
- ECG
- 24-h Holter monitoring: done twice prior to skeletal myoblast transplantation
- Studies within 3 weeks prior to CABG: echocardiography; magnetic resonance imaging (MRI); PET or SPECT perfusion scan.

Source of skeletal muscle biopsy
Approximately 5 weeks prior to surgery, a skeletal muscle biopsy was obtained from the arm or leg. The goal of the biopsy was to obtain a 5-g piece of muscle, from which autologous myoblasts were generated. The biopsies were then transported to the Diacrin facility for cell isolation and expansion.

Cell dosage
Expanded myoblasts were shipped to the clinical site at a concentration of no more than 1.6×10^8 cells/ml, so that up to 32 injections of 60–100 µl each were required to deliver the highest planned dose of 300 million cells.

Transplantation procedure
The goal of the study was to inject cells in the target infarct zone that was determined prior to surgery and based on a baseline MRI evaluation of the left ventricle. Each surgeon was supplied with a diagram of the target injection area. Ideally, injections were equally spaced along a linear array pattern. The pattern was designed so that the entire area of the target infarct zone was covered by injections. Skeletal myoblast transplantation was

298

performed after completion of CABG, and was done either on or off cardiac bypass, at the discretion of the surgeon. The goal was to perform a slow injection in the target infarct region. The injection needle was kept in place for up to 15 s after each injection in order to minimize reflux of cells out of the injection track.

Follow-up

Timing

Follow-up began the day following skeletal myoblast transplantation and continued daily until hospital discharge. Follow-up then occurred 1, 2, 3, 6, 9 and 12 weeks and 6, 9, 12, 18 and 24 months post-transplantation. Specific adverse events that were of concern in the periprocedural period included arrhythmias, ventricular fibrillation during the surgery and injection of the cells, bleeding from the injection sites and infection.

Studies

Primary safety endpoints were determined by physical examination, ECG, Holter monitor and blood tests (Table 21.2). The recovery of myocardial function and perfusion was determined by echocardiography, MRI and PET/SPECT (Table 21.2). It is important to remember that all patients received CABG along with skeletal myoblast transplantation; therefore, based on study design, it is difficult to separate out the efficacy of skeletal myoblast transplantation from CABG.

Table 21.1 Study design

Population	Post-MI with LV dysfunction and undergoing surgical revascularization
Design	Open-label, non-randomized, dose-escalating study; 10 to 300 million total cells injected via multiple injections of ~10 million cells/injection
Cell type studied	Autologous skeletal myoblasts
Endpoint	Two-year follow-up or cardiac transplantation
Primary goal	Safety and efficacy of skeletal myoblast transplantation in patients undergoing CABG
Secondary goal	Begin to accrue data on myocardial response to skeletal myoblast transplantation
Injection site	Transmural myocardial scar
Follow-up	Two years
Measures used:	In all patients, survival, echocardiography, MRI and/or PET. For those patients who went on to cardiac transplantation: immunohistochemistry to identify engrafted cells

MI, myocardial infarction; LV, left ventricular; CABG, coronary artery bypass grafting.

Table 21.2 Follow-up tests and schedule

Test or procedure	Follow-up Visit windows: weekly visits (±3 days); monthly visits (±7 days)													
	D1	D2–6	W1	W2	W3	W6	W9	W12	M6	M9	M12	M18	M24
Physical examination	X		X	X	X	X	X	X	X	X	X	X	X
ECG	X	X	X	X	X	X	X	X	X	X	X	X	X
Echocardiography		X		X	X	X	X	X		X	X		X
24 h Holter		X		X				X		X			X
MRI			X			X	X		X	X			
PET/SPECT scan								X					

Study

To date, 12 patients have been enrolled in the trial. Follow-up is not yet complete for any of the enrolled patients. The demographics of these patients are shown in Table 21.3. The average age of the population treated and being actively followed was 55 years (range: 33–75 years) with an average ejection fraction of 23% (range: 17–32%). The dose of cells delivered was increased after every three patients. The initial dose was 10 million cells, and the dose was escalated during the study to 30 million, 100 million and 300 million cells. The percentage of viable cells injected was 92% ± 3% with, on average, 76% ± 18% of the cells injected being skeletal myoblasts. There was no significant difference in the percentage of viable cells or percentage of skeletal myoblasts between the different doses. An additional six patients were enrolled and underwent skeletal myoblast transplantation at the time of LV assist device (LVAD) placement as part of a separate study.

The study was initially designed to exclude patients undergoing left ventricular remodeling (LVR) surgery; following Diacrin approval, two patients had LVR at the time of CABG and skeletal myoblast transplantation. Patients who received 10 million or 30 million cells all received three injections each, whereas patients who received 100 million or 300 million cells received 10 and 30 injections each, respectively. No procedure-related adverse events, including ventricular fibrillation, ventricular tachycardia, infection or bleeding from the injection sites, were observed in any of the patients studied to date.

As discussed above, it is difficult to assess the efficacy of skeletal myoblast transplantation in this population, since all patients received CABG. One

300

Table 21.3 Patient demographics

	Age (year) at transplantation	% Transmural scar	% Hibernating tissue	Baseline EF (%)
1	61	40–45	<20	19
2	52	45	15	25
3	56	45	<5	15
4	33	40	<5	15
5	63	?	Significant	27
6	69	?	Significant	27.5
7	75	30–40	<5	17
8	53	30–40	<5	20
9	54	?	Significant	32
10	58	30–40	10	28
11	45	20–30	<5	25
12	47	20–30	<5	28
Average	55±11			23±6

EF, ejection fraction.

could hypothesize that the increased improvement in cardiac function in the patients who received larger doses (100 million or 300 million cells) of skeletal myoblasts compared to those who received small doses (10 million or 30 million cells) could represent efficacy of skeletal myoblast transplantation. However, such an analysis is difficult, due to the small number of patients in this trial, as well as the fact that the analysis is premature, due to the limited follow-up available to date for those patients who received large doses of skeletal myoblasts. Figure 21.1 depicts all follow-up ejection fractions as measured by echocardiography at baseline, 6 weeks and 6 and 12 months that were available as of spring 2003. Those patients who received concomitant LVR[15] at the time of skeletal myoblast transplantation are identified by an asterisk in the legend.

As mentioned above, an additional six patients received skeletal myoblast transplantation at the time of LVAD implantation. Of these, to date, five have had their LVAD explanted and immunohistochemistry performed on the explanted heart to identify the presence of engrafted skeletal myoblasts. Of

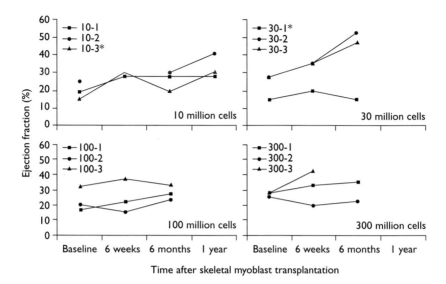

Figure 21.1 *Baseline and follow-up ejection fractions as measured by echocardiography at 6 weeks, 6 months and 1 year after skeletal myoblast transplantation. Patients are stratified by the dose of skeletal myoblasts that they received. *Patients who also underwent a left ventricular remodeling procedure at the time of skeletal myoblast transplantation.*

the three patients who received 300 million cells, evidence of the presence of skeletal myoblast engraftment was found at 5 days and 3, 4 and 6 months after skeletal myoblast transplantation. In the one patient who received 2.2 million cells, perhaps not surprisingly, no evidence of skeletal myoblast engraftment was found. Further details of the findings in these patients have recently been reported.[16]

Summary

The first in man study of skeletal myoblast transplantation in the USA has demonstrated short-term safety and feasibility in a population of patients who are relatively young (mean age 55 years) and with significant LV dysfunction (mean ejection fraction of 23%). Importantly, at least for a dose up to 300 million cells, skeletal myoblast transplantation does not appear to be arrhythmogenic. While this is obviously an important concern, recent studies would indicate that virtually all the patients enrolled in this trial would be eligible for and benefit from implantation of internal cardiac defibrillators.[17] A great deal of data related to the potential efficacy of skeletal myoblast transplantation is yet to be derived from these patients. While these analyses will undoubtedly be hindered due to the small number of patients in this phase 1 trial, the unqualified success of this study with respect to feasibility and safety supports future phase 2 trials in which efficacy can be a primary endpoint.

References

1. Penn MS, Francis GS, Ellis SG et al. Autologous cell therapy for the treatment of damaged myocardium. Prog Cardiovasc Dis 2002; 45: 21–32.

2. Scorsin M, Hagege A, Vilquin JT et al. Comparison of the effects of fetal cardiomyocyte and skeletal myoblast transplantation on postinfarction left ventricular function. J Thorac Cardiovasc Surg 2000; 119(6): 1169–75.

3. Etzion S, Battler A, Barbash IM et al. Influence of embryonic cardiomyocyte transplantation on the progression of heart failure in a rat model of extensive myocardial infarction. J Mol Cell Cardiol 2001; 33(7): 1321–30.

4. Taylor DA, Atkins BZ, Hungspreugs P et al. Regenerating functional myocardium: improved performance after skeletal myoblast transplantation. Nat Med 1998; 4(8): 929–33.

5. Askari AT, Unzek S, Popovic ZB et al. Effect of stromal-cell-derived factor-1 on stem cell homing and tissue regeneration in ischaemic cardiomyopathy. Lancet 362: 697–703, 2003.

6. Leor J, Patterson M, Quinones MJ et al. Transplantation of fetal myocardial tissue into the infarcted myocardium of rat. A potential method for repair of infarcted myocardium? Circulation 1996; 94(9 suppl): II-332–6.

7. Ngo TH, Hoylaerts MF, Knockaert I et al. Identification of a target site in plasminogen activator inhibitor-1 that allows neutralization of its inhibitor properties concomitant with an allosteric up-regulation of its antiadhesive properties. J Biol Chem 2001; 276(28): 26243–8.

8. Menasche P, Hagege AA, Scorsin M et al. Myoblast transplantation for heart failure. Lancet 2001; 357(9252): 279–80.

9. Murry CE, Wiseman RW, Schwartz SM, Hauschka SD. Skeletal myoblast transplantation for repair of myocardial necrosis. J Clin Invest 1996; 98(11): 2512–23.

10. Li RK, Jia ZQ, Weisel RD et al. Smooth muscle cell transplantation into myocardial scar tissue improves heart function. J Mol Cell Cardiol 1999; 31(3): 513–22.

11. Jain M, DerSimonian H, Brenner DA et al. Cell therapy attenuates deleterious ventricular remodeling and improves cardiac performance after myocardial infarction. Circulation 2001; 103(14): 1920–7.

12. Rajnoch C, Chachques JC, Berrebi A et al. Cellular therapy reverses myocardial dysfunction. J Thorac Cardiovasc Surg 2001; 121(5): 871–8.

13. Atkins BZ, Hueman MT, Meuchel JM et al. Myogenic cell transplantation improves in vivo regional performance in infarcted rabbit myocardium. J Heart Lung Transplant 1999; 18(12): 1173–80.

14. Atkins BZ, Hueman MT, Meuchel J et al. Cellular cardiomyoplasty improves diastolic properties of injured heart. J Surg Res 1999; 85(2): 234–42.

15. Franco-Cereceda A, McCarthy PM, Blackstone EH et al. Partial left ventriculectomy for dilated cardiomyopathy: is this an alternative to transplantation? J Thorac Cardiovasc Surg 2001; 121(5): 879–93.

16. Pagani FD, DerSimonian H, Zawadzka A et al. Autologous skeletal myoblasts transplanted to ischemia-damaged myocardium in humans. Histological analysis of cell survival and differentiation. J Am Coll Cardiol 2003; 41(5): 879–88.

17. Moss AJ, Zareba W, Hall WJ et al. Prophylactic implantation of a defibrillator in patients with myocardial infarction and reduced ejection fraction. N Engl J Med 2002; 346(12): 877–83.

22. ADIPOSE STROMAL CELL THERAPY FOR CARDIOVASCULAR DISEASE

Jalees Rehman and Keith L March

Cell transplantation for therapeutic angiogenesis

Coronary artery disease (CAD) is a major cause of morbidity and mortality, requiring bypass surgery or angioplasty in almost 1 000 000 patients/year in the USA. While some of these patients form collateral vessels as alternative pathways for blood supply, thus ameliorating or preventing ischemic myocardial damage, many are not able to develop adequate vascular networks to compensate for the loss of the original blood supply. Accordingly, many patients could be helped by the development of practical approaches that would accelerate the natural processes of postnatal collateral vessel formation. Such approaches are broadly referred to as 'therapeutic angiogenesis', and encompass both angiogenesis (which, strictly speaking, refers to capillary sprouting) and arteriogenesis (the maturation and enlargement of existing vessels).[1,2] Within this chapter, angiogenesis is used in the broad sense to refer to collateral vessel formation at all stages.

An emerging therapeutic approach is the use of stem and progenitor cell transplantation to improve angiogenesis. Endothelial progenitor cells (EPCs) are cells present in bone marrow or peripheral blood which co-express stem and progenitor cell markers such as CD34 or AC133 as well as endothelial markers such as VE-cadherin and vascular endothelial growth factor (VEGF)-receptor-2 (KDR).[3] EPCs and hematopoietic stem cells (HSCs) are thought to be derived from a common 'hemangioblast' precursor.[4–6] Interestingly, the cell surface marker CD34 is only found on either hematopoietic stem/progenitor cells or endothelial cells,[3] which may be a reflection of the common origin of these two cell lineages. In addition to the shared 'hemangioblastic' ancestry between HSCs and endothelial cells, HSCs have also been suggested to transdifferentiate into either endothelial progenitor cells or mature endothelial cells.[7–9] The recent discovery of circulating smooth muscle progenitor cells and the potential of HSCs to differentiate into smooth muscle cells[10,11] suggests yet another novel and intriguing link between the hematopoietic and vascular cell lineages, now in the context of smooth muscle cells.

Animal studies using hindlimb ischemia or myocardial ischemia models in immunodeficient rodents have demonstrated that transplantation of about 10^6 peripheral blood-derived EPCs[12,13] can result in increased angiogenesis. Remarkably, labeled peripheral blood-derived EPCs appear to home preferentially to ischemic areas and incorporate into foci of neovascularization.[12,13] In addition to the above-mentioned studies on peripheral blood-derived cells, EPCs derived from bone marrow, unpurified bone marrow mononuclear cells and HSCs have also been shown to enhance angiogenesis or show endothelial differentiation in vivo in a variety of animal models of ischemia.[14–19]

While the concept of using autologous peripheral blood-derived EPCs in patients seems attractive, based on animal studies, one would need 12 liters of blood from a patient to isolate enough cells to achieve a pro-angiogenic effect.[20] This amount of blood is not readily available in a clinical setting. Human studies that have used bone marrow cell transplantation in ischemic patients[21,22] suggest that human angiogenic cell therapy requires at least cell numbers of $10^7–10^9$, depending on the degree of stem cell purity as well as the optimal delivery method.

Pluripotency of adipose stromal cells

The discovery of pluripotent cells in the adipose tissue[23] has revealed a novel source of cells that may be used for autologous cell therapy to regenerate tissue. These pluripotent cells are found in the 'stromal' or 'non-adipocyte' fraction of the adipose tissue. Adipose stromal cells (ASCs) primarily consist of microvascular endothelial cells,[24] but this cell fraction also contains smooth muscle-like cells and pre-adipocytes. It is not yet known whether each of these ASC subsets possesses pluripotentiality, but multiple studies have confirmed a wide differentiation potential for the total ASC fraction. Zuk et al were able to establish the differentiation of such subcutaneous human ASCs in vitro into adipocytes, chondrocytes and myocytes.[23] These findings were extended in a study by Erickson et al, which showed that human ASCs could differentiate in vivo into chondrocytes[25] following transplantation into immunodeficient mice. More recently, it was demonstrated that human ASCs were able to differentiate into neuronal cells.[26] The key benefits of using pluripotent ASCs for autologous cell therapy are the ease with which they can be isolated and their relative abundance. Approximately $10^5–10^6$ cells can be isolated from 5–10 g of subcutaneous tissue. Considering that the simple outpatient procedure of liposuction can often yield 1 liter of fat tissue even in non-obese patients, $10^8–10^9$ ASCs can be isolated from an individual with little or no expansion.

Adipose stromal cells for cardiovascular cell therapy

The need for large numbers of autologous cells for multiple cardiovascular applications has led to the investigation of the therapeutic potential of autologous ASCs in the setting of cardiovascular disease. Several such studies focused on using the endothelial fraction of ASCs. For example, coating of stents with the microvascular endothelial cell fraction of ASCs has been shown to improve stent patency in an animal model.[27] ASC pluripotency and other aspects of ASC function have opened new avenues for cardiovascular applications of ASCs. Our preliminary data suggest that ASC transplantation can augment angiogenesis in the setting of ischemia, possibly by supplying additional endothelial cells or smooth muscle-like cells resident in the ASC fraction and also by ASC secretion of angiogenic growth factors.[28] Furthermore, ASCs also appear to have the potential of differentiating into cardiomyocytes and may thus have a role in treating cardiomyopathies. Recent experiments have also demonstrated that ASCs can be successfully transfected with mammalian expression plasmids (Rehman and March, unpublished results).

Conclusion

Cardiovascular cell therapy ideally requires large numbers of cells to improve neovascularization and replace damaged tissue. Subcutaneous adipose tissue may be able to provide the required number of autologous ASCs, probably containing a mixture of pluripotent and lineage-committed cells. Recent data suggest that these cells have significant therapeutic potential for patients with cardiovascular disease.

References

1.   Isner JM, Asahara T. Angiogenesis and vasculogenesis as therapeutic strategies for postnatal neovascularization. J Clin Invest 1999; 103: 1231–6.

2.   van Royen N, Piek JJ, Buschmann I et al. Stimulation of arteriogenesis; a new concept for the treatment of arterial occlusive disease. Cardiovasc Res 2001; 49: 543–53.

3.   Rafii S. Circulating endothelial precursors: mystery, reality, and promise. J Clin Invest 2000; 105: 17–19.

4.   Ribatti D, Vacca A, Roncali L, Dammacco F. Hematopoiesis and angiogenesis: a link between two apparently independent processes. J Hematother Stem Cell Res 2000; 9: 13–19.

5. Choi K. The hemangioblast: a common progenitor of hematopoietic and endothelial cells. J Hematother Stem Cell Res 2002; 11: 91–101.

6. Eichmann A, Pardanaud L, Yuan L, Moyon D. Vasculogenesis and the search for the hemangioblast. J Hematother Stem Cell Res 2002; 11: 207–14.

7. Kang HJ, Kim SC, Kim YJ et al. Short-term phytohaemagglutinin-activated mononuclear cells induce endothelial progenitor cells from cord blood CD34+ cells. Br J Haematol 2001; 113: 962–9.

8. Quirici N, Soligo D, Caneva L et al. Differentiation and expansion of endothelial cells from human bone marrow CD133(+) cells. Br J Haematol 2001; 115: 186–94.

9. Gehling UM, Ergun S, Schumacher U et al. In vitro differentiation of endothelial cells from AC133-positive progenitor cells. Blood 2000; 3106–12.

10. Sata M, Saiura A, Kunisato A et al. Hematopoietic stem cells differentiate into vascular cells that participate in the pathogenesis of atherosclerosis. Nat Med 2002; 8: 403–9.

11. Simper D, Stalboerger PG, Panetta CJ et al. Smooth muscle progenitor cells in human blood. Circulation 2002; 106: 1199–204.

12. Kawamoto A, Gwon HC, Iwaguro H et al. Therapeutic potential of ex vivo expanded endothelial progenitor cells for myocardial ischemia. Circulation 2001; 103: 634–7.

13. Kalka C, Masuda H, Takahashi T et al. Transplantation of ex vivo expanded endothelial progenitor cells for therapeutic neovascularization. Proc Natl Acad Sci USA 2000; 97: 3422–7.

14. Kocher AA, Schuster MD, Szabolcs MJ et al. Neovascularization of ischemic myocardium by human bone-marrow-derived angioblasts prevents cardiomyocyte apoptosis, reduces remodeling and improves cardiac function. Nat Med 2001; 7: 430–6.

15. Shintani S, Murohara T, Ikeda H et al. Augmentation of postnatal neovascularization with autologous bone marrow transplantation. Circulation 2001; 103: 897–903.

16. Fuchs S, Baffour R, Zhou YF et al. Transendocardial delivery of autologous bone marrow enhances collateral perfusion and regional function in pigs with chronic experimental myocardial ischemia. J Am Coll Cardiol 2001; 37: 1726–32.

17. Kamihata H, Matsubara H, Nishiue T et al. Implantation of bone marrow mononuclear cells into ischemic myocardium enhances collateral perfusion and regional function via side supply of angioblasts, angiogenic ligands, and cytokines. Circulation 2001; 104: 1046–52.

18. Orlic D, Kajstura J, Chimenti S et al. Mobilized bone marrow cells repair the infarcted heart, improving function and survival. Proc Natl Acad Sci USA 2001; 98: 10344–9.

19. Jackson KA, Majka SM, Wang H et al. Regeneration of ischemic cardiac muscle and vascular endothelium by adult stem cells. J Clin Invest 2001; 107: 1395–402.

20. Iwaguro H, Yamaguchi J, Kalka C et al. Endothelial progenitor cell vascular endothelial growth factor gene transfer for vascular regeneration. Circulation 2002; 105: 732–8.

21. Strauer BE, Brehm M, Zeus T et al. Intracoronary, human autologous stem cell transplantation for myocardial regeneration following myocardial infarction. Dtsch Med Wochenschr 2001;126: 932–8.

22. Tateishi-Yuyama E, Matsubara H, Murohara T et al. Therapeutic angiogenesis for patients with limb ischaemia by autologous transplantation of bone-marrow cells: a pilot study and a randomised controlled trial. Lancet 2002; 360: 427–35.

23. Zuk PA, Zhu M, Mizuno H et al. Multilineage cells from human adipose tissue: implications for cell-based therapies. Tissue Engineering 2001; 7: 211–28.

24. Williams SK, Wang TF, Castrillo R, Jarrell BE. Liposuction-derived human fat used for vascular graft sodding contains endothelial cells and not mesothelial cells as the major cell type. J Vasc Surg 1994; 19: 916–23.

25. Erickson GR, Gimble JM, Franklin DM et al. Chondrogenic potential of adipose tissue-derived stromal cells in vitro and in vivo. Biochem Biophys Res Commun 2002; 290: 763–9.

26. Safford KM, Hicok KC, Safford SD et al. Neurogenic differentiation of murine and human adipose-derived stromal cells. Biochem Biophys Res Commun 2002; 294: 371–9.

27. Williams SK, Rose DG, Jarrell BE. Microvascular endothelial cell sodding of ePTFE vascular grafts: improved patency and stability of the cellular lining. J Biomed Mater Res 1994; 28: 203–12.

28. Rehman J, Li J, Williams CA et al. Human adipose stromal cells express the angiogenic factor VEGF and its receptor VEGFR-2. Arteriosclerosis Thrombosis and Vascular Biology (online abstract supplement for the 3rd Annual Conference on Arteriosclerosis, Thrombosis and Vascular Biology) 2002; 22: 878–a819.

23. Intramyocardial Gene and Cellular Delivery for Myocardial Angiogenesis and Regeneration

Ran Kornowski

Gene transfer for myocardial angiogenesis

Direct transfer of genes holds promise for the sustained delivery of therapeutic proteins to treat cardiovascular diseases. This can be accomplished by several approaches, including use of adenoviral vectors and naked plasmid DNA vectors.[1] Animal studies have shown the feasibility of enhancing collateral perfusion and function by direct intramyocardial delivery of angiogenic factors injected into the myocardium.[2] There is a theoretical advantage of direct intramyocardial injection of the therapeutic agent versus its infusion into the coronary arteries. During intracoronary injection, a significant amount of the drug may not be taken up by the myocardium and therefore will be delivered to systemic organs. With direct intramyocardial injection, it is more likely that less of the drug will be delivered systemically. This mode of delivery would therefore: (1) limit exposure to non-target organs; (2) minimize the likelihood of systemic toxicity and adverse hemodynamic effects; (3) enable high intramyocardial concentration while limiting total dose; and (4) allow precise localization to ischemic and peri-ischemic myocardial regions.

The intramyocardial injection approach has been used successfully in experimental models of chronic ischemia using an adenoviral vector containing the vascular endothelial growth factor transgene (Ad.VEGF121), which was directly injected into ischemic myocardium during open chest thoracotomy.[3] Several trials employed intramyocardial injection of angiogenic proteins,[4] naked DNA (VEGF165 transgene) via a minimally invasive chest wall incision,[5] or Ad.VEGF121 administered during conventional bypass surgery and Ad.VEGF121 administered as 'sole' treatment.[6] These experiences have demonstrated the safety and feasibility characteristics of the angiogenic gene delivery approach. In addition, preliminary results suggest that improved myocardial perfusion and function have been obtained in response to surgical-based intramyocardial angiogenic gene transfer.[7,8]

311

Transendocardial gene delivery in experimental models

Although of potential clinical importance, the practical application of the surgical transepicardial strategy for therapeutic angiogenesis is clearly limited, due to the risks and expenses incurred by the invasive nature of the procedure. The goal of catheter-based intramyocardial injection is to achieve a comparable effect to that achieved by transepicardial injection during thoracotomy. The catheter-based approach may be equally effective as surgery without the need for a thoracotomy and general anesthesia. In addition, it enables access to areas not approachable with surgical approaches (e.g. the ventricular septum and the posterior wall) and, because it is considerably less invasive, provides opportunities for multiple treatment sessions. The feasibility of various catheter-based systems for percutaneous intramyocardial injection of marker and angiogenic transgenes has been demonstrated primarily in animal models.[9–13]

The potential advantage of catheter-based injection using a left ventricular mapping system for guidance is that it allows precise localization of gene transfer directed towards ischemic myocardial regions while avoiding multiple same-site injections and also injections into infarct regions[12] (Figure 23.1). In one study,[13] successful gene delivery (calculated per injection site and

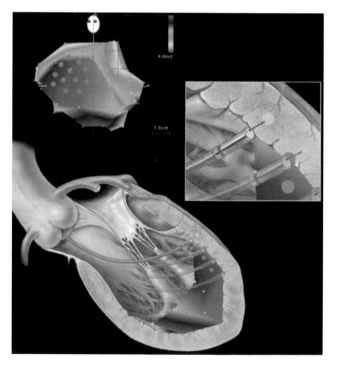

Figure 23.1

Schematic illustration of catheter-based intramyocardial delivery of therapeutic compound using three-dimensional guidance for left ventricular navigation.

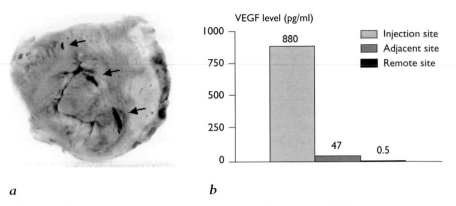

a   b

Figure 23.2 *Intramyocardial reporter gene transfer (a) and VEGF production at
24 h following catheter-based transendocardial gene transfer at injection, adjacent and
remote sites (b).*

identified by co-injection of fluorescentic beads) was achieved in
approximately 95% of cases using either the ß-galactosidase marker gene (ß-
gal) or Ad.VEGF121 transgene to detect gene expression in injected and
adjacent sites. Levels of either VEGF or ß-gal, signifying enhanced tissue
expression at 24–48 h following catheter-based transendocardial gene delivery,
were reproducibly high, while detectable levels were negligible and rarely
found in control right ventricular or remote myocardial samples (Figure
23.2). Another study tested the levels and duration of expression of genes
induced after injection of a specific plasmid vector, using the left ventricular
guidance and catheter-based delivery platform.[14] Measurements of luciferase
activity were performed 3 and 7 days following transendocardial injection.
The results showed high levels of expression of luciferase gene in ischemic
and non-ischemic regions that were comparable to levels achieved using direct
injection of the plasmids into peripheral muscular tissue or using a surgical
thoracotomy. Control non-injected samples from the left and right ventricles
contained no detectable luciferase activity. Another group reported similar
results using the ß-gal reporter plasmid via an identical catheter-based
transendocardial delivery technique.[10]

Technical limitations

The use of catheter-based approaches for transendocardial injection of
recombinant genes or growth factors to enhance myocardial collateral blood
vessel function may represent a relatively novel approach to the treatment of
ischemic cardiovascular disease. However, it should be recognized that the

field of intramyocardial gene transfer in general, and catheter-based transendocardial gene delivery in particular, is in its infancy and may undergo rapid stages of evolution.[15,16] Currently, most catheters for transendocardial gene delivery are either crude in design or require sophisticated manipulation, and technical modifications are expected to ensure better catheter handling and torque response characteristics while optimizing needle stability in beating heart conditions with a minimal amount of myocardial trauma. One study assessed the stability and precise localization parameters during left ventricular-guided catheter-based intramyocardial injection of transgenes and found the catheter tip to be highly stable on the endocardial surface throughout the cardiac cycle.[17] Currently, it is unclear whether similar results could be obtained for other delivery systems.

The potential deleterious effects of overexpression of local angiogenic transgenes following direct myocardial injection should not be underestimated. Potential deleterious effects included the occurrence of myocardial inflammation, fibrosis and angioma formation (Figure 23.3). These deleterious effects should be excluded in appropriate safety preclinical studies before its use in patients. Also, the level and time course of protein expression following local intramyocardial gene delivery should be studied and well defined. Systemic distribution of transgene and/or secreted proteins may still become apparent following local transendocardial gene delivery, especially with suboptimal injection techniques. Maintenance of DNA integrity when it is passing through the injection catheter should be confirmed in order to avoid significant attenuation of transgene activity when using the catheter-based technique.[18] Also, it remains to be determined whether the catheter-based approach would result in equivalent efficacy in terms of delivering therapeutic agents into the myocardium compared to surgical-based

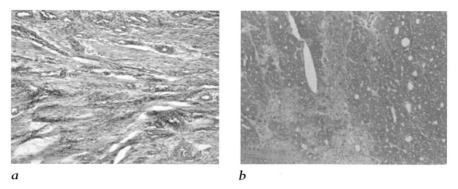

a   b

Figure 23.3 *Potential hazards associated with excessive intramyocardial injection of VEGF (a; angioma and edema formation, H & E × 200) or fibroblast growth factor (FGF) (b; fibrotic tracks, H & E × 100).*

314

techniques. Preliminary data suggested that the catheter-based approach indeed offers a similar degree of VEGF angiogenic gene expression compared to transepicardial open chest surgical injections.[13] However, the catheter-based technique may carry a higher variability of protein expression, potentially due to catheter-induced transgene attenuation and inconsistent procedural techniques.

Clinical experiences using angiogenic gene transfer

Safety and feasibility studies using a catheter-based transendocardial injection technique for either VEGF2 plasmid were recently completed.[19,20] Percutaneous intramyocardial injection of replication-deficient adenovirus containing the VEGF121 transgene was tested in 12 patients in a safety and feasibility study, but results have not yet been reported. These studies were designed to test the feasibility and safety aspects of such catheter-based approaches for transendocardial angiogenic gene delivery. These studies included 'sham controls', while patients were blinded to the actual treatment. In addition, preliminary efficacy endpoints have been assessed following the intramyocardial VEGF gene transfer procedure in patients by including objective measures to assess the impact of treatment on exercise tolerance, quality of life and myocardial ischemia. One small study investigated the safety of percutaneous catheter-based gene transfer of naked plasmid DNA encoding for VEGF2 to left ventricular myocardium in a randomized, placebo-controlled, dose-escalating study of inoperable patients with severe angina.[20] Patients were randomized in a double-blind fashion to receive six injections of placebo or VEGF2 plasmid at doses of either 200, 800 or 2000 μg guided by electromechanical mapping. Overall, the procedure was found to be safe. Endpoint analysis at 12 weeks disclosed a statistically significant improvement in angina scores and a positive change in exercise duration in VEGF-treated versus placebo-treated patients. This study provided preliminary data that support the safety and potential efficacy of VEGF2 catheter-mediated myocardial gene transfer. The Euroinject 1 study is a European multicenter randomized double-blind placebo-controlled gene treatment study using the gene encoding VEGF165 in patients with severe refractory myocardial ischemia. Eighty patients were recruited, and preliminary data confirmed the safety of the procedure, although complete data as well as efficacy endpoints are still pending.

These studies, as well as others that are likely to follow, will aim to establish the role of catheter-based transendocardial angiogenic gene delivery in patients with chronic refractory ischemic heart disease. Nonetheless, it should be emphasized that intracoronary injection of replication-deficient viral vectors is an alternative investigational therapeutic approach to the treatment of patients sustaining chronic myocardial ischemia.[21] A recent study indicated that a single intracoronary infusion of replication-deficient viral vectors containing fibroblast growth factor-4 (Ad.FGF4) may offer improved exercise tolerance in patients with stable mild to moderately symptomatic angina compared to control patients.[21] Currently, the preferred route for intramyocardial gene transfer (e.g. 'direct' intramyocardial or intracoronary delivery) is yet to be determined and may also depend upon the particular tested compound.

Intramyocardial cellular transplantation

Better understanding of the proper formation of blood vessels and myocyte differentiation, and a series of cell-based experiments, have raised hopes that intramyocardial cell transplantation will improve myocardial function in ischemic cardiomyopathic syndromes.[22,23] Novel vascular progenitors have been identified in the embryo and also in the adult bone marrow and peripheral blood. These cells may become candidates for intramyocardial cell transplantation. Transplantation studies revealed that these precursors and other bone marrow-derived cells contribute to the growth of endothelium-lined vessels (angiogenesis) and the expansion of pre-existing collaterals (arteriogenesis).[24] Myocardial contractility was improved in some studies using autologous cell lines for transplantation, which may indicate a positive myogenic response.[25] Also, recent in vitro observations showed that human embryonic stem cells differentiate into cardiomyocytes.[26] Intramyocardial cell transplantation builds upon these observations, proposing to deliver cellular compounds to the myocardium via multiple routes in an effort to enhance myocardial function and have therapeutic benefit in ischemic and/or myocardial infarction syndromes. Theoretically, the goals of cell transplantation are as follows:

- replacing dysfunctional cardiomyocytes with new functional cells, thereby decreasing infarct size and improving cardiac work
- increasing the number of contractile elements
- promoting local angiogenesis and collateralization by EPCs and/or induction of prolonged local delivery of vascular growth factors.

In order to achieve these goals, the choice of the particular cell type will be dictated largely by the pathology being treated and the desired therapeutic effect.

316

Utilization of cells for myocardial regeneration and angiogenesis

Several investigators have shown that animal embryonic stem cells can be induced to develop into tissue-specific cells by bioengineering techniques.[27] EPCs have been isolated from peripheral blood and bone marrow, and shown to be incorporated into sites of physiologic and pathologic neovascularization in vivo.[28,29] In contrast to the case with differentiated endothelial cells, transplantation of progenitor cells successfully enhanced vascular development by in situ differentiation and proliferation within ischemic organs.[30] Endothelial cell progenitors, angioblasts, have been shown to incorporate into the endothelium of newly forming blood vessels in pathologic and non-pathologic conditions.[25,31] Since bone marrow is a natural source of multiple angiogenic growth factors and because of the essential involvement of several bone marrow-derived cells, including vascular progenitors, one group has investigated whether catheter-based intramyocardial transplantation of the entire bone marrow or specific progenitor-enriched cell populations, or their direct implantation into ischemic tissues, would enhance tissue vascularization and function.[32] With the use of freshly aspirated bone marrow cells, catheter-based intramyocardial injection of autologous bone marrow cells was shown to promote collateral development in ischemic porcine myocardium.[32] Moreover, angiogenic cytokine concentrations in vitro increased progressively over time and induced endothelial cell proliferation (Figure 23.4). Another group has shown that bone marrow-derived progenitor cell lines could reduce infarct size and improve myocardial function, as progenitor cells may differentiate into cardiomyocytes following direct transplantation into infarcted and peri-infarction regions.[33] Transplantation of skeletal myoblasts (mainly satellite cells) into cryo-infarcted myocardium of the same animal is another technique that holds promise for myocardial regeneration.[34] Islands of different sizes comprising elongated, striated cells that retained characteristics of both skeletal and cardiac cells were found in scar regions in a rabbit model of cryo-infarction.

Those observations have established the rationale for autologous intramyocardial injection of bone marrow-derived progenitor cells or autologous myoblast cell transfer using techniques similar to those that had been previously described for intramyocardial gene transfer. The feasibility and safety of catheter-based intramyocardial transfer of cellular elements (either progenitor cells or myogenic cells) using left ventricular mapping guidance have been tested and established in experimental models.[32,35]

317

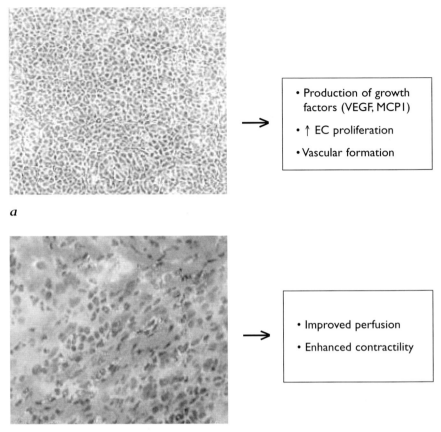

Figure 23.4 *The rationale involving intramyocardial injection of autologous bone marrow cells: vascular effects in vitro (a) and potential myogenic/vascular effects in vivo (b) following intramyocardial transfer in a porcine model.*[32]

Cell transplantation experiences in patients

Several groups have initiated clinical studies with autologous bone marrow-derived cells. A group at Yamaguchi University, Japan initiated in 1999 a clinical trial in five patients in an attempt to induce myocardial angiogenesis by local implantation of autologous bone marrow cells concomitant with bypass surgery.[36] The cells were implanted into the non-graftable areas, and postoperative cardiac scintigraphy showed specific improvement in coronary perfusion in a few patients. Other groups have started to perform percutaneous implantation of autologous bone marrow cells using catheter-based left ventricular-guided transendocardial delivery. Preliminary data suggest that the procedure is feasible and safe, and a larger study is likely to follow in order to test the clinical efficacy of this technique.

A group at Hôpital Bichat, Paris recently initiated a study of autologous myoblast implantation in patients.[37] Soon thereafter, another group at the Thorax-Center in Rotterdam, The Netherlands started to deliver expanded autologous myoblasts percutaneously using an intramyocardial injection catheter for cellular delivery. Although those experiments created waves of public excitement, realistically one should acknowledge that these clinical investigations are premature, since the full scope of the cellular biological effects of these cells is still unknown, as are the potential hazards that may be associated with these techniques. The biomechanical and electrical properties of the implanted cells should be explored prior to proceeding with larger clinical trials with intramyocardial myoblast transplantation.

Conclusion

The intramyocardial transfer of proteins, genes or cells is feasible using either surgical or catheter-based approaches. The effects of direct intramyocardial injection of angiogenic factors and/or cellular transplantation on collateral function and myocardial regeneration have been reported to occur in experimental models and, anecdotally, among treated patients. Nonetheless, there is a need for further understanding of the biological effects of the transplanted compounds, whether therapeutic genes or cells, and to accept the likelihood that unexpected side-effects may occur as these agents are transferred to the diseased myocardium. This awareness, coupled with a rigorous scientific analysis of carefully conducted experimental and clinical studies, will lead to a risk–benefit analysis of these novel, and potentially extremely important, therapeutic interventions.

References

1. Kornowski R, Fuchs S, Leon MB, Epstein SE. Delivery strategies to achieve therapeutic myocardial angiogenesis. Circulation 2000; 101: 454–8.

2. Freedman SB, Isner JM. Therapeutic angiogenesis for coronary artery disease. Ann Intern Med 2002; 136: 54–71.

3. Mack CA, Patel SR, Schwartz EA et al. Biologic bypass with the use of adenovirus-mediated gene transfer of the complementary deoxyribonucleic acid for VEGF-12, improves myocardial perfusion and function in the ischemic porcine heart. J Thorac Cardiovasc Surg 1998; 115: 168–77.

4. Schumacher B, Pecher P, von Specht BU, Stegman T. Induction of neoangiogenesis in ischemic myocardium by human growth factors. First clinical results of a new treatment of coronary heart disease. Circulation 1998; 97: 645–50.

5. Losordo DW, Vale PR, Symes JF et al. Gene therapy for myocardial angiogenesis: initial clinical results with direct myocardial injection of phVEGF165 as sole therapy for myocardial ischemia. Circulation 1998; 98: 2800–4.

6. Rosengart TK, Lee LY, Patel SR et al. Angiogenesis gene therapy: phase I assessment of direct intramyocardial administration of an adenovirus vector expressing VEGF121 cDNA to individuals with clinically significant severe coronary artery disease. Circulation 1999; 100: 468–74.

7. Vale PR, Losordo DW, Milliken CE et al. Left ventricular electromechanical mapping to assess efficacy of phVEGF(165) gene transfer for therapeutic angiogenesis in chronic myocardial ischemia. Circulation 2000; 102: 965–74.

8. Rosengart TK, Lee LY, Patel SR et al. Six-month assessment of a phase I trial of angiogenic gene therapy for the treatment of coronary artery disease using direct intramyocardial administration of an adenovirus vector expressing the VEGF121 cDNA. Ann Surg 1999; 230: 466–70.

9. Li JJ, Ueno H, Pan Y et al. Percutaneous transluminal gene transfer into canine myocardium in vivo by replication-defective adenovirus. Cardiovasc Res 1995; 30: 97–105.

10. Vale PR, Losordo DW, Tkebuchava T et al. Catheter-based myocardial gene-transfer utilizing nonfluoroscopic electromechanical left ventricular mapping. J Am Coll Cardiol 1999; 34: 246–54.

11. Sanborn TA, Hackett NR, Lee LY et al. Percutaneous endocardial transfer and expression of genes to the myocardium utilizing fluoroscopic guidance. Catheter Cardiovasc Intervent 2001; 52: 260–6.

12. Kornowski R, Fuchs S, Tio FO et al. Evaluation of the acute and chronic safety of the biosense injection catheter system in porcine hearts. Catheter Cardiovasc Intervent 1999; 48: 447–53.

13. Kornowski R, Leon MB, Vodovotz Y et al. Electromagnetic-guidance for catheter-based trans-endocardial injection: a platform for myocardial angiogenesis therapy: results in normal and ischemic porcine model. J Am Coll Cardiol 2000; 35: 1031–9.

14. Kornowski R, Fuchs S, Epstein SE et al. Catheter-based plasmid-mediated transfer of genes into ischemic myocardium using the pCOR plasmid. Coron Artery Dis 2000; 11: 615–19.

15. Epstein SE, Kornowski R, Fuchs S, Dvorak HF. Angiogenesis therapy: amidst the hype, the neglected potential for serious side effects. Circulation 2001; 104: 115–19.

16. Kornowski R. Catheter-based transendocardial gene delivery for therapeutic myocardial angiogenesis. Int J Cardiovasc Intervent 2000; 3: 67–70.

17. Lessick J, Kornowski R, Fuchs S, Ben-Haim SA. Assessment of NOGA catheter stability during the entire cardiac cycle by means of a special needle-tipped catheter. Catheter Cardiovasc Intervent 2001; 52: 400–6.

18. Kuliszewski MA, Kutryk MB, Sandhu R et al. DNA integrity and transgene expression after passage through the NOGA needle catheter used for therapeutic myocardial angiogenesis. Int J Cardiovasc Intervent 2000; 3: 167–72.

19. Vale PR, Losordo DW, Milliken CE et al. Randomized, single-blind, placebo-controlled pilot study of catheter-based myocardial gene transfer for therapeutic angiogenesis using left ventricular electromechanical mapping in patients with chronic myocardial ischemia. Circulation 2001; 103: 2138–43.

20. Losordo DW, Vale PR, Hendel RC et al. Phase 1/2 placebo-controlled, double-blind, dose-escalating trial of myocardial vascular endothelial growth factor 2 gene transfer by catheter delivery in patients with chronic myocardial ischemia. Circulation 2002; 105: 2012–18.

21. Grines CL, Watkins MW, Helmer G et al. Angiogenic Gene Therapy (AGENT) trial in patients with stable angina pectoris. Circulation 2002; 105: 1291–7.

22. Anversa P, Nadal-Ginard B. Myocyte renewal and ventricular remodelling. Nature 2002; 415: 240–3.

23. Luttun A, Carmeliet G, Carmeliet P. Vascular progenitors: from biology to treatment. Trends Cardiovasc Med 2002; 12: 88–96.

24. Carmeliet P. Mechanism of angiogenesis and arteriogenesis. Nat Med 2000; 6: 389–95.

25. Tomita S, Li RK, Weisel RD et al. Autologous transplantation of bone marrow cells improves damaged heart function. Circulation 1999; 100: II-247–56.

26. Kehat I, Kenyagin-Karsenti D, Snir M et al. Human embryonic stem cells can differentiate into myocytes with structural and functional properties of cardiomyocytes. J Clin Invest 2001; 108: 407–14.

27. Makino S, Fukuda K, Miyoshi S et al. Cardiomyocytes can be generated from marrow stromal cells in vitro. J Clin Invest 1999; 103: 697–705.

28. Kocher AA, Schuster MD, Szabolcs MJ et al. Neovascularization of ischemic myocardium by human bone marrow derived angioblasts prevents cardiomyocyte apoptosis, reduces remodeling and improves cardiac function. Nat Med 2001; 7: 430–6.

29. Orlic D, Kajstura J, Chimenti S et al. Mobilized bone marrow cells repair the infarcted heart, improving function and survival. Proc Natl Acad Sci USA 2001; 938: 221–9.

30. Jackson KA, Majka SM, Wang H et al. Regeneration of ischemic cardiac muscle and vascular endothelium by adult stem cells. J Clin Invest 2001; 107: 1395–402.

31. Malouf NN, Coleman WB, Grisham JW et al. Adult derived stem cells from the liver become myocytes in the heart in vivo. Am J Pathol 2001; 158: 1929–35.

32. Fuchs S, Baffour R, Zhou YF et al. Transendocardial delivery of autologous bone marrow enhances collateral perfusion and regional function in pigs with chronic experimental myocardial ischemia. J Am Coll Cardiol 2001; 37: 1726–32.

33. Orlic D, Kajstura J, Chimenti S et al. Bone marrow cells regenerate infarcted myocardium. Nature 2001; 410: 701–5.

34. Taylor DA, Atkins BZ, Hungspreugs P et al. Regenerating functional myocardium: improved performance after skeletal myoblast transplantation. Nat Med 1998; 4: 929–33.

35. Oron U, Halevy O, Yaakobi T et al. Technical delivery of myogenic cells through an endocardial injection catheter for myocardial cell implantation. Int J Cardiovasc Intervent 2000; 4: 227–30.

36. Hamano K, Nishida M, Hirata K et al. Local implantation of autologous bone marrow cells for therapeutic angiogenesis in patients with ischemic heart disease: clinical trial and preliminary results. Jpn Circ J 2001; 65: 845–7.

37. Menasche P. Cell transplantation for the treatment of heart failure. Semin Thorac Cardiovasc Surg 2002; 14: 157–66.

24. The Vast Potential of the Coronary Venous System for Drug and Biological Interventions

Mehrdad Rezaee, Eric T Price, Peter J Fitzgerald,
Paul G Yock and Alan C Yeung

Introduction and background

The concept of 'retrograde' venous myocardial delivery has evolved over time. William Harvey first described the closed circulatory system, and correctly noted the relationship between coronary arteries and veins,[1] and in the early eighteenth century anatomists and physiologists expanded the understanding of this complex vascular system.[2,3] However, it was not until 1897 that F. H. Pratt first proposed and investigated the potential 'nutritive significance of regurgitation ... into the coronary veins'.[4] The first human 'arterialization of the coronary sinus' was performed in 1947, although it was quickly abandoned due to excessive myocardial damage, and associated mortality.[5] Unwilling to sacrifice this potential avenue to the heart, many investigators have expanded and improved coronary venous interventions for intermittent coronary sinus occlusion, retroperfusion of oxygenated blood and retroinfusion of myocardially active substances.[6–9] The combined work in this field over the past five decades has produced coronary venous techniques that remain in surgical use today.[10,11] The major applications include retroinfusion of cardioplegia in the arrested heart, which is now a well-established clinical technique, intermittent coronary sinus occlusion during antegrade cardioplegic delivery in the arrested heart, and in the early reperfusion period after surgical revascularization.

Cardiac electrophysiologists were the first to explore percutaneous applications of the coronary venous system (CVS). Percutaneous cannulation of the coronary sinus has been a main route for interrogation of the bundle of His and ablation of the left-sided bypass tracks.[12] More recently, left-sided pacing lead placement in the coronary sinus and its tributaries has been shown to be feasible.[12,13] Advances in both devices and techniques have now positioned coronary venous lead placement as a superior option for many types of electrophysiologic therapy. A recent review has supported the practicality and reproducibility of lead placement with this technique, with high rates of success in accessing targeted areas.[14] Electrophysiologic applications using the coronary sinus remain an active area of investigation and will pave the way for many other applications using this route of entry to the heart.

There is growing interest in using the coronary veins for delivering biologically active agents to the myocardium. According to theory and preliminary practice, this method carries obvious advantages, which include minimal invasiveness, low resistance access to many regional areas of myocardium and minimal potential short- and long-term complications (Table 24.1). Investigations to date have focused on coronary venous delivery of pharmacologic agents, free-radical-targeted enzymes and genetic factors.[15–18] In this chapter, we will summarize the current state of knowledge and future directions for optimal use of this novel technique.

Table 24.1 Properties of ideal and existing local delivery strategies

	Ease	Safety	Critical concentration	Regionality	Systemic exposure
Ideal	++	++	++	++	−
CVS	+	+	++	++	+/−
IV	++	++	+/−	−	++
IC	+	+	+/−	−	++
IP	+/−	+/−	+	++	−
EPI IMD	+/−	+/−	+	++	+/−
PER IMD	+	+	+	++	+

CVS, coronary venous system; IV, intravenous; IC, intracoronary; IP, intrapericardial.

Anatomy of the coronary veins

Harvey's original model of arteries draining into veins accurately but incompletely defines the human coronary circulation. Eventually, the presence of an alternative route for drainage of coronary arterial blood back into the chambers of the heart was described;[2] these thebesian vessels or sinusoids play a major role in drainage of the coronary arteries, but an even potentially greater role in retrograde venous delivery. While an estimated 60–90% of antegrade coronary arterial flow passes through capillary beds (nutrient flow),[19,20] only 5–45% of retrograde coronary flow passes through the capillary system,[21] with the remainder traversing either venovenous

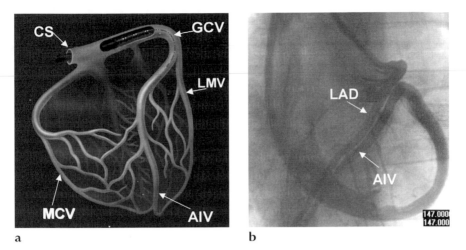

Figure 24.1 *Coronary venous anatomy. (a) The network of venous plexuses which
drain into major venous branches: middle cardiac vein (MCV), anterior intraventricular
vein (AIV) and lateral marginal vein (LMV). The blood from these flows into the great
cardiac vein (GCV), which finally drains into the coronary sinus (CS).*
*(b) Co-injection of the left anterior descending artery (LAD) and AIV demonstrates the
proximity of the epicardial arteries to their corresponding venous branch.*

anastomoses (collaterals) or thebesian conduits. The multiple potential routes
for retrograde venous flow may in part account for limits in retrograde
perfusion, and must be considered with all retrograde coronary venous
delivery.[22] Even with these anatomic caveats, primary circulatory principles
remain, and specific coronary veins drain regional areas of myocardium that
are fed by specific coronary arteries.[23]

Our current understanding of the CVS results from a composite of
information gained from various techniques, mostly venous angiograms (Figure
24.1). The major vessels consistently identified in humans are: the coronary
sinus (CS), which drains the middle cardiac vein (MCV) and also the great
cardiac vein (GCV), which in turn drains the posterior interventricular vein,
lateral marginal veins (PIV/LMV) and the anterior interventricular vein (AIV).
While there is significant variability in PIV and LMV vessel diameter, there is
consistent presence (>99%) of all the major branches.[14]

Venous delivery for local and regional treatment

Regional access to the myocardium can be accomplished through selective
cannulation and retroinfusion of the sub-branches of the CS. A catheter-based

325

approach with the use of routine right heart cardiac catheterization procedures can be applied for therapeutic application of this modality. In this section, the feasibility and preclinical efficacy studies that have led to the development of this topic will be reviewed. This will be followed by a description of the current, state-of-the-art applications of the CVS for biological treatment of cardiac disease.

One of the original investigations in this field demonstrated the efficacy of retrograde coronary venous delivery of procainamide for the management of ventricular tachycardia.[15] In this study, selective retrograde injection of procainamide was accomplished through an autoinflatable balloon catheter placed in the GCV. This therapy was significantly more effective than systemic intravenous injection against spontaneous ventricular tachycardia after coronary artery occlusion. Lower doses of procainamide were used with retroinfusion as compared with systemic administration. Myocardial tissue procainamide levels measured in infarcted and ischemic zones of the left anterior ventricular wall were up to 100 times higher after GCV retroinfusion than after systemic injection. This study demonstrated that regional coronary venous procainamide retroinfusion in infarcted dog hearts is more effective than systemic intravenous injection. Efficacy was also demonstrated in the spatial distribution of retrogradely infused felodipine during regional myocardial ischemia. The drug was specifically delivered into the ischemic myocardium, where it exerted a myocardial protective effect in isolated rat hearts subjected to 60 min of regional ischemia followed by 60 min of reperfusion.[16] Similarly, in pigs subjected to 60 min of LAD occlusion, pretreatment with diltiazem by retrograde coronary vein infusion was more effective than intravenous drug administration in providing myocardial protection.[17] The observed efficacy in these studies appears to be primarily related to the selectively increased delivery of drugs to ischemic myocardial sites inaccessible to intravenous or intracoronary delivery that was accomplished safely by the coronary venous route.

In order to prevent reperfusion injury, superoxide dismutase and catalase were delivered through the CVS in dogs with 90 min of LAD occlusion. In the group that received superoxide dismutase (2.5 mg/kg) and catalase (2.5 mg/kg) through a bolus injection in the GCV immediately before reperfusion, infarct size was significantly smaller, and regional function of the ischemic zone exhibited significantly greater recovery after 3 h of reperfusion. Moreover, there were significantly fewer post-reperfusion ventricular arrhythmias in the treated group. These data demonstrate the efficacy of the CVS for treatment of myocardium with biologically active (proteins) reagents.[24]

Most recent work in this area has concentrated on: (1) developing an efficient delivery modality; and (2) optimizing the application of

retroinfusion/perfusion/injection for targeted regional delivery of biological
agents (i.e. proteins, genetic factors, cells).

Development of treatment modalities through the coronary venous system

The complexity of cardiac venous drainage, significant differences in
microvascular flow and branching between the arterial and venous systems
and the variable effects of cardiac cycle on venous flow have limited the
widespread application of CVS delivery for myocardial treatment.[25] Based on
these findings, several unique approaches for intramyocardial delivery via
coronary venous retroinfusion/injection have been devised.

Simple injection into the CS or GCV results in poor efficiency of delivery
unless sufficiently high pressure is applied to overcome that of the venous
drainage. With application of adequate pressure, venous flow is not only
reversed but is also a disruption of small venous plexuses; this can be
accomplished without damage to the larger and potentially clinically
significant branches. Extravasation through the smaller channels results in
access to the adjoining myocardial interstitial space and individual
cardiomyocytes. Flow pathways in CVS retroperfusion were first analyzed by
examining the distribution of retroinfusate premixed with radionuclide-labeled
15-μm microspheres in ischemic canine hearts; these were injected into the
CS without occlusion.[25] The results showed that 95% of the injected material
bypassed the intramyocardial microcirculation to directly enter the right heart
chamber. Potential bypass routes included significant backflow into the CS,
venovenous collaterals and entry into the parallel thebesian vascular system.
Of the 5% of retroinfusate that passed the intramyocardial microcirculation, a
majority localized to the ischemic area (LAD), with a subendocardial to
subepicardial distribution ratio of up to 1.79 ± 0.21.[26] Thereafter, balloon
occlusion of the venous flow has been utilized to limit backflow via the
coronary sinus.

The effects of proximal coronary venous occlusion have been shown to be
dependent primarily on the site of occlusion (i.e. non-selective placement
within the CS or selective placement within a tributary branch). In a study
by Punzengruber et al, retrograde administration of contrast into the GCV of
dogs resulted in systolic/diastolic blood pressure readings in the GCV of
$7 \pm 3/1 \pm 0.6$ mmHg without balloon occlusion, and $29 \pm 11/5 \pm 3$ mmHg after
CS occlusion, with an increase to $55 \pm 2.3/15 \pm 12$ mmHg during injection.[27]
The effects of AIV occlusion are presented in Table 24.2. In these

327

experiments, the balloon tip catheter was advanced to the distal (anteriobasal region) AIV, and intraluminal pressures were recorded both during balloon occlusion of venous flow and during the delivery of contrast. As shown, there were no significant hemodynamic changes, including left ventricular end diastolic pressure or coronary arterial (LAD) flow.[28]

Table 24.2 Hemodynamic results after AIV occlusion and delivery

		MAP	LVEDP	Coronary WP	AIV
Proximal	Before	98±12	7±4	5±2	17±6
	After	101±20	7±3	7±4	28±9
Mid/distal	Before	98±12	9±3	6.2±3	19±5
	After	90±18	5±2	7±3.8	50±21

A balloon-tipped wedge catheter was placed at the takeoff of the anterior intraventricular vein (AIV) from the GCV (proximal) or mid-AIV (mid/distal). Pressure measurements were performed through the distal end of the catheter and/or via a pressure wire placed in the AIV or LAD. Simultaneous mean arterial pressure (MAP) and left ventricular end diastolic pressure (LVEDP) (through the pig tail placed in the LV) were measured. Before and after refer to PA catheter balloon inflation to occlude AIV drainage into the GCV. Coronary wedge pressure (WP) measurements through the pressure wire were performed as described in the materials and methods.

The functional benefit (improvement in ischemia) attainable with AIV retroperfusion has also been investigated. In ischemic pigs, regional myocardial function increased linearly with increasing retroperfusion flow rates, averaging 62% of control values, at a retroperfusion rate equal to 200% of arterial flow. At this retroperfusion rate, intraluminal pressures within the AIV increased up to 132 ±57 mmHg. In the same study, retrograde injection of silicone elastomer at different retroperfusion pressures (50, 75 and 100 mmHg), resulted in well-visualized capillaries, complete filling of small venules and prominent intramyocardial venous anastomotic connections only at the highest retroperfusion pressure (100 mmHg).[29] This observation was significant for not only demonstrating recovery of regional myocardial function with low capillary bloodflow but also for visualization of retrograde capillary filling with a rich venous network, providing support for oxygen delivery via the intramyocardial venous plexus.

Because of the mechanical effects of cardiac contraction on venous flow, a retroperfusion system was developed to augment retrograde delivery during diastole and facilitate coronary venous drainage in systole.[30,31] In this and other similar systems, an electrocardiogram-synchronized, gas-actuated pump propels retroperfusate through an autoinflatable balloon catheter whose tip is placed within the regional coronary vein that drains the ischemic myocardium. This approach resulted in localization of delivery material within the ischemic region, as demonstrated by injection of monastral blue dye, which had a three-fold higher content in capillaries of ischemic anterior wall than in the non-ischemic posterior aspects of the left ventricle.[32] Retroinfusion of oxygenized blood in dogs with coronary (LAD) occlusion via synchronized retroperfusion resulted in significantly improved ventricular systolic and diastolic functions, decreased ischemia and reduction in the size of ischemic injury.[6]

In contrast to the elaborate device discussed above, it has been shown that simple manual retroperfusion of oxygenated blood into the CVS also reduces the infarct size.[33] Our own work has consistently demonstrated that single 'high' pressure selective injection into a CS branch provides an efficient method for regional intramyocardial delivery. This requires selective branch balloon occlusion, and injection can be accomplished at delivery rates of 0.5–1.0 ml/min, with application pressures of 100–200 mmHg, without any acute or chronic clinical consequences. As described above, this amount of pressure allows for disruption of small, low-resistance venous plexus, without damage to larger major branches (Figure 24.2). By use of this approach with proximal balloon occlusion, venous injection of radiographic contrast selectively infiltrates targeted myocardial regions, with videodensitometric evidence of radiographic contrast persistence for at least 30 min.[23] Unlike other systems, where the pressure of infusion is set to prevent inadvertent

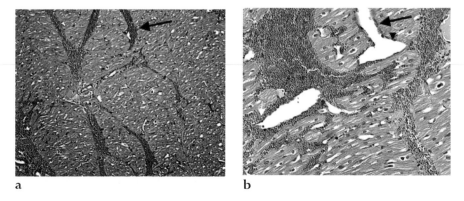

a   b

Figure 24.2 *Intramyocardial hematoma after high-pressure retrograde delivery. After high-pressure injection of contrast into the AIV, hearts were collected and samples of the anterior wall were subjected to histologic analysis, which demonstrated intact myocardial architecture. There were small, diffuse areas of hematoma, as shown in (a) (arrow). These resolve by 7 days after the injection. (b) Under higher magnification, the major venous branches are intact, and the extravasation of blood results in damage to the microvasculature.*

capillary injury, the current technique is designed to incorporate controlled venocapillary disruption. This relatively simple procedure is designed to require only a few minutes (rather than the several hours associated with other methods), to be suitable for ambulatory patients and to be applicable for repeated treatments if necessary. Further studies are underway to identify the appropriate range of injection pressures and further define its efficiency.

Another approach to utilize the CVS stems from the proximity of major venous branches to epicardial arteries in a given myocardial territory. A catheter-based system for arterializing the anterior cardiac vein has been developed. This system has a composite catheter (phased-array ultrasound imaging system mounted on a catheter with extendable nitinol needle) to allow for the development of a fistula between the proximal segment of the occluded artery and the coronary vein. The proximal vein is then blocked to force retroperfusion of the anterior wall. This system has been tested in a small number of patients and is currently under clinical investigation.[34] The same needle-based system can be used to inject biological reagents directly from the venous system into the myocardium using a superfine infusion catheter through the nitinol needle. Preliminary animal work has been done to show its feasibility.

Localized and regionalized intramyocardial delivery of biologically active reagents through the coronary venous system

Applications of angiogenic factors and mammalian cells for transplantation have emerged as potential adjunctive modalities for the treatment of non-functional myocardium.[35–37] These studies suggest that the route of delivery of these factors may play a major role in achieving efficacy in terms of angiogenesis and functional improvement. Effective delivery modalities must result in a critical local concentration of reagents with an acceptable safety profile. The current methods for local delivery of reagents into the myocardium include intracoronary injection, pericardial delivery, direct epicardial injection through surgical procedures or intramyocardial injections via a catheter within the left ventricular cavity. While the feasibility of these modalities has been demonstrated, their general application may be limited by procedural complexity and/or the low efficiency rate afforded by a particular delivery system (<1.0% of total delivered basic fibroblast growth factor (bFGF) is retained within the myocardium after intracoronary delivery) (Figure 24.3).[38,39]

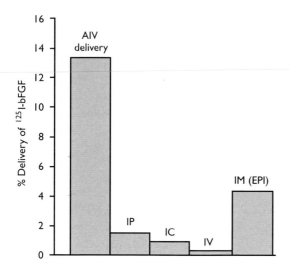

Figure 24.3 *Coronary venous high-pressure injection provides efficient regional delivery of bFGF. ^{125}I-labeled bFGF was delivered through the AIV, and acute myocardial retention (expressed as the percentage of the total amount delivered) was quantified and compared to the levels achieved by other delivery modalities.[39] IP, intrapericardial; IC, intracoronary; IV, intravenous; IM (EPI), intramyocardial by epicardial injection.*

The distribution and efficiency of protein delivery through high-pressure injection into coronary veins has been studied. In an ischemic pig model, the acute efficiency of bFGF delivery was 13.4%.[28] This approach resulted in high tissue-specific activity, with >80% of the detected bFGF localized to the ischemic myocardium. This amount of retention correlated moderately with a single low-dose delivery of bFGF. In a pig model of LAD ischemia, there was an average 21% improvement in flow within the ischemic myocardium as compared to the placebo-treated group 3 weeks after treatment with 180 μg of bFGF.[28]

As with protein delivery, an efficient delivery system is a prerequisite for myocardial gene therapy. Among the various procedures studied so far, catheter-based percutaneous gene delivery to the myocardium through the coronary venous vessels has been studied. To examine this, a formulation of plasmid encoding for the angiogenic factor Del-1 with the non-ionic PINC (Protective, Interactive, Non-Condensing) was used.[40] CVS delivery to the left ventricle was accomplished via balloon occlusion of the AIV followed by infusion of the formulated plasmid under high pressure. Seven days post-delivery, transgene expression was examined by quantitative RT-PCR. AIV delivery of 1–10 mg of hDel-1 polymer-formulated plasmid was well tolerated and resulted in levels of hDel-1 mRNA in pig myocardium similar to those shown to elicit increases in capillary density in hindlimb muscles of mice. Assay of other organs (e.g. liver, kidney and spleen) and non-treated regions of the heart by PCR and RT-PCR indicated that plasmid distribution and transgene expression were essentially confined to the treated area of myocardium. These data showed percutaneous retrograde injection to be an efficient method for transgene delivery, with localized expression isolated to targeted regions of myocardium. Boekstegers et al have demonstrated that selective retrograde AIV gene delivery (using the synchronized retroinfusion system described above) substantially increased reporter gene expression in the targeted ischemic myocardium when compared with intracoronary delivery.[18]

Finally, the applicability of high-pressure CVS injection for mammalian cellular transplantation has recently been evaluated (Figure 24.4) (unpublished results). In this study by our group, fibroblasts ($2–3 \times 10^6$) prelabeled with iron oxide nanoparticles were delivered to porcine hearts (by single injection at 100–200 mmHg) through the AIV. In acute studies, transplanted cells (detected using Prussian blue (iron) staining) were localized to infarcted

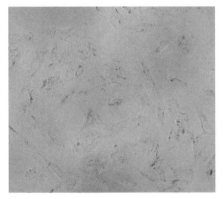

a

b

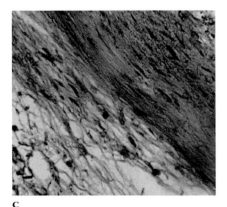

c

Figure 24.4 Regional cellular transplantation through coronary venous high-pressure injection. Cultured porcine fibroblasts were prelabeled with MRI-compatible iron oxide particles. (a) Iron staining of cultured cells (blue): $1–2 \times 10^6$ of these prelabeled cells were delivered through the AIV at 100 mmHg, in a pig model of anterior wall infarct. (b) The labeled fibroblasts within the infarct zone 21 days after delivery. (c) Of these cells, 35–45% are BrdU positive, demonstrating proliferative activity.

myocardium. With a linear computational model, the efficiency of this modality was determined to be $14.0 \pm 16.6\%$, with all transplanted cells identified in the LAD territory (82.8% within the anterior wall, 17.2% within the septum and 86.9% within a 4-cm span in the longitudinal axis). In chronic studies with LAD infarction, 97.6% of identified cells were within the LAD territory, in a similar longitudinal distribution from the AIV. Of the original transplanted cells, an estimated 15.7 ± 11.6 were identified at 21 days, all within definitive areas of infarct. Bromodeoxyuridine (BrdU) staining demonstrated proliferation of a subpopulation of transplanted cells. These data suggest that high-pressure selective coronary venous delivery can provide an efficient means of delivering cells to targeted areas of infarcted myocardium, without significant dissemination after 21 days. Future studies will examine device and technique modifications for improving delivery efficiency, as well as transplantation of other cell types for efficacy in providing myocardial protection and functional improvement after infarction.

In conclusion, better understanding of the pathophysiology of cardiovascular disease, and availability of potent biologically active agents, require significant advancement of delivery modalities. For example, in the case of cellular transplantation for cardiomyopathy, where morbidity and mortality are related to a large area of necrosis and not focal myocardial damage, a regional treatment, encompassing an entire epicardial artery territory, has tremendous clinical potential. As presented above, selective coronary venous high-pressure injection fits many of the profiles for a desired delivery modality. It is relatively simple, safe, has a good track record and provides efficient regional coverage regardless of the reagent material. Further work to better determine the optimal rate and pressure of delivery, improvements in delivery devices and selection of the optimal biological agent for delivery may advance this exciting modality for treating a wide range of cardiovascular diseases.

References

1. Harvey W. Exercitatio anatomica de motu cordis et sanguinis in animalibus. Frankfurt, 1628.

2. Thebesius A. De circulo sanguines in corde. Leiden, 1708.

3. Viesussens R. Nouvelles de couvertes sur le coeur. 1706.

4. Pratt FH. The nutrition of the heart through the vessels of Thebesius and the coronary veins. Am J Physiol 1897; 1: 86 103.

5. Beck CS. Revascularization of the heart. Surgery 1949; 26: 82–8.

6. Farcot JC, Meerbaum S, Lang TW et al. Synchronized retroperfusion of coronary veins for circulatory support of jeopardized ischemic myocardium. Am J Cardiol 1978; 41(7): 1191–201.

7. Meerbaum S. Coronary venous retroperfusion delivery of treatment to ischemic myocardium. Herz 1986; 11(1): 41–54.

8. Mohl W. Retrograde cardioplegia via the coronary sinus. Ann Chir Gynaecol 1987; 76(1): 61–7.

9. Mohl W. The momentum of coronary sinus interventions clinically. Circulation 1988; 77(1): 6–12.

10. Ruengsakulrach P, Buxton BF. Anatomic and hemodynamic considerations influencing the efficiency of retrograde cardioplegia. Ann Thorac Surg 2001; 71(4): 1389–95.

11. Mohl W. The relevance of coronary sinus interventions in cardiac surgery. Thorac Cardiovasc Surg 1991; 39(5): 245–50.

12. Gabriele OF. Pacing via coronary sinus. N Engl J Med 1969; 280(4): 219.

13. Hunt D, Sloman G. Long-term electrode catheter pacing from coronary sinus. BMJ 1968; 4(629): 495–6.

14. Meisel E, Pfeiffer D, Engelmann L et al. Investigation of coronary venous anatomy by retrograde venography in patients with malignant ventricular tachycardia. Circulation 2001; 104(4): 442–7.

15. Karagueuzian HS, Ohta M, Drury JK et al. Coronary venous retroinfusion of procainamide: a new approach for the management of spontaneous and inducible sustained ventricular tachycardia during myocardial infarction. J Am Coll Cardiol 1986; 7(3): 551–63.

16. Uriuda Y, Wang QD, Li XS et al. Coronary venous drug infusion in the ischaemic-reperfused isolated rat heart. Cardiovasc Res 1996; 31(1): 82–92.

17. Tadokoro H, Miyazaki A, Satomura K et al. Infarct size reduction with coronary venous retroinfusion of diltiazem in the acute occlusion/reperfusion porcine heart model. J Cardiovasc Pharmacol 1996; 28(1): 134–41.

18. Boekstegers PvDG, Giehrl W, Heinrich D et al. Myocardial gene transfer by selective pressure-regulated retroinfusion of coronary veins. Gene Ther 2000; 7(3): 232–40.

19. Kar S, Nordlander R. Coronary veins: an alternate route to ischemic myocardium. Heart Lung 1992; 21(2): 148–57.

20. Hochberg MS, Austen WG. Selective retrograde coronary venous perfusion. Ann Thorac Surg 1980; 29(6): 578–80.

21. Menasche P, Piwnica A. Cardioplegia by way of the coronary sinus for valvular and coronary surgery. J Am Coll Cardiol 1991; 18(2): 628–36.

22. Pakalska E, Kolff WJ. Anatomical basis for retrograde coronary vein perfusion. Venous anatomy and veno-venous anastomoses in the hearts of humans and some animals. Minn Med 1980; 63(11): 795–801.

23. Herity NA, Lo ST, Oei F et al. Selective regional myocardial infiltration by the percutaneous coronary venous route: a novel technique for local drug delivery. Catheter Cardiovasc Intervent 2000; 51(3): 358–63.

24. Hatori N, Miyazaki A, Tadokoro H et al. Beneficial effects of coronary venous retroinfusion of superoxide dismutase and catalase on reperfusion arrhythmias, myocardial function, and infarct size in dogs. J Cardiovasc Pharmacol 1989; 14(3): 396–404.

25. Villanueva FS, Spotnitz WD, Glasheen WP et al. New insights into the physiology of retrograde cardioplegia delivery. Am J Physiol 1995; 268(4 Pt 2): H1555–66.

26. Chen SG, Chang BL, Meerbaum S et al. The pattern of delivery and distribution of coronary venous retroinfusate in canine hearts. Proc Chin Acad Med Sci Peking Union Med Coll 1989; 4(1): 19–25.

27. Punzengruber C, Maurer G, Chang BL et al. Factors affecting penetration of retrograde coronary venous injections into normal and ischemic canine myocardium: assessment by contrast echocardiography and digital angiography. Basic Res Cardiol 1990; 85(1): 21–32.

28. Rezaee M, Herity N, Lo S et al. Therapeutic angiogenesis by selective delivery of basic FGF in the anterior interventricular vein. J Am Coll Cardiol 2001; 37(2): 47A (abstract).

29. Oh BH, Volpini M, Kambayashi M et al. Myocardial function and transmural blood flow during coronary venous retroperfusion in pigs. Circulation 1992; 86(4): 1265–79.

30. Kar S, Barnett JC, Freedman RJ Jr et al. Synchronized coronary venous retroperfusion. J Am Coll Cardiol 1994; 24(2): 579–81.

31. Farcot JC, Barry M, Bourdarias JP et al. New catheter-pump system for diastolic synchronized coronary sinus retroperfusion. Med Prog Technol 1980; 8(1): 29–37.

32. Chang BL, Drury JK, Meerbaum S et al. Enhanced myocardial washout and retrograde blood delivery with synchronized retroperfusion during acute myocardial ischemia. J Am Coll Cardiol 1987; 9(5): 1091–8.

33. Katircioglu SF, Yucel D, Saritas Z et al. Simplified retroperfusion system preserves the myocardial function during acute coronary artery occlusion. Thorac Cardiovasc Surg 1998; 46(1) 1–6.

34. Oesterle SN, Reifart N, Hauptmann E et al. Percutaneous in situ coronary venous arterialization: report of the first human catheter-based coronary artery bypass. Circulation 2001; 103(21): 2539–43.

35. Lazarous DFSM, Scheinowitz M, Hodge E et al. Comparative effects of basic fibroblast growth factor and vascular endothelial growth factor on coronary collateral development and the arterial response to injury. Circulation 1996; 94: 1074–82.

36. Banai SJMT, Shou M, Lazarous DF et al. Angiogenic-induced enhancement of collateral blood flow to ischemic myocardium by vascular endothelial growth factor in dogs. Circulation 1994; 89: 2138–89.

37. Laham R, Rezaee M, Post MJ et al. Intrapericardial delivery of fibroblast growth factor-2 induces neovascularization in a porcine model of chronic myocardial ischemia. J Pharmacol Exp Ther 2000; 292: 795–802.

38. Laham R, Rezaee M, Post M et al. Intracoronary and intravenous administration of basic fibroblast growth factor: myocardial and tissue distribution. Drug Metab Dispos 1999; 27: 821–6.

39. Laham R, Rezaee M, Garcia L et al. Tissue and myocardial distribution of intracoronary, intravenous, intrapericardial, and intramyocardial 125I-labeled basic fibroblast growth factor (bFGF) favor intramyocardial delivery. J Am Coll Cardiol 2000; 35(2): 10A (abstract).

40. Earls RHD, Coleman M, Rother E et al. Percutaneous delivery of a plasmid-based Del-1 gene therapy to the myocardium of pigs. Am Soc Gene Ther 2001; 780 (abstract).

25. TRANSVENOUS INTRAMYOCARDIAL INJECTION

Pieter C Smits, Wim J van der Giessen, Craig A Thompson and Patrick W Serruys

Introduction

Pioneering work in cardiac cell and gene transfer has primarily been conducted either surgically[1,2] or through intracoronary infusion.[3,4] While the open surgical approach offers visual feedback for locating and controlling injections, the target patient populations, those with recent myocardial infarction or advanced heart failure, are typically at higher risk for major complications, encountered when conventional surgical approaches and general anesthesia are used. Intracoronary injection is less specific than direct injections. Furthermore, the therapeutic yield may be limited by the presence of advanced coronary disease, which may in fact direct cells to non-target regions of the myocardium. Finally, transendothelial cell migration has yet to be well demonstrated, and with larger cells, such as skeletal myoblasts, the risk of distal embolization is theoretically high. The indications for new therapies such as direct intramyocardial cell and gene therapy might be significantly expanded if a straightforward, repeatable and expeditious percutaneous technique could be identified.

Early efforts in the development of such a technique have focused on endoventricular direct intramyocardial injection.[5–8] Endoventricular methods have limited access to the myocardium in the area of the submitral valve apparatus and may be unstable in the mobile ventricular wall. Additionally, preclinical studies have demonstrated low efficiency and retention in these approaches, and thus the net dose delivered to the tissue may unfortunately be low.[9–12] This low efficiency may theoretically be a result of either bleedback through the 4–8-mm needle tract,[11–13] or simply the fact that injections were not made into myocardium but instead into the dense matrix of endocardial trabeculae.

A compelling alternative approach to endoventricular injection is transvenous intramyocardial injection.[14,15] In this technique, a needle injection catheter resides stably in an epicardial vein, and injections are made tangentially across the septum or free walls of the ventricle. Clinical surgical injection of skeletal myoblasts into infarcted tissue has yielded promising results.[1,2] Investigators have used similar surgical techniques, injecting the cells tangentially, just under the visceral pericardium. Unlike endocardial injection approaches, which direct injections perpendicular to the ventricle wall, transvenous injection allows for cells or therapeutic substances to be deposited in long tracts tangential to the ventricle wall, similar to the surgical approach.[13-15] Additionally, transvenous injections may offer an improvement over the surgical approach because the entire injection is contained within the epicardium, thus precluding the epicardial bleedback seen in the surgical injection approach. Lastly, access via the vein may improve septal wall access.

Technique

Transvenous intramyocardial injection uses the coronary venous system as a 'vascular highway' to access the ventricular myocardium (Figure 25.1). From a percutaneous femoral approach, access to the coronary sinus (CS) is accomplished. Although the approach is from the femoral vein, identification and entry into the CS is very similar to the technique applied in the

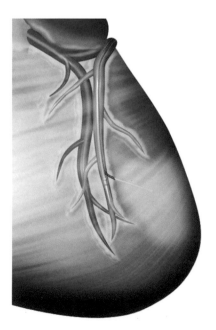

Figure 25.1 *Transvenous myocardial injection, as depicted from an epicardial vein. A TransAccess needle injection catheter (TransVascular, Inc., Menlo Park, CA, USA) is shown residing within the vein, with its needle penetrating the vein wall, gaining purchase to the adjacent myocardium. An integrated intravascular ultrasound (IVUS) transducer (20 MHz; compatible with the JOMED system) allows the operator to orient towards and target the area of treatment. From the deployed needle of the composite catheter, a smaller (27 G) IntraLume microcatheter (TransVascular, Inc., Menlo Park, CA, USA) is advanced through normal and infarcted myocardial tissue. Subsequent injections to remote myocardial locations are accomplished with a syringe attached to the proximal hub of the microcatheter.*

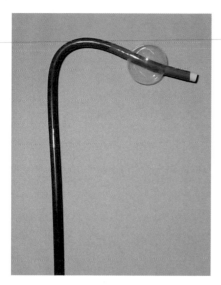

Figure 25.2 *A specially designed balloon occlusion guiding catheter (coronary sinus (CS) balloon occlusion guide catheter (10 Fr)) (TransVascular, Inc., Menlo Park, CA, USA) is used to select and temporarily occlude the CS for venography. The design permits immediate access to distal venous conduits, for the positioning of the TransAccess and IntraLume catheters for intramyocardial injection.*

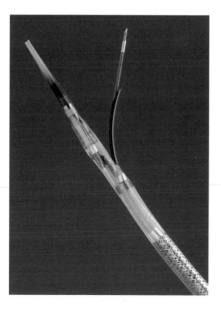

Figure 25.3 *Transvenous intramyocardial injection system: the TransAccess catheter (TransVascular, Inc., Menlo Park, CA, USA) is shown with its 24-gauge (G) needle deployed. The IntraLume microcatheter (27 G) (TransVascular, Inc., Menlo Park, CA, USA), with its radiopaque distal tip marker, is shown extending from the needle. The IntraLume catheter is advanced through the deployed needle and extended deep into myocardial tissue. The gold element located between the deployed needle and the distal tip of the TransAccess catheter is the IVUS phased-array transducer (20 MHz), which is compatible with the JOMED system.*

placement of biventricular pacing leads. A 10-Fr CS balloon occlusion guide catheter (Figure 25.2) is used to cannulate the CS, and a guide wire is advanced into the great cardiac vein (GCV). When the balloon on the guide catheter is inflated, it allows for retrograde venous angiography. A composite needle injection catheter is then advanced into the epicardial vein near the area of treatment. The needle injection catheter (Figure 25.3), known as a

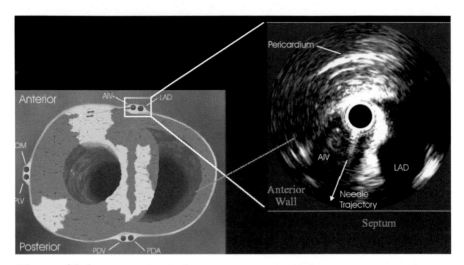

Figure 25.4 *IVUS landmarks for transvenous myocardial injection. Because the injection catheter system is stable within the cardiac vein and the ventricular wall, the needle can be precisely directed tangential to the ventricular targets using IVUS imaging (shown on right). OM, obtuse marginal artery; PLV, posterolateral vein; PDA, posterior descending artery; PDV, posterior descending vein; LAD, left anterior descending artery; AIV, anterior interventricular vein.*

TransAccess catheter (TransVascular, Inc., Menlo Park, CA, USA), is composed of an integrated intravascular ultrasound (IVUS) imaging probe and a precisely oriented needle. With the use of IVUS and fluoroscopy, the catheter is directed towards the myocardium (Figure 25.4) and the 24-gauge needle is deployed. From within the needle, the 27-gauge IntraLume microcatheter (TransVascular, Inc.) is extended deeper into the myocardium. Because the injection catheter is stable within the vein and ventricle wall, the needle can be precisely directed tangential to the ventricle free wall or septum. In such a way, an entire tract of cells or therapeutic substance may be injected from a single needle deployment. It has recently been shown that a contiguous tract of cells may foster the growth of a myocardial syncytium and that this may be necessary for proper engraftment and function.[16] Thus, the catheter's ability to track tangentially may be an essential aspect of its utility.

Recently, a new version of the TransAccess catheter has been designed to allow for a much larger territory of myocardium to be treated from a single access point (Figure 25.5). The needle of this device has a much larger curvature and maximum extension. As can be seen from Figure 26.6, the needle sets the injection trajectory, while the IntraLume penetrates linearly from that access point. The figures show a schematic of injections that cover

340

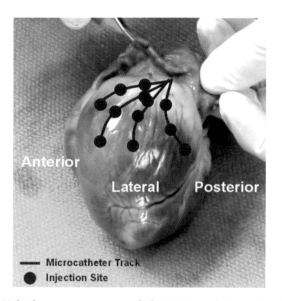

Figure 25.5 *Multiple transvenous myocardial injection technique. Anterior, lateral and posterior tangents can be achieved from a single position in the great cardiac vein (GCV). Here, the injection catheter system was used in the intact heart of a juvenile pig. With varying needle curvature and extension distance, the subsequent passage of the IntraLume microcatheter was directed to different injection depths, to cover several myocardial targets from a single injection plane. —, Microcatheter track; •, injection site.*

the anterolateral, lateral and posterolateral surfaces of the left ventricle from a single catheter location. Recent experience in biventricular pacing has brought attention to coronary venous anatomy.[17] This work has demonstrated that significant variation occurs in human venous anatomy in the lateral and posterolateral walls of the left ventricle. However, given the versatility and reach of the transvenous intramyocardial injection system described above, there exists a more than adequate set of alternative venous access points from which delivery to the myocardium can be achieved.

Clinical and preclinical studies

One of the unique aspects of the TransAccess system is that the same catheter has applications that extend beyond transvenous intramyocardial injection. The system was first used clinically in a procedure called percutaneous in situ coronary venous arterialization (PICVA).[18] Targeted at end-stage cardiovascular disease, the PICVA procedure allows for the perfusion of chronically ischemic

341

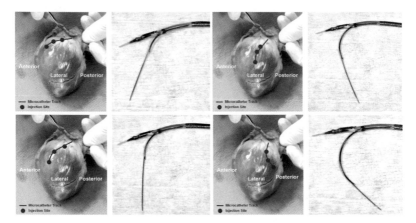

Figure 25.6 *Tangential vectors vary as functions of both needle curvature and needle extension distance. Panel sequence demonstrates: anterior projection of microcatheter (top, left); anterolateral projection (bottom, left); lateral projection (top, right); and posterior projection (bottom, right). –, Microcatheter track; •, injection site.*

myocardium via a percutaneously arterialized epicardial vein. For PICVA, the TransAccess system is used to facilitate the orientation, targeting, access and passage of a guide wire between the target arterial and venous epicardial vessels. Clinical studies on a new version of the system for this application are currently underway in Europe.[19,20] The system is also currently commercially available for use in several peripheral applications in the USA and Europe. Peripheral applications of the TransAccess catheter include: (1) controlled re-entry into the distal true lumen of a chronically occluded vessel during accidental or intentional subintimal entrapment of the guide wire; (2) controlled access between the true and false lumens of an aortic dissection to facilitate aortic fenestration;[21] and (3) creation of a new completely percutaneous femoral–popliteal bypass procedure where the catheter is used to exit the proximal stump vessel and re-enter distally, facilitating the placement of a percutaneously deployable covered graft.[22]

The transvenous intramyocardial injection system has been developed and studied in several animal studies under the direction of investigators such as Alan Yeung (Stanford University Hospital and Clinics, Stanford, CA, USA), Stephen Oesterle, Moto Hayase and Reginald Low (University of California, Davis, CA, USA), Craig Thompson (Massachusetts General Hospital, Boston, MA, USA), Camille Brasselet (Hôpital European Georges Pompidou, Paris, France), Philippe Menasché (Assistance Publique-Hôpitaux de Paris, Department of Cardiovascular Surgery B, Hôpital Bichat, Paris, France) and Patrick Serruys, Willem J. van der Giessen and Pieter Smits (Thoraxcenter, Erasmus Medical Center, Rotterdam, The Netherlands).

Utilizing a unique real-time assay developed at the Thoraxcenter at Erasmus Medical Center (Rotterdam, The Netherlands), Smits et al demonstrated that the transvenous intramyocardial injection system could provide superior efficiency and retention characteristics compared with two of the leading endoventricular-based systems. These data, first presented at the EuroPCR 2002 (Paris, France), demonstrated that the TransAccess transvenous intramyocardial injection system had a 1-min efficiency of 63.5% ±26% using a radiolabeled vascular endothelial growth factor (VEGF) substrate. This compared very favorably with the results of the NOGA (Biosense) and fluoroscopy-guided (MicroHeart) endoventricular systems, which demonstrated efficiencies of 26% ±23% and 25% ±18%, respectively.[9] While the retention of injected proteins decreased over time in all cases, the transvenous intramyocardial injection approach maintained a ×2.5 advantage after 3 h. Thompson et al initially validated safety, targeting accuracy and proof-of-concept of this method for cell delivery in a normal-heart swine model with subpopulations of bone marrow-derived cell lines (Figure 25.7).[23] Brasselet et al demonstrated similar feasibility with skeletal myoblast cell sources.[24] Transvenous, direct myocardial delivery has been demonstrated to be safe and feasible in infarcted tissue as well with recovery of prelabeled, viable cells from infarcted tissue at 6–8 weeks (Figure 25.8) (Thompson et al unpublished data). Having shown the initial feasibility and safety of the system, as well as cellular viability and engraftment acutely and chronically with several cell types, many of these investigators will be mounting clinical efforts with the device in the coming months.

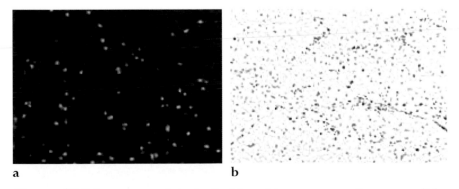

a   b

Figure 25.7 *Bone marrow-derived cells delivered by transvenous, direct myocardial injection. Two week post-cell transplant histologic preparation of VSV-transduced, GFP⁺ bone marrow-derived cells: (a) direct fluorescence of GFP⁺ cells with fluorescein isothiocyanate (FITC) conjugate; and (b) corresponding H & E stain (×200 magnification). GFP, green fluorescence protein; VSV, vesiculostomatitis virus. (Reproduced with permission from the American College of Cardiology.)*

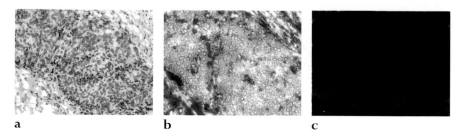

a   b   c

Figure 25.8 Cell survival analysis in myocardial scar tissue. Histologic analysis of rhodamine-conjugated bone marrow-derived cells 6 weeks post-transplantation deep within myocardial scar: (a) H & E, (b) Trichrome and (c) direct fluorescence (red) confirming rhodamine-conjugated cells. Magnification ×200.

The transvenous intramyocardial injection system is currently part of two clinical protocols focused on the treatment of congestive heart failure. The first, under the direction of Serruys, van der Giessen and Smits in Rotterdam, is focused on the safety and feasibility of injecting autologous skeletal myoblasts expanded by a proprietary process (BioHeart, Inc., Weston, FL, USA). Professor Tomasz Siminiak is leading another clinical effort utilizing autologous skeletal myoblasts, processed by the Hematology Department at the District Hospital, Poznan, Poland. Additionally, the transvenous intramyocardial injection system is part of a clinical protocol focused on the treatment of no-option angina patients under the direction of Antonio Colombo (EMO Centro Cuore Columbus, Milan, Italy), utilizing filtered autologous bone marrow, both alone and in combination with VEGF. Initial results from these studies should be available soon.

Conclusion

The transvenous intramyocardial injection system has the potential to be a key tool for interventionalists in the rapidly evolving field of angiogenesis and myogenesis. The transvenous intramyocardial injection system's superior efficiency compared to several transendocardial approaches and its trajectory and stability characteristics hold promise for enhancing the effectiveness of local intramyocardial cell and drug delivery. Furthermore, the method may reduce required injection volumes and cell counts and thus may limit potential systemic side-effects and reduce the costs of these therapies as they enter broader clinical application. Clinical studies investigating the safety and feasibility of the transvenous intramyocardial cell transplantation procedure are ongoing.

References

1. Menasché P, Hagège AA, Vilquin JT et al. Autologous skeletal myoblast transplantation for severe post-infarction left ventricular dysfunction. J Am Coll Cardiol 2003; 41: 1078–83.

2. Siminiak T. Transplantation of autologous skeletal myoblasts in the treatment of patients with post-infarction heart failure: one-year experience. Presented at the American College of Cardiology 52nd Scientific Sessions, Late-Breaking Clinical Trials, Chicago, IL, 2003.

3. Taylor DA, Silvestry SC, Bishop SP et al. Delivery of primary autologous skeletal myoblasts into rabbit heart by coronary infusion: a potential approach to myocardial repair. Proc Assoc Am Physicians 1997; 109: 245–53.

4. Assmus B, Schachinger V, Teupe C et al. Transplantation of progenitor cells and regeneration enhancement in acute myocardial infarction (TOPCARE-AMI). Circulation 2002; 106: 3009–17.

5. Laham R, Rezaee M, Garcia L et al. Tissue and myocardial distribution of intracoronary, intravenous, intraperitoneal, and intramyocardial 125I-labeled basic fibroblast growth factor (bFGF) favor intramyocardial delivery. J Am Coll Cardiol 2000; 35(suppl): 10a (abstract).

6. Rezaee M, Yeung AC, Altman P et al. Evaluation of percutaneous intramyocardial injection for local myocardial treatment. Catheter Cardiovasc Intervent 2001; 53: 271–6.

7. Kornowski R, Leon MB, Fuchs S et al. Electromagnetic guidance for catheter-based transendocardial injection: a platform for intramyocardial angiogenesis therapy. Results in normal and ischemic pig models. J Am Coll Cardiol 2000; 35: 1031–9.

8. Lederman RJ, Guttman MA, Peters DC et al. Catheter-based endomyocardial injection with real-time magnetic resonance imaging. Circulation 2002; 105: 1282–4.

9. Smits PC, van der Giessen WJ, Reys AE et al. Comparison in efficiency between a NOGA and fluoroscopy guided transendomyocardial injection catheter. AHA Abstract: Scientific Conference on Therapeutic Angiogenesis & Myocardial Laser Revascularization, 2001.

10. Smits PC, van der Giessen WJ, Reys AE et al. Efficiency and retention of percutaneous transendomyocardial injection of VEGF[165] by a fluoroscopy guided injection catheter: a radionuclide study. AHA Abstract: Scientific Conference on Therapeutic Angiogenesis & Myocardial Laser Revascularization, 2001.

11. Smits PC, van Langenhove G, Schaar M et al. Efficacy of percutaneous intramyocardial injections using a nonfluoroscopic 3-D mapping based catheter system. Cardiovasc Drugs Ther 2002; 16(6): 527–33.

345

12. Grossman PM, Han Z, Palasis M. Incomplete retention after direct myocardial injection. Catheter Cardiovasc Intervent 2002; 55: 392–7.

13. Thompson CA, Nasseri BA, Makower J. Percutaneous transvenous cellular cardiomyoplasty: a novel nonsurgical approach for myocardial cell transplantation. J Am Coll Cardiol 2003; 41: 1964–71.

14. Simons M, Post MJ. Angiogenesis. In: Topol E, ed. Textbook of interventional cardiology, 4th edn. Philadelphia: Saunders/Elsevier Science, 2003: 72–3.

15. Menasché P, Hagege AA, Scorsin M et al. Myoblast transplantation for heart failure. Lancet 2001; 357: 279–80.

16. Pagani FD, DerSimonian H, Zawadzka A et al. Autologous skeletal myoblasts transplanted to ischemia-damaged myocardium in humans. Histological analysis of cell survival and differentiation. J Am Coll Cardiol 2003; 41(5): 879–88.

17. Meisel E, Pfeiffer D, Engelmann L et al. Investigation of coronary venous anatomy by retrograde venography in patients with malignant ventricular tachycardias. Circulation 2001; 104: 442–7.

18. Oesterle SN , Reifart N, Hauptmann E et al. Percutaneous in situ coronary venous arterialization. Report of the first human catheter-based coronary artery bypass. Circulation 2001; 103: 2539–43.

19. Oesterle SN, Reifart N, Hayase M et al. Catheter-based coronary bypass: a development update. Catheter Cardiovasc Intervent 2003; 58: 212–18.

20. Thompson CA, Burkhoff D, Oesterle S. Percutaneous bypass surgery. In: Topol E, ed. Textbook of interventional cardiology, 4th edn. Philadelphia: Saunders/Elsevier Science, 2003: 781–93.

21. Saketkhoo RR, Razavi MK, Padidar A et al. A novel intravascular ultrasound guided method to create transintimal arterial communications: initial experience in peripheral occlusive disease and an aortic dissection. Circulation (in press).

22. Haskal ZJ, Razavi M, Lamson T. Percutaneous creation of extra-vascular and in-situ arterio-veno-arterial infrainguinal and infrapopliteal bypasses using the Transvascular Guidance System (abstract). Presented at Annual Meeting of the Society of Cardiovascular and Interventional Radiologists, 2002.

23. Thompson CA, Nasseri BA, Makower J et al. Percutaneous transvenous cellular cardiomyoplasty: a novel approach for myocardial cell transplantation. J Am Coll Cardiol 2003; 41: 1964–71.

24. Brasselet C et al. The coronary sinus: a safe and effective route for percutaneous myoblast transplantation. ACC Abstract: American College of Cardiology Conference, April 2003.

26. Perivascular Endothelial Cell Tissue Engineering

Helen M Nugent and Elazer R Edelman

Introduction

The normal blood vessel is a complex structure composed of three concentric tunics, the tunica intima, tunica media and tunica adventitia (Figure 26.1). The intima, located at the blood vessel wall–lumen interface, is lined by a single layer of endothelial cells supported by a basement membrane, below which resides a sparse layer of vascular smooth muscle cells.[1] The media, located in the middle of the blood vessel wall, consists of smooth muscle cells in lamellar units bound by elastic bands or lamina. The contraction and relaxation of these units allow the artery to constrict or dilate, regulating bloodflow.[1] The adventitia, located at the outer layer of the blood vessel, is composed of a loose fibrous network of fibroblasts. The vessels that nourish the blood vessel wall and the nerves that supply neural control are also found in the adventitia.[1] The physical continuity of these cells and tissues provides structural integrity to the blood vessel wall while also maintaining homeostasis through biochemical regulation. The complexity of this system renders it extremely sensitive to inflammation, injury or infection and

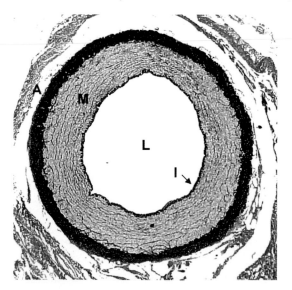

Figure 26.1 Histologic cross-section of a normal porcine carotid artery stained with Verhoeff's elastin stain (magnification ×20). L, lumen; I, intima; M, media; A, adventitia.

susceptible to significant complications after mechanical manipulation. Angioplasty,[2–4] arteriovenous shunts and fistulae[5–7] and organ transplantation,[8] may bypass or treat blood vessel obstructions but they also elicit a sequence of events that induces inflammation, stimulates smooth muscle cell proliferation and culminates in intimal hyperplasia and luminal occlusions.[9,10]

The vascular endothelium is central to understanding vascular biology and critical to maintaining vascular health. The endothelial monolayer that normally lines blood vessels forms a continuous, selectively permeable, thromboresistant surface that regulates local biology to prevent luminal obstructions and ensure uninterrupted distal bloodflow and adequate distal tissue perfusion.[11] This level of control is achieved throughout the blood vessel by an array of endothelial cell-derived biologically active compounds that regulate virtually every aspect of vascular biology, including thrombosis, vasomotor tone, smooth muscle cell proliferation and migration, lipid infiltration, and leukocyte adhesion or diapedesion.[10,12–16] Endothelial state and cell density determine what compounds will be secreted. While confluence breeds quiescence, monolayer disruption signals growth promotion and accompanying phenomena.[17–21] As a natural consequence of these observations, many have tried to isolate and infuse single endothelial products to regulate vascular disease,[22–26] and when this has failed, to restore denuded or repair dysfunctional endothelium.[27–29] As a result of these studies, several questions have arisen. Must one recapitulate the ordered architecture of the blood vessel to restore endothelial health? Might structure and function be defined as a continuum, so that restoration of only part of the structure is required for restoration of part of the function? Does one need to completely reconstruct a blood vessel or can one find an intermediate state that will restore health, and does this intermediate state necessitate that we place the cells where they would naturally reside or simply in direct contact with the blood vessel?

Innovative studies have been performed with autologous endothelial cell transplantation,[30–32] implantation of endothelial cell-seeded grafts[33] or endovascular stents.[34] But the answer to our questions required that we place endothelial cells in positions other than at the luminal–vessel wall interface. Tissue engineering provided a means to achieve this. Proposed primarily as a solution to the limited supply of transplantable autologous tissue, tissue-engineered constructs may also be used as a tool to examine structure–function relationships for specific cell and tissues. Methods of tissue engineering can be used to implant endothelial cells at sites distant to or in different configurations from their original state, providing an opportunity to examine their autocrine, paracrine and endocrine functions independent of their barrier function. We have demonstrated, through the use of tissue-engineered endothelial cells, that the biological effect of these cells on vascular repair is maintained even when they are implanted at a distance from their original location at the lumen.[35–39] Endothelial cells were cultured in three-dimensional polymer matrices and implanted in the perivascular space of injured rat or porcine blood vessels. In this chapter, we will discuss the results of implantation of perivascular endothelial cells in several animal models of vascular injury.

Perivascular delivery devices

Polymer-based controlled drug delivery systems offer the potential of sustained and controlled release of specific drugs.[40] These systems present distinct advantages over pumps that deliver substances from a reservoir into the intra- or extravascular spaces. Polymer delivery systems can handle compounds in their dry state and as such can be smaller, markedly decrease potential drug degradation, prolong shelf-life and enable administration of compounds in minute concentrations. Such devices have been used to maintain euglycemia in diabetic rats,[41] preserve and release unstable growth factors[42,43] and inhibit or stimulate angiogenesis.[44] Controlled release of compounds from polymer matrices in the perivascular space is also an efficient means of administering drugs to deal with vascular disease.[45–49]

Heparin, a potent smooth muscle cell inhibitor, can cause serious side-effects such as uncontrolled bleeding if administered systemically. When controlled-release matrices containing dry heparin were placed adjacent to injured rat carotid arteries (Figure 26.2), the drug was solubilized slowly and eluted out.[45] Systemic levels of the drug were not detectable, as perivascular

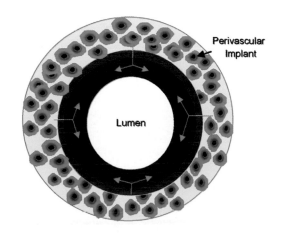

Figure 26.2 *A perivascular implant wrapped around a denuded blood vessel. Antiproliferative compounds released from endothelial cell implants may move throughout the blood vessel wall in a manner similar to the controlled adventitial delivery of single endothelial cell-derived compounds such as heparin and fibroblast growth factor (FGF-2)*

heparin did not elevate activated partial thromboplastin time, yet the perivascular administration produced the greatest inhibition of intimal hyperplasia compared to intravenous or subcutaneous administration. Controlled perivascular release reduced intimal hyperplasia $83.0 \pm 2.6\%$ with anticoagulant heparin and $68.3 \pm 3.7\%$ with non-anticoagulant heparin. Perivascular delivery was also found to be far more efficient than intravenous delivery at depositing fibroblast growth factor (FGF-2), a potent smooth muscle cell stimulator with a short half-life, within the arterial wall.[47] FGF-2 was rapidly cleared following intravenous injection and deposited within both solid organs and the walls of blood vessels. The in vivo half-life of FGF-2 has been estimated to be in the range of 2–4 min, and this growth factor is prone to denaturation and degradation. Peak serum FGF-2 levels were detected within 1 min of injection, and the growth factor was cleared thereafter with a half-life of almost 3 min. In contrast, when FGF-2 was delivered by polymeric controlled-release devices in the perivascular space, deposition within the blood vessel wall was rapidly distributed circumferentially and was substantially greater than that observed following intravenous injection (Figure 26.2). The amount of FGF-2 deposited in arteries adjacent to the release devices was 40 times greater than that deposited in arteries in animals following intravenous injection. Therefore, FGF-2 is most effective when administered in the perivascular region of the injured blood vessel rather than in a manner that would require transport through the entire vascular system first. Based on these results, we reasoned that perhaps perivascular tissue-engineered endothelial cells could provide physiologic control by the local delivery of all the cell-based products without the need for pharmacologic dosing with isolated compounds (Figure 26.2).

Perivascular tissue-engineered endothelial cells

The isolation and subsequent transplantation of endothelial cells onto polymeric surfaces were first reported by Herring et al as a means to improve the long-term patency of small-diameter bypass grafts.[50] Since this study, research in numerous laboratories has focused on improving endothelial cell attachment, growth and function on polymer surfaces.[51–63] Seeding endothelial cells at the luminal surface of a blood vessel or graft is technically difficult to achieve in practice, applies a limited number of endothelial cells during periods of intense injury and vascular response and may not be necessary for the production and secretion of biologically active compounds from the endothelial cells. To address these issues, we cultured endothelial cells on three-dimensional polymer matrices (Gelfoam) with retention of viability, normal growth kinetics and biochemical activity. Matrices containing cells were then placed in the perivascular space of injured blood vessels.

Seeding of endothelial cells in Gelfoam matrices has been described in detail.[35–39] Briefly, sterile Gelfoam was cut into blocks of specific dimensions, hydrated and seeded with approximately 1.25×10^5 cells/cm^3 Gelfoam (exact cell density will vary depending on cell type). The cell-seeded Gelfoam blocks were then incubated for up to 2 weeks to allow the cells to reach confluence within the polymer matrices. The number of cells attached to the Gelfoam was determined after digestion with collagenase, and cell viability was assessed by trypan blue exclusion. The state of the endothelial cells, whether they are confluent or proliferating, will determine the nature of their control over vascular biology, specifically smooth muscle cell biology.[64] We have demonstrated in vitro that conditioned medium from post-confluent endothelial cells inhibits cultured smooth muscle cell proliferation; however, conditioned medium from sparse, proliferating endothelial cells stimulates smooth muscle cell growth.[64] It was determined that this effect results not from a difference in heparin-like compounds, as both sparse and confluent endothelial cells produce heparan sulfate proteoglycans that are inhibitory to smooth muscle cell proliferation, but rather from a difference in the non-proteoglycan proteins that interact with the heparan sulfates. Therefore, to ensure that the tissue-engineered endothelial cells produce optimal amounts of inhibitory compounds once implanted in vivo, cell-seeded Gelfoam sponges were implanted approximately 3 days after reaching confluence.

Bovine aortic endothelial cells (BAEs) cultured in Gelfoam matrices lined the interstices of the three-dimensional sponge and followed a growth pattern similar to that obtained on tissue culture-treated polystyrene.[35,36] Viability, evaluated by trypan blue exclusion and a LIVE/DEAD cytotoxicity assay, remained $\geq 95\%$ throughout the 2-week culture period. Endothelial cells cultured on Gelfoam also retained their biological potency and ability to take up acetylated low-density lipoprotein (LDL) (Figure 26.3). BAEs cultured in Gelfoam produced nearly identical amounts of total sulfated glycosaminoglycan ($4.1 \pm 0.3 \,\mu$g per 10^6 cells per day) and heparan sulfate ($1.2 \pm 0.05 \,\mu$g per 10^6 cells per day) to that produced by cells cultured on standard polystyrene dishes.[35] In addition, conditioned medium from BAEs on Gelfoam inhibited binding of ^{125}I-FGF-2 to heparan sulfate proteoglycan and the mitogenic effect of FGF-2 on smooth muscle cells in a dose-dependent fashion.[35] Porcine aortic endothelial cells (PAEs) were also grown in Gelfoam matrices and found to follow a similar growth curve, remain viable and produce nearly identical amounts of heparan sulfate and transforming growth factor-beta$_1$ (TGF-ß$_1$) compared to BAEs cultured in Gelfoam.[36,38] Perivascular implantation of BAE–Gelfoam scaffolds around balloon-denuded rat carotid arteries reduced

Figure 26.3 *The preservation of endothelial cell identity is verified by uptake of acetylated low-density lipoprotein (Ac-LDL). BAEs were cultured in Gelfoam matrices and incubated with 1,1'-dioctadecyl-3,3,3',3'-tetramethyl-indo-carbocyanine perchlorate (DiI)–Ac-LDL. Confocal laser-scanning microscopy was used to visualize positive cells within the matrices after 2 weeks in culture. Red cells indicate positive Ac-LDL uptake (magnification ×200). Empty control Gelfoam matrices do not stain positively for Ac-LDL.*

intimal hyperplasia by 88% when compared to balloon-injured controls.[35] Control Chinese hamster ovary (CHO-745) cells engrafted in Gelfoam and placed adjacent to the injured arteries had no significant effect on intimal hyperplasia compared to balloon injury alone or empty control Gelfoam matrices. Heparin has been identified as a potent inhibitor of smooth muscle cell proliferation both in vitro and in animal models, mainly because it resembles endothelial-derived heparan sulfate proteoglycan. As expected, the perivascular delivery of heparin from controlled-release devices reduced intimal hyperplasia in this animal study by 60%. However, this result was 3.2-fold less effective than the inhibition observed with the perivascular endothelial cells, despite the fact that the rate of release of heparin from the polymer devices was twice the calculated rate of release of heparan sulfate from the endothelial implants. These experiments supported the hypothesis that endothelial control over vascular repair is derived from the secretion of endothelial cell-based products and need not emanate from the luminal surface. Unfortunately, there is usually a lack of correlation between small animal models and human vascular disease. These observations may stem from the increased complexity of the lesions with increased injury or higher species. Therefore, in experiments designed to exploit tissue-engineered endothelial cells as a tool to further elucidate the fundamental issues of vascular biology, we performed studies in more complex models of vascular injury.

Porcine models of vascular injury

Vascular injury of pig carotid or femoral arteries as experimental models of acute and chronic vascular injury offered advantages over other models for our studies. The carotid arteries were accessible by standard catheterization techniques and both the carotid and femoral arteries were easily accessible to surgical manipulation. In addition, compared with smaller animal models, the pig has more in common with humans with respect to platelet coagulation[65] and histologic characteristics.[66–68]

Short-term study

BAEs and PAEs were grown in Gelfoam and implanted around balloon-injured porcine carotid arteries.[36] One month postoperatively, both BAE and PAE implants significantly reduced intimal hyperplasia by 46% and 54%, respectively (Figure 26.4). Perivascular heparin devices, formulated to release

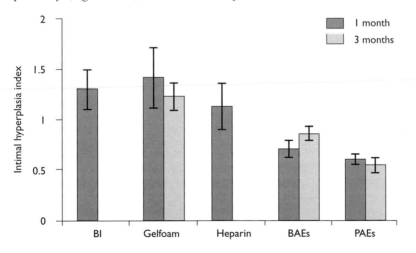

Figure 26.4 *The effects of BAEs and PAEs on intimal thickening in balloon-injured porcine carotid arteries 1 and 3 months postoperatively. Both BAEs and PAEs significantly reduced intimal thickening when compared to either heparin-treated, balloon injury (BI) or Gelfoam controls (P < 0.05). (Modified from Nugent et al[36] and Nugent and Edelman.[38])*

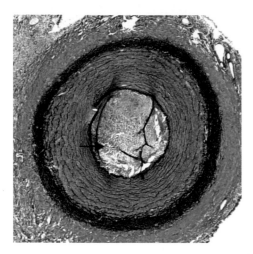

Figure 26.5 Histologic cross-section of a control balloon-injured porcine carotid artery stained with Verhoeff's elastin stain (magnification ×20). The artery is completely occluded with organized thrombus 1 month postoperatively. Arrow points to organized thrombus.

heparin at twice the rate of release of heparan sulfate from the endothelial cell implants, produced an insignificant reduction of 25% when compared to control balloon-injured arteries. BAEs and PAEs also reduced occlusive thrombosis compared to control and heparin-release devices. Extensive occlusive organized thrombosis (Figure 26.5) was observed in 40% of the arteries treated with empty control Gelfoam, in 33% of the control balloon-injured arteries, in 25% of the heparin-treated arteries and in none (0%) of either the BAE- or PAE-treated arteries (Figure 26.6). The increasing appreciation of the potential of tissue-engineered constructs necessitated an investigation of host immune responses to both the allogeneic (porcine) and xenogeneic (bovine) implants. The ability to use either allogeneic or xenogeneic cells in a clinical setting would greatly enhance the potential applications of tissue-engineered implants. The BAE implants elicited both a cell-mediated and a humoral immune response in pigs. Leukocytes, consisting mainly of T lymphocytes, and macrophages, were found within and surrounding the BAE implants at 1 month. Lymphocytes were also found within the PAE implants, although there were markedly fewer infiltrating cells compared to the BAE implants. Sera obtained at 28 days from pigs implanted with BAE cells displayed an increase in circulating antibodies to the transplanted cells. No humoral response was detected in the animals that received PAE implants. Interestingly, although there was a significant difference in the immune responses between pigs that were implanted with bovine or porcine cells, there was no difference in biological effects between BAE or PAE implants. These data suggested that the tissue-engineered implants were able to affect thrombus formation, cellular recruitment and subsequent smooth muscle cell proliferation that led to intimal hyperplasia at 28 days before undergoing rejection or cell loss from other causes.

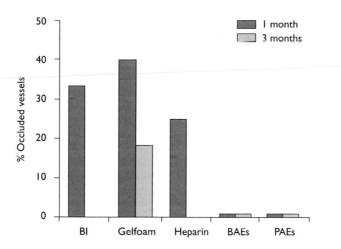

Figure 26.6 *Bar graph shows a decrease in occlusive thrombosis in balloon-injured porcine carotid arteries treated with either BAEs or PAEs 1 and 3 months postoperatively. Controlled perivascular release of heparin did not have a significant effect compared to controls. BI, balloon injury. (Modified from Nugent et al[36] and Nugent and Edelman.[38])*

Long-term study

A 3-month study was performed to determine whether tissue-engineered endothelial implants provide long-term control of vascular homeostasis, or if they simply delay lesion formation.[37] An important issue in the development of potential therapies to treat accelerated arteriopathies relates to the extent of the observed effects. Many compounds that inhibit intimal hyperplasia lose effect as soon as the therapy is discontinued. For example, in a study where animals were made transiently thrombocytopenic after balloon denudation, intimal proliferation was inhibited during the period of platelet suppression but returned in full as soon as platelet function was allowed to recover.[69] Removing the critical elements necessary for intimal proliferation temporarily provided a beneficial effect. However, if blood vessel homeostasis is not established by the time the critical elements return, neointimal formation is only delayed and will eventually return in full. We hypothesized that because perivascular endothelial implants not only inhibit intimal hyperplasia and thrombotic occlusion but also enable vascular healing and restore homeostasis, a permanent implant would not be necessary to achieve lasting benefits. To test this hypothesis, we investigated the biological effects of the endothelial implants 3 months after angioplasty, approximately 2 months after implant degradation or destruction had occurred. Gelfoam is a marketed surgical sponge with a typical in vivo degradation rate of approximately 4–6 weeks.

355

Three months postoperatively, neither Gelfoam nor the transplanted endothelial cells could be detected at the implant site, and yet both bovine and porcine implants inhibited occlusive thrombosis and intimal hyperplasia. Extensive occlusive organized thrombosis was observed in 18% of the arteries treated with empty control Gelfoam, and in none (0%) of either the BAE- or PAE-treated arteries (Figure 26.6). PAE and BAE implants also significantly reduced intimal thickening compared to controls by 56% and 31%, respectively (Figure 26.4). In contrast to the 1-month study, implants containing allogeneic cells were almost two-fold more effective at inhibiting intimal thickening at 3 months than those containing xenogeneic cells. Staining for endothelial cells at the lumen interface revealed that arteries in all treatment groups were completely re-endothelialized at 3 months, supporting the idea that the beneficial effects of the endothelial implants were permanent, since significant intimal formation would not be expected after regeneration of the luminal endothelium.

The differential effects of the bovine and porcine cells on intimal thickening at 3 months suggested a relationship between the biological and immunologic responses. Serial serum samples from animals implanted with bovine cells demonstrated an increase in cytotoxic antibodies to the BAEs beginning 4 days after injury and resolving at approximately 40 days. No significant increase in cytotoxic antibodies to PAE was observed during the course of the 3-month study in animals implanted with porcine cells. Because thrombus formation occurs within minutes to hours after vascular injury, an increase in antibodies to the bovine cells 4–40 days postoperatively did not impact on the implants' inhibitory effects on occlusive thrombosis. However, an increase in cytotoxic antibodies occurring after day 4 did affect the BAE implants' influence on the late proliferative phase that occurs days to months after injury. Thus, while the choice of cell type in our studies was less important for the thrombotic complications of vascular injury, it was crucial for maximum control of the late proliferative response that led to intimal hyperplasia at 3 months.

Coupling of perivascular endothelial cell transplantation with molecular modification technology

Techniques of tissue engineering also enable the implantation of cells that have been genetically modified to produce more or less specific compounds. Perivascular implants bearing genetically modified endothelial cells could then be used to dissect the components critical in the vascular response to injury. Perlecan, a heparan sulfate proteoglycan, has been suggested to be important in the regulation of vascular repair.[70–73] Perlecan is a major proteoglycan secreted by cultured endothelial cells and is a potent inhibitor of smooth muscle cell proliferation in vitro.[72,73] Perlecan has been proposed to bind to heparin-binding mitogens, such as FGF-2, and prevent them from stimulating smooth muscle cells[16,74] Endothelial cell-secreted perlecan probably plays a major role in vascular repair after injury in vivo. We generated stably transfected clones of BAEs that expressed high levels of an antisense vector targeting domain III of perlecan.[37] Transfected cells produced significantly less perlecan in vitro, and showed a reduced ability to inhibit FGF-2 binding to and mitogenic activity in cultured smooth muscle cells. When Gelfoam matrices containing transfected endothelial cells were implanted adjacent to injured porcine carotid arteries, an interesting divergence of biological effects was observed.[37] Endothelial cell implants with reduced perlecan expression (BAE-AP) were less effective than implants containing endothelial cells transfected with vector only (BAE-NEO) at inhibiting intimal hyperplasia, yet showed a complete loss of the antithrombotic effect observed with the non-transfected cellular implants. BAE-NEO reduced intimal thickening by 42% ($P < 0.05$) compared to control arteries, while BAE-AP reduced intimal thickening by only 25% ($P = NS$). Extensive organized thrombus was also observed in a significant number of the arteries treated with BAE-AP (22%), comparable to that observed in control arteries. In contrast, occlusive thrombus was not observed in any of the arteries treated with BAE-NEO. These results demonstrated that endothelial control over intimal thickening results from a combination of perlecan and other secreted cell-based products. When one important factor (perlecan) that directly interacted in these processes was removed, the implanted cells were completely ineffective at preventing occlusive thrombosis and displayed a decreased ability to reduce intimal thickening. These observations may explain why single endothelial cell-derived products, usually aimed at a single cellular event thought to be involved in either thrombosis or smooth muscle cell proliferation, do not lead to full control of vascular homeostasis. Tissue engineering offers new tools to gain added insight into vascular biology and, when coupled with molecular modification technology, is invaluable as a method to further dissect the complex mechanism of vascular repair.

Arteriovenous fistula study

We have demonstrated that perivascular endothelial cell implants are effective at inhibiting intimal thickening following acute balloon injury in rats and pigs. We then sought to determine if these implants could provide a similar benefit in the chronic and more complex injury model of arteriovenous anastomoses. Vascular access failure is the greatest cause of morbidity in hemodialysis patients in the United States, and a satisfactory long-term pharmacologic means of preventing failure due to intimal hyperplasia does not yet exist.[75,76]

Although endothelial injury most likely plays a role in both balloon and anastomotic injury, the exact causes of intimal hyperplasia at the anastomotic site of arteriovenous fistulae are not completely understood. Isolation of veins and arteries followed by exposure of the vein segment to arterial blood flow and pressure, as well as subsequent surgical manipulation such as suturing, can result in direct trauma to the endothelium and smooth muscle cells in both the veins and arteries.[5,77] The question remained whether the complexity of these types of lesions would render them resistant to therapies found to be effective in the simpler, acute balloon injury models of vascular injury.

Side-to-side femoral artery–femoral vein anastomoses were created in pigs. The biological and immunologic responses to PAE implants were investigated 3 days and 1 and 2 months postoperatively.[39] Four weeks after implantation, PAE implants had reduced intimal hyperplasia at the anastomotic site by 35% compared to controls ($P = NS$). Between 4 and 8 weeks, the extent of intimal hyperplasia remained essentially unchanged in PAE-treated anastomoses, while there was an almost two-fold increase in control animals during this same time period. PAE implants significantly reduced intimal hyperplasia at the anastomotic sites by 68% when compared to control matrices at 2 months (Figure 26.7). We also demonstrated that the reduction observed in intimal formation was not due to an early recovery of luminal endothelial cells in

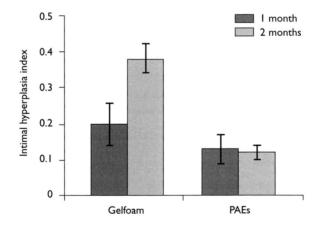

Figure 26.7 *The effects of PAEs on intimal thickening of porcine femoral arteriovenous fistulae 1 and 2 months postoperatively. PAEs decreased the intimal hyperplasia index by 35% ($P = NS$) compared to Gelfoam controls at 1 month. Two months after implantation, the extent of intimal thickening remained unchanged in treated fistulae, while there was an almost two-fold increase in control animals during this time period. PAE implants significantly reduced the intimal hyperplasia index compared to controls by 68% ($P < 0.05$) at 2 months.*[39]

treated animals, as the completely denuded endothelium regenerated at similar rates in both groups. Analysis of tissue sections from animals euthanized at 3 days revealed less neutrophil inflammation at the lumen–vessel wall interface of the arterial and venous segments of PAE-treated anastomoses compared to control segments. A previous study had shown that neutrophil infiltration preceded neointimal thickening in injured rabbit iliac arteries.[78] The study also demonstrated a correlation between inhibition of neutrophil infiltration and inhibition of smooth muscle cell proliferation. The data from our arteriovenous study in pigs suggested that the perivascular tissue-engineered endothelial cells, or compounds released by the cells, may control intimal formation by influencing early events such as neutrophil infiltration into the blood vessel wall. Tissue sections of anastomotic sites from animals euthanized at 3 days and stained for endothelial cells showed a denuded luminal endothelium and confluent endothelial cells lining the perivascular Gelfoam (Figure 26.8).

A humoral immune response to the allogeneic endothelial cells was detected in only 3 of the 14 treated animals 22 days after implantation. Sera from the same three animals also tested positive for antibodies to porcine T cells (PTCs) (Figure 26.9). On average, the increased levels of antibodies were not statistically significant, and only one pig remained positive at 2 months. Although the antigenic specificity of the humoral response remains as

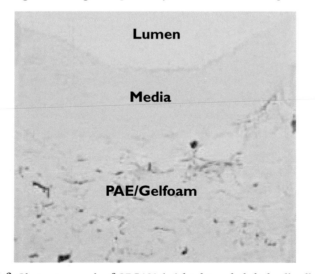

Figure 26.8 Photomicrograph of PECAM-1 (platelet endothelial cell adhesion molecule) staining of a section of a porcine femoral arteriovenous fistula 3 days postoperatively (magnification ×100). Brown cells are PECAM-1 positive. Gelfoam containing PAE stained positive for PECAM-1. Control Gelfoam showed no positive staining. (Modified from Nugent et al.[39])

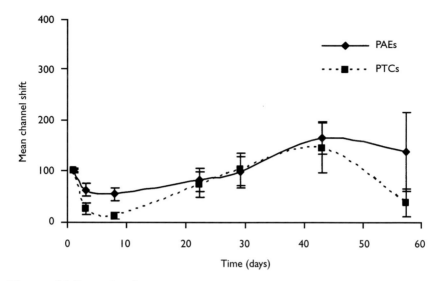

Figure 26.9 *Graphs of average humoral responses in pigs implanted with perivascular allogeneic endothelial cells. Sera were collected on day 1 (presurgery), and 3 days, 1 week, 3 weeks, 1 month, 6 weeks and 2 months postoperatively, and tested against the strain of PAE used in the implants and against PTCs pooled from domestic pigs. On average, an insignificant increase in antibodies binding to PAE was detected 6 weeks and 2 months postoperatively. A similar increase in antibodies binding to PTC was detected at 6 weeks but not at 2 months. (Modified from Nugent et al.[39])*

yet unclear, the activity is probably attributable to cell surface antigens common to both endothelial and T cells, such as swine leukocyte antigen. There was no correlation between the effects on intimal hyperplasia and the humoral response in animals with increased levels of circulating antibodies, suggesting that the implants were able to influence vascular repair and control homeostasis before eliciting effective immune responses.

Conclusion

The technology of endothelial cell tissue engineering has provided an invaluable technique to aid in our current understanding of vascular physiology and cardiovascular diseases. Many of the pathologic events associated with vascular disease arise from endothelial injury or dysfunction.[2-9,17,18] When isolated endothelial compounds are placed back into experimental models of vascular injury, they provide the maximal control over smooth muscle cell proliferation and intimal hyperplasia.[15,45,79,80]

However, infusion of these compounds either fails or produces inconsistent results in clinical trials.[23-26,81-83] It is possible that we have yet to define the exact combination of agents and/or conditions under which endothelial control over vascular homeostasis is achieved. Perivascular tissue-engineered endothelial cells offered a model with which to answer many of the questions regarding endothelial cell control over vascular repair following injury. These cells can serve as viable devices for the local delivery of cell-based products, thereby maximizing local effects and minimizing systemic toxicity. Coupling this technology with genetic modification techniques has provided a new approach for dissecting the role of specific endothelial factors within the complex environment that exists after vascular injury. Further exploration into the control mechanisms of endothelial implants would provide additional insight and support the design of drug delivery devices, tissue-engineered systems and novel pharmacologic therapies for vascular proliferative diseases.

References

1. Burkitt HG, Young B, Heath JW. Wheater's functional histology: a text and colour atlas, 3rd edn. New York: Churchill Livingstone, 1993.

2. Fischell TA, Derby G, Tse TM, Stadius ML. Coronary artery vasoconstriction routinely occurs after percutaneous transluminal coronary angioplasty. Circulation 1988; 78: 1323–34.

3. El-Tamimi H, Davies GJ, Hackett D et al. Abnormal vasomotor changes early after coronary angioplasty. A quantitative arteriographic study of their time course. Circulation 1991; 84: 1198–202.

4. Castaneda-Zuniga WR, Formanek A, Tadavarthy M et al. The mechanism of balloon angioplasty. Radiology 1980; 135: 565–71.

5. Chervu A, Moore WS. An overview of intimal hyperplasia. Surgery 1990; 171: 433–47.

6. Sivanesan S, How TV, Black RA, Bakran A. Flow patterns in the radiocephalic arteriovenous fistula: an in vitro study. J Biomech 1999; 32: 915–25.

7. Sullivan KL, Besarab A, Bonn J et al. Hemodynamics of failing dialysis grafts. Radiology 1993; 186: 867–72.

8. Yamani MH, Tuzcu EM, Starling RC et al. Myocardial ischemic injury after heart transplantation is associated with upregulation of vitronectin receptor (alpha(v)beta3), activation of the matrix metalloproteinase induction system, and subsequent development of coronary vasculopathy. Circulation 2002; 105: 1955–61.

9. Edelman ER, Nugent MA, Smith LT, Karnovsky MJ. Basic fibroblast growth factor enhances the coupling of intimal hyperplasia and proliferation of vasa vasorum in injured rat arteries. J Clin Invest 1992; 89: 465–73.

10. Casscells W. Migration of smooth muscle and endothelial cells. Critical events in restenosis. Circulation 1992; 86: 723–9.

11. Rubanyi GM. The role of endothelium in cardiovascular homeostasis and diseases. J Cardiovasc Pharmacol 1993; 22: S1–14.

12. Furchgott RF, Zawadzki JV. The obligatory role of endothelial cells in the relaxation of arterial smooth muscle by acetylcholine. Nature 1980; 288: 373–6.

13. Autio I, Maol-Ranta RU, Kallioniemi OP, Nikkari T. Cultured bovine aortic endothelial cells secrete factor(s) chemotactic for aortic smooth muscle cells. Artery 1989; 16: 72–83.

14. Cybulsky MI, Gimbrone MA. Endothelial expression of a mononuclear leukocyte adhesion molecule during atherogenesis. Science 1991; 251: 788–91.

15. Castellot JJ, Addonizio ML, Rosenberg RD, Karnovsky MJ. Cultured endothelial cells produce a heparin-like inhibition of smooth muscle growth. J Cell Biol 1981; 90: 372–9.

16. Nugent MA, Karnovsky MJ, Edelman ER. Vascular cell-derived heparan sulfate shows coupled inhibition of basic fibroblast growth factor binding and mitogenesis in vascular smooth muscle cells. Circ Res 1993; 73: 1051–60.

17. Blankenberg FG, Wen P, Dai M et al. Detection of early atherosclerosis with radiolabeled monocyte chemoattractant protein-1 in prediabeteic Zucker rats. Pediatr Radiol 2001; 31: 827–35.

18. Hafer-Macko CE, Ivey FM, Gyure KA et al. Thrombomodulin deficiency in human diabetic nerve microvasculature. Diabetes 2002; 511: 957–63.

19. Nabel EG. Biology of the impaired endothelium. Am J Cardiol 1991; 68: 6C–8C.

20. Furchgott RF, Vanhoutte PM. Endothelium-derived relaxing and contracting factors. FASEB J 1989; 3: 2007–18.

21. Gertler JP, Abbott WM. Prothrombic and fibrinolytic function of normal and perturbed endothelium. J Surg Res 1992; 52: 89–95.

22. Liu MW, Roubin GS, Robinson KA et al. Trapadil in preventing restenosis after balloon angioplasty in the atherosclerotic rabbit. Circulation 1990; 81: 1089–93.

23. Pepine CJ, Hirshfeld JW, Macdonald RG et al. A controlled trial of corticosteroids to prevent restenosis after coronary angioplasty. Circulation 1990; 81: 1753–61.

24. Ellis SG, Roubin GS, Wilentz J et al. Effect of 18- to 24-hour heparin administration for prevention of restenosis after uncomplicated coronary angioplasty. Am Heart J 1989; 117: 777–82.

25. Whitworth HB, Roubin GS, Hollman J et al. Effect of nifedipine in recurrent stenosis after percutaneous coronary angioplasty. J Am Coll Cardiol 1986; 8: 1271–6.

26. Laskey MA, Deutsch E, Hirshfeld JW Jr et al. Influence of heparin therapy on percutaneous transluminal coronary angioplasty outcomes in patients with coronary arterial thrombus. Am J Cardiol 1990; 65: 179–82.

27. Fishman JA, Ryan GB, Karnovsky MJ. Endothelial regeneration in the rat carotid artery and the significance of endothelial denudation in the pathogenesis of myointimal thickening. Lab Invest 1975; 32: 339–51.

28. Schwartz SM, Stemerman MB, Benditt EP. The aortic intima. II. Repair of the aortic lining after mechanical denudation. Am J Pathol 1975; 81: 15–42.

29. Bjornsson TD, Dryjski M, Tluczek J et al. Acidic fibroblast growth factor promotes vascular repair. Proc Natl Acad Sci USA 1991; 88: 8651–5.

30. Nabel EG, Plautz G, Boyce FM et al. Recombinant gene expression in vivo within endothelial cells of the arterial wall. Science 1989; 244: 1342–4.

31. Messina LM, Podrazik RM, Whitehill TA et al. Adhesion and incorporation of lacZ-transduced endothelial cells into the intact capillary wall in the rat. Proc Natl Acad Sci USA 1992; 89: 12018–22.

32. Conte MS, Birinyi LK, Miyata T et al. Efficient repopulation of denuded rabbit arteries with autologous genetically modified endothelial cells. Circulation 1994; 23: 2161–9.

33. Wilson JW, Birinyi LK, Salomon RN et al. Implantation of vascular grafts lined with genetically modified endothelial cells. Science 1989; 244: 1344–6.

34. Dichek DA, Neville RF, Zwiebel JA et al. Seeding of intravascular stents with genetically engineered endothelial cells. Circulation 1989; 80: 1347–53.

35. Nathan A, Nugent MA, Edelman ER. Tissue engineered perivascular endothelial cell implants regulate vascular injury. Proc Natl Acad Sci USA 1995; 92: 8130–4.

36. Nugent HM, Rogers C, Edelman ER. Endothelial implants inhibit intimal hyperplasia after porcine angioplasty. Circ Res 1999; 84: 384–91.

37. Nugent MA, Nugent HM, Lozzo RV et al. Perlecan is required to inhibit thrombosis after deep vascular injury and contributes to endothelial cell-mediated inhibition of intimal hyperplasia. Proc Natl Acad Sci USA 2000; 97: 6722–7.

38. Nugent HM, Edelman ER. Endothelial implants provide long-term control of vascular repair in a porcine model of arterial injury. J Surg Res 2001; 99: 228–34.

39. Nugent HM, Groothuis A, Seifert P et al. Perivascular endothelial implants inhibit intimal hyperplasia in a model of arteriovenous fistulae: a safety and efficacy study in the pig. J Vasc Res 2002; 39: 524–33.

40. Langer R. New methods of drug delivery. Science 1990; 249: 1527–33.

41. Brown L, Munoz C, Siemer L et al. Controlled release of insulin from polymer matrices. Control of diabetes in rats. Diabetes 1986; 35: 692–7.

42. Murray JB, Brown L, Langer R, Klagsburn M. A micro sustained release system for epidermal growth factor. In Vitro 1983; 19: 743–8.

43. Edelman ER, Mathiowitz E, Langer R, Klagsbrun M. Controlled and modulated release of basic fibroblast growth factor. Biomaterials 1991; 12: 619–26.

44. Langer R, Murray J. Angiogenesis inhibitors and their delivery systems. Appl Biochem Biotechnol 1983; 8: 9–24.

45. Edelman ER, Adams DH, Karnovsky MJ. Effect of controlled adventitial heparin delivery on smooth muscle cell proliferation following endothelial injury. Proc Natl Acad Sci USA 1990; 87: 3773–7.

46. Edelman ER, Karnovsky MJ. Contrasting effects of the intermittent and continuous administration of heparin in experimental restenosis, Circulation 1994; 89: 770–6.

47. Edelman ER, Nugent MA, Karnovsky MJ. Perivascular and intravenous administration of basic fibroblast growth factor: vascular and solid organ deposition. Proc Natl Acad Sci USA 1993; 90: 1513–17.

48. Rogers C, Karnovsky MJ, Edelman ER. Inhibition of experimental neointimal hyperplasia and thrombosis depends on the type of vascular injury and the site of drug administration. Circulation 1993; 88: 1215–21.

49. Edelman ER, Nathan A, Katada M et al. Perivascular graft heparin delivery using biodegradable polymer wraps. Biomaterials 2000; 21: 2279–86.

50. Herring M, Gardner A, Glover J. A single staged technique for seeding vascular grafts with autologous endothelium. Surgery 1978; 84: 498–504.

51. van Wachem PB, Hogt AH, Beugeling T et al. Adhesion of cultured human endothelial cells onto methacrylate polymers with varying surface wettability and charge. Biomaterials 1987; 8: 323–8.

52. McAuslan BR, Johnson G. Cell responses to biomaterials I: adhesion and growth of vascular endothelial cells on poly(hydroxyethyl methacrylate) following surface modification by hydrolytic etching. J Biomed Mat Res 1987; 21: 921–35.

53. Ramires PA, Mirenghi L, Romano AR et al. Plasma-treated PET surfaces improve the biocompatibility of human endothelial cells. J Biomed Mater Res 2000; 51: 535–9.

54. Absolom DR, Hawthorn LA, Chang G. Endothelialization of polymer surfaces. J Biomed Mat Res 1988; 22: 271–85.

55. McAuslan BR, Johnson G, Hannan GN et al. Cell responses to biomaterials II: endothelial cell adhesion and growth on perfluorosulfonic acid. J Biomed Mat Res 1988; 22: 963–76.

56. Steele JG, Johnson G, Norris WD, Underwood PA. Adhesion and growth of cultured human endothelial cells on perfluorosulphonate: role of vitronectin and fibronectin in cell attachment. Biomaterials 1991; 12: 531–9.

57. Brunstedt MR, Ziats NP, Rose-Caprara V et al. Attachment and proliferation of bovine aortic endothelial cells onto additive modified poly(ether urethane ureas). J Biomed Mat Res 1993; 27: 483–92.

58. Zhang JC, Wojta J, Binder BR. Growth and fibrinolytic parameters of human umbilical vein endothelial cells seeded onto cardiovascular grafts. J Thor Card Surg 1995; 109: 1059–65.

59. Storck J, Razek H, Zimmerman ER. Effect of polyvinyl chloride plastic on the growth and physiology of human umbilical vein endothelial cells. Biomaterials 1996; 17: 1791–4.

60. Cenni E, Granchi D, Ciapetti G et al. Expression of adhesion molecules on endothelial cells after contact with knitted Dacron. Biomaterials 1997; 18: 489–94.

61. Massia SP, Hubbell JA. Human endothelial cell interactions with surface-coupled adhesion peptides on a nonadhesive glass substrate and two polymeric biomaterials. J Biomed Mat Res 1991; 25: 223–42.

62. Holland J, Hersh L, Bryhan M et al. Culture of human vascular endothelial cells on an RGD-containing synthetic peptide attached to a starch-coated polystyrene surface: comparison with fibronectin-coated tissue culture grade polystyrene. Biomaterials 1996; 17: 2147–56.

63. Hubbell JA, Massia SP, Desai NP, Drumheller PD. Endothelial cell-selective materials for tissue engineering in the vascular graft via a new receptor. Biotechnology 1991; 9: 568–72.

64. Ettenson DS, Koo EWY, Januzzi JL, Edelman ER. Endothelial heparan sulfate is necessary but not sufficient for control of vascular smooth muscle cell growth. J Cell Physiol 2000; 184: 93–100.

65. Leach CM, Thorburn GD. A comparative study of collagen-induced thromboxane release from platelets of different species: implications for human atherosclerosis models. Prostaglandins 1982; 24: 47–59.

365

66. Bonan R, Paiement P, Scortichini D et al. Coronary restenosis: evaluation of a restenosis injury index in a swine model. Am Heart J 1993; 126: 1334–40.

67. Steele PM, Chesebro JH, Stanson AW et al. Balloon angioplasty. Natural history of the pathophysiological response to injury in a pig model. Circ Res 1985; 57: 105–12.

68. Karas SP, Gravanis MB, Santoian C et al. Coronary intimal proliferation after balloon injury and stenting in swine: an animal model of restenosis. J Am Coll Cardiol 1992; 20: 467–74.

69. Sirois MG, Simons M, Kuter DJ et al. Rat arterial wall retains myointimal hyperplasia potential long after arterial injury. Circulation 1997; 96: 1291–8.

70. Noonan DM, Fulle A, Valente P et al. The complete sequence of perlecan, a basement membrane heparan sulfate proteoglycan, reveals extensive similarity with laminin A chain, low density lipoprotein-receptor, and the neural cell adhesion molecule. J Biol Chem 1991; 266: 22939–47.

71. Iozzo RV. Matrix proteoglycans: from molecular design to cellular function. Annu Rev Biochem 1998; 67: 609–52.

72. Kojima T, Leone CW, Marchildon GA et al. Isolation and characterization of heparan sulfate proteoglycans produced by cloned rat microvascular endothelial cells. J Biol Chem 1992; 267: 4859–69.

73. Benitz WE, Kelley RT, Anderson CM et al. Endothelial heparan sulfate proteoglycan. Inhibitory effects on smooth muscle cell proliferation. Am J Respir Cell Mol Biol 1990; 2: 13–24.

74. Forsten KE, Courant NA, Nugent MA. Endothelial proteoglycans inhibit FGF-2 binding and mitogenesis. J Cell Physiol 1997; 172: 209–20.

75. Windus DW. Permanent vascular access: a nephrologist's view. Am J Kidney Dis 1993; 21: 457–71.

76. Dixon BS, Novak L, Fangman BS. Hemodialysis vascular access survival: upper-arm native arteriovenous fistula. Am J Kidney Dis 2002; 39: 1–15.

77. Bourassa MG. Long-term vein graft patency. Curr Opin Cardiol 1994; 9: 685–91.

78. Welt FP, Edelman ER, Simon DI, Rogers C. Neutrophil, not macrophage, infiltration precedes neointimal thickening in balloon-injured arteries. Arterioscler Thromb Vasc Biol 2000; 20: 2553–8.

79. Castellot JJ, Cochran DL, Karnovsky MJ. Effect of heparin on vascular smooth muscle cells. I. Cell metabolism. J Cell Physiol 1985; 124: 21–8.

80. Clowes AW, Karnovsky MJ. Suppression by heparin of smooth muscle cell proliferation in injured arteries. Nature (Lond) 1977; 265: 625–6.

81. Clowes AW, Karnovsky MJ. Failure of certain antiplatelet drugs to affect myointimal thickening following arterial endothelial injury in the rat. Lab Invest 1977; 36: 452–64.

82. Powell JS, Clozel JP, Muller RK et al. Inhibitors of angiotensin-converting enzyme prevent myointimal proliferation after vascular injury. Science 1989; 245: 187–9.

83. Lundergan CF, Foegh ML, Ramwell PW. Peptide inhibition of myointimal proliferation by angiopeptin, a somatostatin analogue. J Am Coll Cardiol 1991; 17: 132B–6B.

27. TISSUE-ENGINEERED SMALL VESSEL GRAFTS

Briain D MacNeill and Stephen N Oesterle

Introduction

Atherosclerotic disease of small-diameter vessels remains the commonest cause of premature mortality in the Western world, with more than two of every five Americans dying of a cardiovascular event. The incidence of myocardial infarction is estimated at over a million cases annually in the USA alone, while the prevalence of stable angina is 16 500 000. Current treatment strategies include aggressive risk factor modification, lifestyle adjustment and pharmacologic intervention; however, increasing numbers of patients require revascularization necessitating coronary artery bypass grafting (CABG) or percutaneous coronary intervention (PCI).

Surgical revascularization, which employs autologous arteries and veins to bypass atherosclerotic coronary arteries, results in approximately 600 000 CABG procedures annually in the USA. The use of autologous arteries is, however, complicated by the need for a harvest procedure and by a paucity of suitable harvest sites. Similarly, autologous vein grafts demonstrate limited long-term patency as a result of graft atherosclerosis, in part due to lack of vasomotor tone and manual handling at the time of harvest.[1] Furthermore, graft sites are prone to infection and poor healing, particularly in diabetic patients. Although large-caliber arterial bypass with synthetic grafts has long reached clinical application, the same cannot be said for small-diameter vessels (<6 mm), where the use of synthetic materials as conduits has yielded little success. Advances in tissue engineering have therefore led investigators to search for a biologically engineered functional substitute for vascular conduits.

In 1986, Weinberg and Bell reported the first tissue-engineered blood vessel created from collagen gels combined with bovine endothelial cells, fibroblasts and smooth muscle cells.[2] Subsequent modifications in technique have expanded the potential[3–5] to such an extent that large-caliber tissue-engineered vessels have reached clinical application.[6] As with other areas of tissue engineering, the essential elements in the development of small-caliber blood vessels include graft design, cells, signaling, extracellular matrix and evaluation.

Graft design

The ideal small-caliber arterial substitute incorporates physiologic and mechanical characteristics to support its normal function. Biocompatibility is necessary to reduce thrombogenicity, promote healing and diminish the immune response. Vasoreactivity and permeability are necessary for normal blood supply, while mechanical strength is required to permit suturing and to withstand prolonged arterial pressures.

Normal arteries have a trilamellar structure in which each layer plays an important role in arterial function. The tunica intima, or endothelial layer, operates as a transport barrier, a filter and a regulator of vascular tone, and prevents thrombosis. The tunica media, or medial layer, is formed from smooth muscle cells, collagen, elastin and proteoglycans that together confer mechanical strength and vasoreactivity. The tunica adventitia, or adventitial layer, comprises fibroblasts and extracellular matrix and is important in supporting the vasa vasorum and vascular innervation. Given the significance of each layer, it is not surprising that most designs have attempted to replicate the normal trilamellar arterial architecture (Table 27.1).

Table 27.1 Basic stages in graft development

Stage	Comment
1. Cell harvest	Potential sources include autologous artery, vein, skin scrapings, adipose tissue, bone marrow or circulating progenitor cells
2. Cell culture	A variety of combinations of culture media, antibiotics, growth factors and supplements have been suggested
3. Scaffold seeding	Some investigators do not use scaffolds. Possible scaffold components include PLLA, PGA, PLGA and P4HB
4. Bioreactor	Variables include flow rate, pressure and frequency of culture exchange
5. Vessel growth	A variety of culture times have been used, ranging from 2 weeks to 8 weeks, with variable results in graft morphology and mechanics
6. Graft evaluation	In vivo evaluation includes clinical, Doppler and angiographic testing. Ex vivo evaluation includes microscopic, pharmacologic and mechanical
7. Implantation	Various animal models have been used, including rat, rabbit, dog and pig

PLLA, poly-L-lactic acid; PGA, polyglycolic acid; PLGA, poly-DL-lactic-co-glycolic acid; P4HB, poly-4-hydroxybutyrate.

As with other tissue-engineering techniques, the design of an arterial graft often requires a scaffold to serve as a three-dimensional template for cell attachment, proliferation and maintenance of differentiated function. A scaffold acts as an exogenous extracellular matrix to mimic the architecture of the normal tissue and to support structured growth of cultured cells. Materials such as collagen and polyglycolide were initially used; however, as the tissue develops, it rapidly outgrows the nutrient supply, unlike branched microporous polymers, which maximize surface area and thus nutrient supply.[7] Currently, most polymer scaffolds include poly-L-lactic acid (PLLA), polyglycolic acid (PGA), poly-DL-lactic-co-glycolic acid (PLGA) or poly-4-hydroxybutyrate (P4HB) (Figures 27.1 and 27.2).

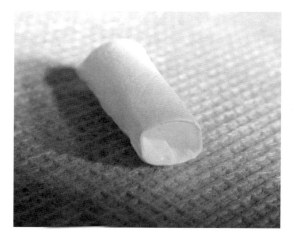

Figure 27.1 *An example of a biodegradable polymer scaffold designed to support structured cell growth and facilitate nutrient diffusion to growing cells.*

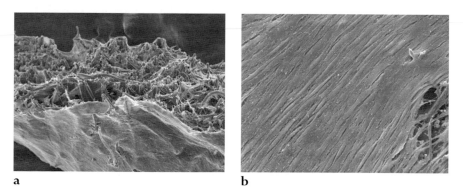

a   b

Figure 27.2 *(a) Scanning electronmicrograph (SEM) of a transverse section of a polymer scaffold (PGA) seeded with smooth muscle cells after 7 days of culture. The obvious porosity of the polymer allows diffusion of cellular nutrients while maintaining overall structure. (b) SEM of the luminal surface of a construct seeded with smooth muscle cells after 10 days of culture, demonstrating a confluent sheet of organized cells.*

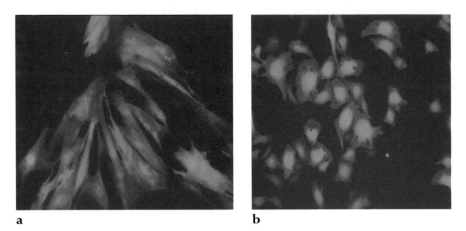

a   b

Figure 27.3 *GFP labeling of smooth muscle cells (a) and endothelial cells (b) (magnification ×20), highlighting not only the ability to tag harvested cells for later identification but also the potential to transfect harvested cells to promote characteristics beneficial to the construct development.*

Historically, the use of biomaterials in medicine has been confined to functional or non-biological roles: facilitating sliding, transmitting loads or filling spaces, roles that require the material used to be durable and thus bioinert. Ideally, however, a vascular scaffold should degrade on completion of its role as a structural support, yet should not stimulate an immune response during degradation. Consequently, a small vessel scaffold requires 'controlled reactivity', structural integrity to withstand implantation and subsequent physiologic pressure, and porous interconnectivity to allow adequate nutrient supply to the developing tissue.

Compliance matching in synthetic vascular grafts has been shown to promote long-term graft patency.[8] Compliance mismatch results in altered flow, increasing shear rates and downstream turbulence; over time, this gives rise to endothelial damage and intimal hyperplasia.[9] Furthermore, the stress–strain relationship is dependent not only on the scaffold type but also on the seeded cells, demonstrating that the mechanical and the biological features of the graft are interdependent.[10]

Techniques other than traditional scaffolds have also been used (Table 27.2).[3,11,12] Branched grafts have been constructed using a tubular mold of smooth muscle cells and collagen followed by thermal gelation.[11] The addition of an adventitial layer enabled the development of a construct composed exclusively of cultured human cells without the use of a scaffold, with microscopic and pharmacologic properties similar to those of a native

Table 27.2 Comparison of methods used for in vivo evaluation in various trials[3,5,12]

Cells	Technique	Evaluation	Comment
Human cells cultured without scaffold implanted in a canine model[3]	Constructs 3 × 5cm in length, implanted. No endothelial layer used	Doppler and angiography displayed patency rate of 50% at 7 days	Mechanical properties similar to those of normal vessel. High rate of thrombosis assumed to relate to lack of endothelial layer
Bovine and pig cells, cultured on a PGA scaffold, implanted in the saphenous artery of miniswine[5]	Autologous and xenograft vessels cultured under pulsatile and static conditions	Doppler and digital subtraction angiography. Ex vivo contraction studies and histologic analysis	Patency preserved in grafts cultured under pulsatile conditions. Non-pulsed grafts developed thrombosis at 3 weeks. Significantly less inflammatory response noted in autologous grafts
Silastic tubing implanted in the peritoneal cavity. At 2 weeks, it had become covered by myofibroblasts, collagen matrix and a layer of mesothelium[12]	Tubing removed, and tissue was everted (10–20 mm long) and grafted by end-to-end anastomoses into the severed carotid artery or aorta of the same animal	Clinical evaluation, histologic analysis and contractile studies were carried out. Overall patency rates were 67%	A novel technique of autologous culture with resultant grafts resembling normal blood vessels. Patency up to 4 months noted

vessel.[3] Finally, intraperitoneal culture on silastic tubing created a layer of mesothelial cells which, after removal of the tubing, could be everted and fashioned into an arterial conduit.[12]

Cells

Although initially considered a simple protective barrier, endothelial cells serve to regulate vascular healing, vasomotor tone and thromboresistance of the arterial surface.[13–18] The discovery of the paracrine release of vasoactive substances such as prostacyclin, prostaglandins and nitrous oxide in addition to angiotensin-converting enzyme (ACE), anticoagulants and antifibrinolytics signaled the importance of endothelial cell incorporation into graft design.

Endothelial cell harvest was first achieved from human umbilical veins in

1973,[19] and subsequent discovery of growth factors, including endothelial cell growth factor (ECGF), resulted in improved culture techniques.[20] Although endothelialization of vascular grafts was long thought of as a beneficial host response, it was unclear whether it occurred as a result of transanastomotic ingrowth or transmural migration of endothelial cells into the graft body. The observation, however, of complete endothelialization of a Dacron graft after only 7 days, a period too short to allow either significant ingrowth or migration, suggested an alternative source for endothelialization.[21] Accordingly, the potential of circulating stem cells capable of differentiating into vascular cells was examined.

Within the bone marrow, mature blood cells are derived from a small group of primitive hematologic stem cells that bear a unique surface glycoprotein (CD34). CD34-positive cells have been isolated from peripheral blood and demonstrate persistent multipotency. Although the concentration of these circulating precursor cells is low, the development of cellular isolation techniques using unique antigenic properties, such as CD34, permits isolation of a sufficient number of cells for endothelial culture.[22] Decellularized arteries, seeded with these cells and preconditioned in vitro with shear stress, displayed prolonged patency with a non-thrombogenic luminal surface of precursor-derived autologous endothelial cells.[23] Subsequently, alternative sites for adult stem cell retrieval have included bone marrow, epithelial tissues and, more recently, adipose tissue.[24-26] These studies demonstrate the ability to obtain endothelium from peripheral progenitor cells, thereby eliminating the need for an initial arterial harvest.

Endothelial cell characteristics can broadly be categorized as dependent or independent of their origin. Differing replication rate, growth rate, protein synthesis and cellular morphology have been described in endothelium cultured from various donor sites.[27] Similarly, a diverse response to growth factors and vasoactive mediators has been demonstrated.[28] Characteristics that are universal although not unique to endothelial cells are the secretion of ACE and platelet endothelial cell adhesion molecule (PECAM-CD$_{31}$), and the uptake of oxidized low-density lipoproteins.[29] The presence of Weibel–Palade bodies, which secrete P-selectin and Von Willebrand factor, is both unique to endothelial cells and displayed by all endothelial cells regardless of their origin.[30] The potential to incorporate gene therapy into cell lines is actively being sought to further improve tissue-engineered graft design to reduce or prevent disease recurrence (Figure 27.3).[31,32]

Vascular smooth muscle is the sole cell type normally found in the media of human arteries. In the normal state, vascular smooth muscle cells exhibit a contractile phenotype, existing in a non-proliferating differentiated state. In this state, cytoskeletal marker proteins (smooth muscle α-actin, myosin heavy chains and calponin) are expressed, and contract in response to chemical and mechanical stimuli.[33] Vascular smooth muscle cells have been shown to be pleiotropic and capable of phenotypic change associated with the synthesis of several biologically active substances that mediate cell numbers and architecture. In atherosclerosis, for example, the phenotype changes in response to various growth factors to assume a synthetic or secretory phenotype. This change, termed 'modulation', results in proliferation, causing vasculogenesis in the fetus and neointimal hyperplasia or graft stenosis in the adult.[34,35]

Characterization of smooth muscle cells relies on the morphologic 'hill and valley' appearance in culture and the demonstration of α-actin. Other characteristics include the presence of myosin heavy chains and calponin, the latter being confined to functional cells with a contractile phenotype. As with endothelial cells, genetic modification of smooth muscle cells is an attractive concept for concentrated gene delivery at the site of intimal hyperplasia and atherosclerosis. Accordingly, using smooth muscle cells as 'hosts' to express therapeutic recombinant genes may permit modification of their behavior and their role in vascular pathology.[36,37]

The adventitia consists predominantly of fibroblasts and extracellular matrix and augments the structural integrity necessary to withstand hemodynamic insult. Much of the strength of an artery is derived from its adventitial layer.[38] Although several investigators have engineered grafts without including an adventitial layer, the combination of sheets of fibroblasts and smooth muscle cells before seeding with endothelial cells can confer increased mechanical strength such that a supporting scaffold is redundant.[3] Fibroblast harvest is easily achieved from simple skin scrapings, and fibroblast growth is augmented in the presence of sodium ascorbate, the cells eventually growing into malleable sheets. Characterization usually relies on detection of anti-elastin or anti-vimentin antibody.[3]

Signaling

Cultured cells respond to a variety of physical and chemical stimuli that elicit genetic responses governing cellular migration, differentiation and apoptosis. To date, much of the experience of cell culture has been derived from single cell populations grown in two dimensions. The interactions of multiple cell lines grown in a complex architectural lattice is poorly understood. Direct co-culture of smooth muscle cells and endothelial cells, with or without contact, has demonstrated intercellular growth control, secretory activity and cellular responses to mechanical stimuli.[39–41]

Cellular interaction was demonstrated in a multicellular culture incorporating endothelial cells, smooth muscle cells, fibroblasts and collagen. Smooth muscle cells were seen to adopt a circular orientation, particularly in areas where longitudinal forces are minimal. Endothelial cells established a confluent monolayer with several in vivo characteristics. Small cellular anchors were seen to project from the endothelial cells to the adjacent collagen. Moreover, the endothelial cells elongated in parallel to the axis of the vessel, a phenomenon ascribed to endothelial cell modifications produced by smooth muscle cells.[42] The significance of intercellular signaling in response to mechanical stimuli was demonstrated using a bioreactor system exposing the cultured cells to pulsatile pressure. Both collagen content and levels of matrix metalloproteinases type 1 (MMP-1) were shown to be closely related to the rate of pulsation of the bioreactor.[43]

Bioreactors

As with other disciplines of tissue engineering, translation of basic research principles in cell culture and signaling to a clinically applicable and commercially viable product requires the use of large-scale production that is not possible within a simple culture flask (Figure 27.4). For this reason, scientists have concentrated on the development of bioreactors as a means of reliably and reproducibly fabricating constructs. The simplest bioreactor is a spinner flask that augments diffusion of nutrients by continuously circulating both the cultured material and the culture medium.

A more elaborate bioreactor system that exposes cultured cells to cyclical pulsatile flow, similar to that encountered in physiologic conditions, has also been developed, resulting in improved structural integrity and cellular development and ultimately conferring greater mechanical strength to the engineered vessel.[5] This bioreactor design also facilitates assessment of various physiologic parameters, including pressure, pulse rate, radial expansion and laminar flow on the end-product.[43]

Evaluation

Following successful culture of any tissue-engineered graft, the ultimate questions are, first, how well it will function, and second, how well its host will tolerate it. In order to evaluate its functional characteristics, investigators have compared tissue-engineered constructs with normal arteries at the microscopic, biochemical, mechanical and pharmacologic levels. Microscopic

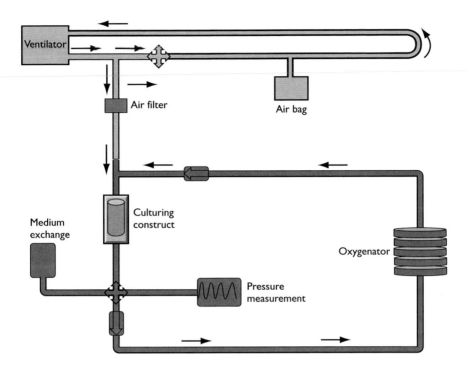

Figure 27.4 *Schematic representation of a biomimetic system. The ventilator generates cyclical pressure changes that are transferred through an air filter into a circulating system filled with culture medium that bathes the growing construct. An integrated pressure manometer allows adjustment of the pressure achieved within the system.*

evaluation, including electronmicroscopy, confirms the trilamellar structure, and the degree of scaffold attachment and degradation, and allows specific staining (Figure 27.3). Biochemical evaluation quantitatively measures the various constituents of the graft. MMPs, which mediate the breakdown of type I and III collagens, can be measured using an ELISA-based assay. With the addition of a radiometric metalloproteinase assay, it is possible to measure not only the levels but also the activity of MMPs and tissue inhibitors of MMPs (TIMPs),[44,45] which is of particular interest given the dynamic relationship between MMPs, TIMPs and the proliferating smooth muscle in the formation of neointimal hyperplasia following graft insertion. The mechanical properties of tensile strength, graft compliance and burst pressure are compared to those of both synthetic grafts and autologous arteries and veins.[3,5] Pharmacologic properties that have been studied include the relaxant effect of cAMP, the role of Ca^{2+}-enhanced contraction and the effect of a variety of pharmacologic interventions.[46] Dose–response curves for tissue-engineered constructs and normal vessels were compared and found to be similar, albeit of a much lower amplitude in tissue-engineered vessels, possibly due to lower numbers of vascular smooth muscle cells in the tissue-engineered grafts.[46,47]

How the host will respond to the tissue-engineered vascular graft is a complex issue, although certainly some degree of host remodeling is to be both expected and desired. Lessons learnt from allograft and xenograft organ transplantation highlight the difficulties that host immunity can pose, even for autologous tissue. To date, experience from in vivo models has raised important issues, such as homogeneity between donor and recipient. Various techniques have been adopted to overcome the problem of immune reaction, with varied success. Tissue-engineered conduits were cultured from human vascular cells and inserted as femoral grafts in a canine model. Acute rejection causing thrombosis was felt to be a high risk, and so the endothelial layer was omitted, being substituted instead with anticoagulation with warfarin; patency rates of only 50% were obtained after 7 days.[3] Autologous and xenograft constructs were inserted into the saphenous artery of Yucatan miniswine, treated with daily aspirin. All implants remained patent for 2 weeks, and autologous grafts that had been cultured under pulsatile conditions remained patent for 4 weeks.[5] Finally, a novel approach to the intraperitoneal culture of vascular constructs, involving their subsequent implantation as interpositional carotid artery grafts into adult rats and rabbits, resulted in graft patency for 4 months, and a structure similar to that of a native vessel developed.[12]

Conclusion

The burden of cardiovascular disease combined with limitations in our ability to adequately treat small vessel atherosclerosis has spurred progress in the tissue engineering of blood vessels. Despite the major advances made, there remain significant hurdles to overcome before this field can move to widespread clinical application. The future challenges include the incorporation of seemingly opposing properties such as elasticity and burst strength. The immune response is also a significant obstacle, particularly the immunogenicity of the endothelial layer, without which graft thrombosis occurs. Finally, greater understanding of the remodeling response following implantation is needed before genetic and pharmacologic control can be developed to positively affect the host response. What is certain is that tissue-engineered small blood vessels have the potential to change the treatment of atherosclerosis.

References

1. Hamada Y, Kawachi K, Yamamoto T et al. Effect of coronary artery bypass grafting on native coronary artery stenosis. Comparison of internal thoracic artery and saphenous vein grafts. J Cardiovasc Surg 2001; 42: 159–64.

2. Weinberg C, Bell E. A blood vessel model constructed from collagen and cultured vascular cells. Science 1986; 231: 397–400.

3. L'Heureux N, Paquet S, Labbe R et al. A completely biological tissue-engineered human blood vessel. FASEB J 1998; 12: 47–56.

4. Seliktar D, Black R, Vito R, Nerem R. Dynamic mechanical conditioning of collagen-gel blood vessel constructs induces remodeling in vitro. Ann Biomed Eng 2000; 28: 351–62.

5. Niklason L, Gao J, Abbott W et al. Functional arteries grown in vitro. Science 1999; 284: 489–93.

6. Hibino N, Imai Y, Shin-oka T et al. First successful clinical application of tissue engineered blood vessel. Kyobu Geka 2002; 55: 368–73.

7. Ma P, Zhang R. Microtubular architecture of biodegradable polymer scaffolds. J Biomed Mater Res 2001; 56: 469–77.

8. Clark R, Apostolou S, Kardos J. Mismatch of mechanical properties as a cause of arterial thrombosis. Surg Forum 1976; 27: 208.

9. Howard A, Alexander R, Nerem R et al. Cyclic strain induces an oxidative stress in endothelial cells. Am J Physiol 1997; 272: C421–7.

10. Greer L, Vito R, Nerem R. Material property testing of a collagen–smooth muscle cell lattice for the construction of a bioartificial vascular graft. Adv Bioeng 1994; 28: 69–70.

11. Kobashi T, Matsuda T. Branched hybrid vessel: in vitro loaded hydrodynamic forces influence the tissue architecture. Cell Transplant 2000; 9: 93–105.

12. Campbell J, Efendy J, Campbell G. Novel vasdcular graft grown within recipient's own peritoneal cavity. Circ Res 1999; 85: 1173–8.

13. Herring M, Gardner A, Glover J. A single-staged technique for seeding vascular grafts with autogenous endothelium. Surgery 1978; 84: 498–504.

14. Herring M, Baughman S, Glover J et al. Endothelial seeding of Dacron and polytetrafluorethylene grafts: the cellular events of healing. Surgery 1984; 96: 745–55.

15. Nathan A, Nugent M, Edelman E. Tissue engineered perivascular endothelial cell implants regulate vascular injury. Proc Natl Acad Sci USA 1995; 92: 8130–4.

16. Dichek D, Neville R, Zwiebel J et al. Seeding of intravascular stents with genetically engineered endothelial cells. Circulation 1989; 80: 1347–53.

17. Nugent H, Rogers C, Edelman E. Endothelial implants inhibit intimal hyperplasia after porcine angioplasty. Circ Res 1999; 84: 384–91.

18. Nugent H, Edelman E. Endothelial implants provide long-term control of vascular repair in a porcine model of arterial injury. J Surg Res 2001; 99: 228–34.

19. Jaffe E, Nachman R, Becker C, Minick C. Culture of human endothelial cells derived from umbilical veins. Identification by morphologic and immunologic criteria. J Clin Invest 1973; 52: 2745–56.

20. Maciag T, Hoover G, Stemerman M, Weinstein R. Serial propagation of human endothelial cells in vitro. J Cell Biol 1981; 91: 420–6.

21. Stump MM, Jordon GJ, De Bakey, Halper B. Endothelium grown from circulating blood on isolated Dacron hub. Am J Pathol 1963; 43: 361–7.

22. Asahara T, Murohara T, Sullivan A et al. Isolation of putative progenitor endothelial cells for angiogenesis. Science 1997; 275: 964–7.

23. Kaushal S, Amiel G, Guleserian K et al. Functional small-diameter neovessels created using endothelial progenitor cells expanded ex vivo. Nat Med 2001; 7: 1035–40.

24. Orlic D, Kajstura J, Chimenti S et al. Bone marrow cells regenerate infarcted myocardium. Nature 2001; 410: 640–1.

25. Toma J, Akhavan M, Fernandes K et al. Isolation of multipotent adult stem cells from the dermis of mammalian skin. Nat Cell Biol 2001; 3: 778–84.

26. Zuk P, Zhu M, Mizuno H et al. Multilineage cells from human adipose tissue: implications for cell-based therapies. Tissue Eng 2001; 7: 211–28.

27. Wagner W, Henderssin R, Hicks H et al. Differences in morphology, growth rate and protein synthesis between cultured arterial and venous endothelial cells. J Vasc Surg 1988; 8: 509–19.

28. D'Amore P. Mechanisms of endothelial growth control. Am J Respir Cell Mol Biol 1992; 6: 1–8.

29. Newman P, Berndt M, Gorski J et al. PECAM-1 (CD31) cloning and relation to adhesion molecules of the immunoglobulin gene superfamily. Science 1990; 247: 1219–22.

30. Wibel EGP. New cytoplasmic components in arterial endothelia. J Cell Biol 1964; 23: 101–10.

31. Rios C, Ooboshi H, Piegors D et al. Adenovirus-mediated gene transfer to normal and atherosclerotic arteries. A novel approach. Arterioscler Thromb Vasc Biol 1995; 15: 2241–5.

380

32. Nicklin S, Reynolds P, Brosnan M et al. Analysis of cell-specific promoters for viral gene therapy targeted at the vascular endothelium. Hypertension 2001; 38: 65–70.

33. Pauly R, Bialto C, Cheng L et al. Vascular smooth muscle cell cultures. London: Academic Press, 1998.

34. Chamley-Campbell JH, Campbell GR, Ross R. The smooth muscle cell in culture. Physiol Rev 1979; 59: 1–61.

35. Campbell J, Campbell G, Kocher O, Gabbiani G. Cell biology of smooth muscle in culture: implications for atherogenesis. Int Angiol 1987; 6: 73–9.

36. Armeanu S, Pelisek J, Krausz E et al. Optimization of nonviral gene transfer of vascular smooth muscle cells in vitro and in vivo. Mol Ther 2000; 1: 366–75.

37. Cable D, Caccitolo J, Caplice N et al. The role of gene therapy for intimal hyperplasia of bypass grafts. Circulation 1999; 100: II-392–6.

38. Cox RH, Bockus Institute, Philadelphia, Pennsylvania. Comparison of carotid artery mechanics in the rat, rabbit, and dog. Am J Physiol 1978; 234: H280–8.

39. Campbell GR, Campbell JH, Manderson JA et al. Arterial smooth muscle. A mutifunctional mesenchymal cell. Arch Pathol Lab Med 1988; 112: 977–86.

40. Castellot JJ Jr, Wright TC, Karnovsky MJ. Regulation of vascular smooth muscle cell growth by heparin and heparan sulfates. Semin Thromb Hemost 1987; 13: 489–503.

41. Ganz P, Davies PF, Leopold JA et al. Short- and long-term interactions of endothelium and vascular smooth muscle in coculture: effects on cyclic GMP production. Proc Natl Acad Sci USA 1986; 83: 3552–6.

42. L'Heureux N, Germain L, Labbe R, Auger FA. In vitro construction of a human blood vessel from cultured vascular cells: a morphologic study. J Vasc Surg 1993; 17: 499–509.

43. Solan A, Prabhakar V, Niklason L. Engineered vessels: importance of the extracellular matrix. Transplant Proc 2001; 33: 66–8.

44. Moses M, Langer R. A metalloproteinase inhibitor as an inhibitor of neovascularization. J Cell Biochem 1991; 47: 230–5.

45. Moses M, Langer R. Metalloproteinase inhibition as a mechanism for the inhibition of angiogenesis. EXS 1992; 61: 146–51.

46. L'Heureux N, Stocklet J, Auger F et al. A human tissue-engineered vascular media: a new model for pharmacological studies of contractile responses. FASEB J 2001; 15: 515–24.

47. Niklason L, Abbott W, Gao J et al. Morphologic and mechanical characteristics of engineered bovine arteries. J Vasc Surg 2001; 33: 628–38.

28. The 'Living Stent': Cell-Based Implantable Vascular Therapy

Robert S Schwartz and Katsumi Miyauchi

Introduction

All forms of percutaneous coronary intervention (PCI) induce marked injury to the coronary or peripheral artery, and the injury response is critical to the long-term success or failure of the procedure.[1-3] The immediate response is platelet and thrombus activation, both of which induce cell activation with migration, proliferation and colonization and matrix synthesis.[4-7] These cellular processes cause subsequent neointimal formation, with accumulation of fibroblasts/myofibroblasts. Figure 28.1 is a high-power view of neointima from a human coronary artery. Neointimal thickening is the principal cause of

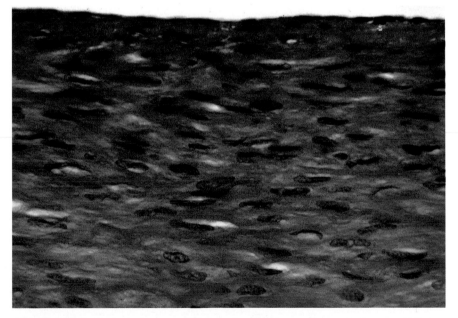

Figure 28.1 *High-power view of human medial tissue. The tissue is very cellular, and these smooth muscle cells probably have functions other than mechanical contraction, since they provide an arterial lining for bloodflow. H & E stain, magnification ×40.*

in-stent restenosis, and may be of varying degrees through mechanisms not understood. Additionally, the adventitia thickens, and may contribute cells to the neointima in some circumstances.[8–10] This latter process frequently causes vessel shrinkage, or negative remodeling, and is a principal cause of restenosis when a stent is not present to resist the constriction.[11–13] With stent placement, neointimal hyperplasia is the determining factor for in-stent restenosis, and is the major target of drug-eluting stents.[14,15]

The intracoronary stent improves long-term minimum luminal diameter and lowers restenosis rates. However, success of the stent is due to the geometric feature of a larger post-procedural lumen, allowing more late loss without causing severe stenoses. A bare (non-drug-eluting) stent possesses essentially no biological activity against neointima and hence does not limit neointimal thickening. Indeed, stenting is associated with increased neointima compared to balloon angioplasty.[6,7] It is only with the advent of brachytherapy and, more recently, drug-eluting stents that restenosis may finally be adequately controlled, through neointimal overgrowth limitation and preventing negative remodeling.

Drug-eluting stents

Drug-eluting stents are attractive to the interventional community as a viable solution to the vexing restenosis problem. Attempts to develop these devices have themselves met substantial difficulties, both in developing biocompatible carriers of pharmacologic agents and in finding agents effective for releasing the drug at local artery sites.[16,17] Prior studies clearly showed problems with synthetic polymers (Figure 28.2). Many polymers considered to be biocompatible for subcutaneous, body cavity, pacing or large vessel implantation proved disappointing when implanted in animal coronary arteries during testing.[18] Serious problems with these implants include inflammation, acute and chronic thrombus formation, and destruction of vessel architecture through inflammatory processes.

Early clinical data from drug-eluting stent trials show impressive results. The SIRIUS trial showed a 23% reduction in 8-month angiographic restenosis, from 32.3% (control stents) to 9.1% (rapamycin-eluting stents). Clinically driven target lesion revascularization (TLR) was reduced by 12%, from 16.7% to 4.7%, between control and rapamycin-eluting stents. Paclitaxel-eluting stents show similar excellent results, with the TAXUS I trial showing 6-month angiographic restenosis rates of 10% compared to 0%, and 27% versus 13% for control versus paclitaxel stents respectively. These outstanding results are being validated and are expected to hold true for larger studies.

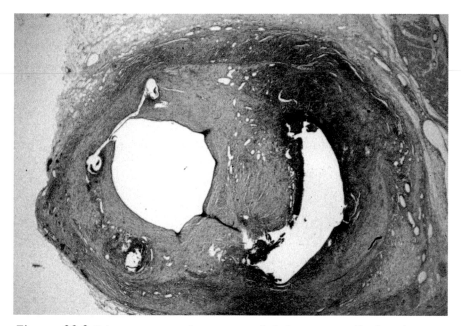

Figure 28.2 *Polymers can stimulate neointimal thickening, typically through inflammatory processes. This polymer created thick neointima in the lumen of a porcine coronary artery. The purple regions are those with significant inflammation. H & E stain, magnification ×10.*

Rapamycin and paclitaxel are agents that inhibit neointimal formation. These agents act at a multiplicity of levels. For example, paclitaxel has activity against cell division (proliferation), motility and migration, activation (inhibiting cytokines and growth factors), secretory processes (matrix metalloproteinases) and signal transduction (e.g. c-fos, c-jun, AP-1), and has cell- and dose-dependent effects (exhibiting different dose effects on different cell types).[9,19–21]

Many agents under consideration for elution from stents can cause cell toxicity if delivered at very high local doses. These effects may be manifested as cell death in the media and adventitia of the artery. Studies using very high temperatures may also cause cell death, which in turn stimulates neointima rather than inhibiting it (Figure 28.3).[10] In the porcine model, very high temperatures are used to generate stenoses for device testing, and these reliably occur with such heat treatment. Based on these and other observations, it is clear that drug-eluting stents must not kill or eliminate arterial cells.

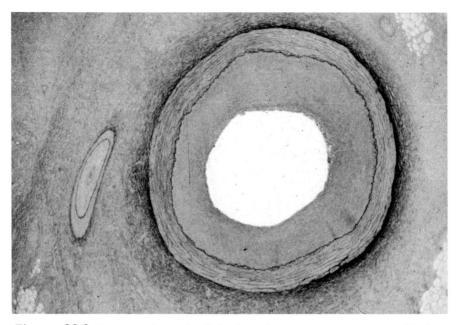

Figure 28.3 *Heat caused medial cell death in this porcine coronary artery, 28 days prior to euthanasia. The loss of medial cells was responsible for prolific neointimal growth. It is reasonable to consider that neointimal cells fulfill the arterial function in this situation. Actin immunostain, magnification ×16.*

A novel concept entails using the body's own cells to populate a stent, under the assumption that such cells, whether externally or internally supplied, populate the system and create a permanent source of cells. This concept has been called 'biomimicry', and involves the implanted cells functioning immediately as arterial cells when implanted by the stent.

Arterial biocompatibility and biomimicry

Biomimicry is an evolving strategy in vascular biology fueled by the biotechnology revolution.[22] It involves the interaction of technology (devices, molecular engineering, nanotechnology) and cells or tissues to promote novel biological functions. It is implicit in designing prosthetic arterial devices such as stents that a 'biocompatible' surface can be strictly passive. Passive refers to devices or materials designed to function as a vascular conduit that is inanimate. This notion of simultaneous biocompatibility and passivity has yet to be proven either in a theoretical or practical context. For example, over

30 years of research into prosthetic arterial grafts has failed to develop a material usable in small-diameter vessels; this is referred to by Buddy Ratner as the 'blood compatibility catastrophe'.[23]

These failures mandate that we reassess the meaning of blood compatibility as required by arterial implant technology. The artery responds to injury as it does to prosthetic implants by forming neointimal hyperplasia, frequently growing thick enough to cause stenosis. Strategies to limit neointimal hyperplasia by killing cells paradoxically stimulates rather than inhibits neointimal growth. Biomimicry takes an alternative approach, instead adopting a strategy to restore normal arterial function more rapidly by assisting the normal healing processes. Neointima forms for a purpose, with neointimal cells probably restoring normal arterial function. The role played by neointimal thickness is uncertain, but thick neointima may be necessary for this purpose. Neointimal function must be understood and a strategy developed to emulate these roles as we mimic arterial function.

The normal coronary artery: more than a passive conduit

The coronary artery appears deceptively simple when viewed only anatomically. Its three substructures are endothelium/intima, media and adventitia. Three cell types comprise these layers: adventitial fibroblasts/myofibroblasts, medial smooth muscle cells and endothelial cells. These arterial structures and cells are only now becoming understood, in large part through research into coronary restenosis.[24]

Endothelium

Vascular endothelium was formerly considered to be a passive blood vessel lining. It is now clear that endothelium is far from passive, and is a source of multiple, highly bioactive substances, and indeed orchestrates complex events that confer 'biocompatibility'. The endothelium itself is not essential for vascular function, at least in the short term; this is supported by several observations. Small blood vessels (coronary arteries) remain patent for years despite endothelial dysfunction or even absence as found in atherosclerosis. Coronary intervention causes complete endothelial denudation, yet such arterial segments still function satisfactorily as blood conduits. This is also illustrated by intervention in normal coronary pig, dog, rabbit or baboon arteries.[25] Simple endothelial denudation causes neither significant neointima nor stenosis. Is thus unclear whether endothelium is a key element of neointimal growth, although this hypothesis remains an open question.

Adventitia

The arterial adventitia is principally connective tissue providing mechanical support to the vessel. It also provides 'back-up' to limit bleeding should the vessel be lacerated or perforated, containing the hemorrhage and promoting potentially life-saving thrombus. The adventitial role for arteries is nourishment and support, with adventitial vasa vasorum supplying oxygen and nutrients to arteries more than 30 cell layers thick. This remarkably delicate and intricate capillary network arises from the main lumen of the coronary artery (Figure 28.4). Longitudinal vasa run parallel to the lumen, and give rise to secondary branches running circumferentially around the lumen, terminating in the outer medial border. In serial studies of these vasa using microscopic computed tomography, the vasa do not penetrate the media of normal coronary arteries. Atherosclerosis causes adventitial angiogenesis, with small capillaries that frequently penetrate from the adventitia through the media and into the atherosclerotic plaque. Normal porcine coronary arteries that are injured develop marked adventitial angiogenesis, in direct proportion to the degree of injury. This is principally in the form of (circumferential) secondary vasa, thus disrupting the normal ratio of primary/secondary vessels.

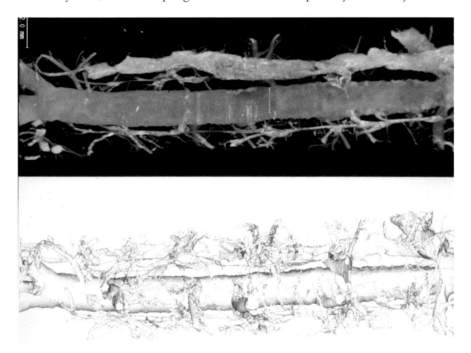

Figure 28.4 *Microscopic computed tomographic image of a normal porcine coronary artery. Note the first-order (longitudinal) and second-order (circumferential) capillaries supplying blood to the vessel.*

The adventia may have a major role in neointimal formation. Removing the adventitia from a normal artery causes non-obstructive neointimal formation, even when no mechanical medial injury occurs.[26] Similarly, placing a tight polymer band around a normal artery also produces neointimal formation. This may result from constriction of adventitial capillaries. However, removing the adventitia but placing a loose polymer collar around a normal artery segment eventuates in a 'pseudo-adventitia' that limits neointimal formation. These studies strongly suggest an important role for the adventitia in metabolically supporting normal arterial function. Adventitial cells also appear to play an important role in healing the injured artery. Studies also suggest that adventitial cells are the source of neointimal cells following mechanical injury.

Media

The arterial media is composed of a smooth muscle cell layer serving as a mechanical structure, giving strength and vasomotor tone in the form of relaxation and constriction to the muscular coronary arteries. The media may have a substantial biological role in limiting neointimal growth. Numerous studies of normal porcine coronary arteries have shown that neointima does not grow following arterial injury unless the internal elastic lamina is fractured and arterial media is injured. Ruptured internal elastic lamina sites are sites of neointima growth. The depth and severity of medial injury generates a proportional neointimal response in both pigs and patients, as appears true for other species as well.

In experimental angioplasty, medial death or absence causes neointimal growth, well illustrated by thermal arterial injury. The normal porcine coronary arterial media is typically killed when subjected to temperatures of 80°C for 30 s. This medial cell death is accompanied by voluminous neointimal formation, principally at sites of dead or missing media. Conversely, where arterial media survive the heat, there is little to no neointimal thickening. This observation appears extendable to human atherosclerotic coronary arteries, in that high-temperature balloon angioplasty following coronary angioplasty markedly raises restenosis rates.

Another example of the importance of the media in preventing or limiting neointimal thickening is directly related to polymers. Impermeable, non-porous polymer stents were implanted in normal porcine coronary arteries. These arteries uniformly developed thick, totally occlusive neointima. A second stent configuration was fabricated identically from a chemically identical polymer, except that the polymer was porous. Neointimal formation on this porous polymer was markedly reduced, with excellent artery patency at 28 days (Figure 28.5). In this case, the polymer porosity allowed

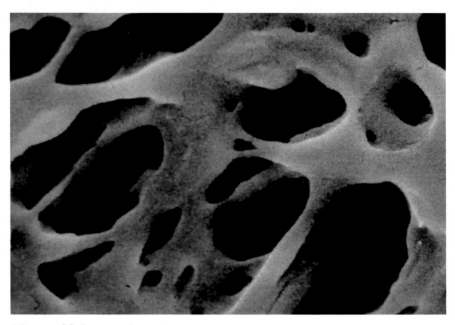

Figure 28.5 *Circumferential porous polymer implant results in widely patent lumen at 28 days in a porcine coronary artery. Cells have populated the polymer structure. Elastic van Gieson stain, magnification ×10.*

biochemical products from the media to affect luminal events, and so did not interfere with homeostatic arterial function.

A unified hypothesis for neointimal inhibition

These examples suggest that healthy media may participate in actively inhibiting neointimal formation. Marked neointimal growth occurs (only) at sites of medial cell death or severe injury. Endothelial cell dysfunction, death or removal causes limited or no neointimal growth. The adventitia does not limit neointima in coronary artery injury, since medial laceration with dissection causes adventitial exposure directly to the lumen, and marked neointima grows. An analogous situation occurs when the media is isolated from the artery lumen by, for example, an impermeable polymer. Voluminous neointima typically occlude such vessels within 28 days, as shown amply in prior animal studies.

These observations thus suggest an important metabolic role for media. Extending the concept, neointimal growth is under constant negative inhibition by diffusable medial products. Medial smooth muscle cells must provide an interface to the lumen to prevent this neointimal growth. Medial absence removes an inhibitory agent, and neointimal growth commences.

Neointimal growth may be 'good' for an injured artery, since these cells may reinstitute inhibitory signaling and prevent thrombotic occlusion. The neointimal cell functions as a substitute arterial cell in both structure and function. Neointima grows until normal or near-normal arterial function is restored, in turn limiting further neointimal formation. Neointima in this respect is a necessary and beneficial outcome of arterial injury, replacing the function of absent media in mechanical and metabolic terms.

Neointimal growth: lumen or tissue dependent?

Is neointimal formation lumen driven or wall driven? This depends on whether forces occurring in the lumen (shear, turbulence, thrombus) or cellular events in the nascent neointima are responsible for deriving neointimal thickness. Heuristically, the question asks whether neointima in a healing artery 'knows' the lumen size, or whether it instead is controlled by events in the artery wall. The logical conclusion is that neointimal growth may be driven by absent, dysfunctional or insensitive lumen-based signals (possibly from endothelium), or perhaps a combination of lumen and wall events. The lumen-based signals which should normally originate from an increasingly tighter stenosis either do not occur, or the target tissues for such signals are inappropriately insensitive and do not stop neointimal thickening, before inappropriate arterial stenosis occurs. Neointimal growth in this paradigm is lumen driven.

An alternative to lumen-driven neointimal growth is neointimal tissue-driven neointimal growth. These two are not mutually exclusive. Neointimal growth may proceed from paracrine signaling. That is, biological signals halting neointimal growth may originate as feedback from the neointima itself. Neointimal growth may be negatively dependent on neointimal mass. Also, neointimal cell maturity/differentiation may govern the ability of a neointimal cell to produce the appropriate growth-inhibiting signals. Restenosis may result from exuberant neointimal growth because appropriate, tissue-based (versus lumen-based) negative feedback is absent.

These paradigms of lumen- or tissue-based neointimal growth and inhibition need not be mutually exclusive. If correct, restenosis might be solved by supplying the appropriate negative signals through 'quality' cells

391

functioning at the angioplasty site as soon as possible after vascular injury. This could be obtained by promoting and accommodating larger masses of neointima, or by stimulating early neointimal cells to produce appropriate feedback inhibition.

What are the practical implications of this hypothesis? If normal arteries require constant and active neointimal inhibition, it explains why no perfect arterial biomaterial has been found and why the 'blood compatibility catastrophe' is real. No biologically passive surface could provide the requisite biological inhibitory signals to limit neointimal growth. The artery must have an active, living lining to prevent neointimal formation or be externally supplied with the inhibition.

Biomimicry in arterial prostheses

Killing arterial cells or interfering with their function exacts a price, generally enhanced neointima. The artery must be supplied with appropriate biochemical or cellular signals to inhibit neointimal formation. This could be accomplished by supplying such signals artificially, or could be done with cells at the local site. Such cells could be implanted at the artery site and could be recombinant through transfection prior to local implant. Several groups have pursued this strategy in the past. Alternatively, local cells could be stimulated to produce the appropriate biological activity.

Biomimicry: a practical implementation

The biomimicry concept underwent a pilot investigation in our laboratory, with the use of two configurations. In the first, a polyurethane sleeve with substantial porosity was fabricated to encase a clinically used metal stent (Figure 28.6). The polymer was made with the intention that placing it in a coronary artery would cause living cells to infiltrate the polymer, yielding a living structure, a hybrid polymer–cellular device. The cells would be infiltrating from the vascular wall, presumably in much the same way as an artery develops neointima. The devices were implanted in normal, uninjured porcine coronary arteries, and left in place for 28 days, when the pigs were euthanized and the stents examined. Figure 28.7 shows the gross and low-power results. They indeed showed neointimal formation within the polymer, as thick as the polymer itself, but with very little neointimal formation outside the polymer in the artery lumen. The cells within the polymer appeared as normal neointima, and the structure had even developed a blood

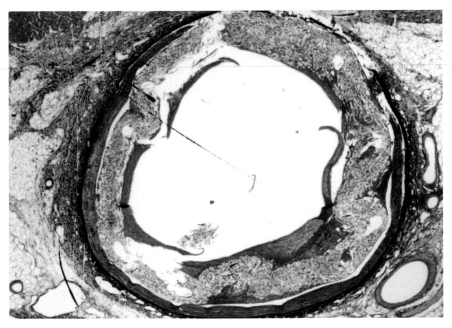

Figure 28.6 *Scanning electronmicroscopy of the porous polyurethane sleeve used for Figure 28.5. This was an experimental stent to test the biomimicry concept. The concept was to allow cells to populate the polymer and to permit the stent to become a hybrid structure.*

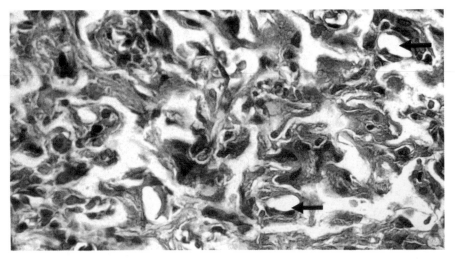

Figure 28.7 *Histopathology results from the porous polymer 28 days after implant. As desired, cells have populated the polymer, and the cells have even developed their own blood supply, as shown by capillaries growing within the structure. H & E stain, magnification ×15.*

supply, as evidenced by capillaries within the polymer porosity structure (Figure 28.7). This configuration may be viable for limiting neointimal thickening outside a polymer sleeve. Importantly, no inflammation was seen to result from the polymer or its coatings.

A second pilot study was performed with a different stent fabrication. A 316L stainless steel screen with small fibers (<0.001 inch) was fashioned into a cylindrical configuration and welded to a commercial stent to facilitate delivery in porcine coronary arteries.[27,28] After the mechanical aspects of the stent screen were developed, the device was coated with fibronectin to allow cell ingrowth in vitro. Porcine smooth muscle cells were harvested and prepared from the carotid arteries. These cells were next transduced (in the laboratory of Dr Noel Caplice) with green fluoresecent protein (GFP) to permit identification as transplanted cells. As its name implies, this protein fluoresces green and is not expressed in any non-altered porcine cell. Thus, any cell expressing GFP must have been exogenously implanted, and its identification in or near the stent proves its origin. Figure 28.8 shows a fluorescent micrograph of the stent at 28 days, with avid fluorescence suggesting survival of the recombinant cells for at least this long. Histopathologic evaluation showed only mild neointimal thickening, without

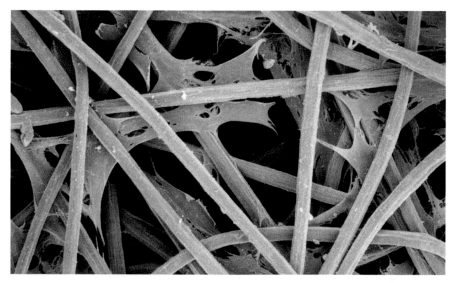

Figure 28.8 Fluorescent microscopy of stent structure with cells populated by green fluorescent protein (GFP) transduced porcine arterial cells. Images show fluorescent cells at 28 days, suggesting that such transduced cells can survive for intermediate times. A key question is whether these cells function as arterial cells. Fluorescent image, magnification ×50.

inflammatory infiltrates. This feasibility study suggests that cells can be reliably implanted within the protective environment of a stent and survive for short periods of time. The biomimicry concept is clearly demonstrated through studies such as this.

Recent studies suggest that some neointimal cells may originate from circulating cells in the blood.[29] Indeed, multiple studies are emerging suggesting a bone marrow origin for neointimal (or endothelial) cells, or utilizing bone marrow therapeutically for injured blood vessels.[30–36] These studies are in their earliest phases, but will probably become more deterministic in the near future.

Summary and conclusion

Biomimicry is in its earliest stages and is being considered in the realm of tissue engineering. If arterial implants are to limit neointimal thickening, purely passive structures cannot succeed. Bioactivity must be present, either by pharmacologic intervention or by fabricating a 'living stent' that contains active cellular material. As tissue engineering evolves, useful solutions will emerge from applying this knowledge directly to vascular biological problems resulting from angioplasty, stenting and vascular prosthesis research.

References

1. Moustapha A et al. Percutaneous and surgical interventions for in-stent restenosis: long-term outcomes and effect of diabetes mellitus. J Am Coll Cardiol 2001; 37(7): 1877–82.

2. Moreno R et al. Long-term outcome of patients with proximal left anterior descending coronary artery in-stent restenosis treated with rotational atherectomy. Catheter Cardiovasc Intervent 2001; 52(4): 435–42.

3. Manolis AS. Reduced incidence of clinical restenosis with newer generation stents, stent oversizing, and high-pressure deployment: single-operator experience. Clin Cardiol 2001; 24(2): 119–26.

4. Glover C, O'Brien ER. Pathophysiological insights from studies of retrieved coronary atherectomy tissue. Semin Intervent Cardiol 2000; 5(4): 167–73.

5. Foo RS et al. Inhibition of platelet thrombosis using an activated protein C-loaded stent: in vitro and in vivo results. Thromb Haemost 2000; 83(3): 496–502.

6. Virmani R, Farb A. Pathology of in-stent restenosis. Curr Opin Lipidol 1999; 10(6): 499–506.

7. Farb A et al. Pathology of acute and chronic coronary stenting in humans. Circulation 1999; 99(1): 44–52.

8. Lafont A et al. Restenosis after experimental angioplasty. Intimal, medial, and adventitial changes associated with constrictive remodeling. Circ Res 1995; 76: 996–1002.

9. Farb A et al. Pathological analysis of local delivery of paclitaxel via a polymer-coated stent. Circulation 2001; 104(4): 473–9.

10. Staab ME et al. Arterial remodeling after experimental percutaneous injury is highly dependent on adventitial injury and histopathology. Int J Cardiol 1997; 58(1): 31–40.

11. Wallner K et al. Adventitial remodeling after angioplasty is associated with expression of tenascin mRNA by adventitial myofibroblasts. J Am Coll Cardiol 2001; 37(2): 655–61.

12. Kobayashi Y et al. Long-term vessel response to a self-expanding coronary stent: a serial volumetric intravascular ultrasound analysis from the ASSURE Trial: A Stent vs. Stent Ultrasound Remodeling Evaluation. J Am Coll Cardiol 2001; 37(5): 1329–34.

13. Christen T et al. Mechanisms of neointima formation and remodeling in the porcine coronary artery. Circulation 2001; 103(6): 882–8.

14. Hoffmann R, Mintz GS. Coronary in-stent restenosis – predictors, treatment and prevention. Eur Heart J 2000; 21(21): 1739–49.

15. Dussaillant GR et al. Small stent size and intimal hyperplasia contribute to restenosis: a volumetric intravascular ultrasound analysis. J Am Coll Cardiol 1995; 26(3): 720–4.

16. van der Giessen WJ et al. Marked inflammatory sequelae to implantation of biodegradable and nonbiodegradable polymers in porcine coronary arteries. Circulation 1996; 94(7): 1690–7.

17. Salzmann DL et al. Healing response associated with balloon-dilated ePTFE. J Biomed Mater Res 1998; 41(3) 364–70.

18. Palmaz JC. Review of polymeric graft materials for endovascular applications. J Vasc Intervent Radiol 1998; 9(1 Pt 1): 7–13.

19. Heldman AW et al. Paclitaxel stent coating inhibits neointimal hyperplasia at 4 weeks in a porcine model of coronary restenosis. Circulation 2001; 103(18): 2289–95.

20. Axel DI et al. Paclitaxel inhibits arterial smooth muscle cell proliferation and migration in vitro and in vivo using local drug delivery. Circulation 1997; 96(2): 636–45.

21. Signore PE et al. Complete inhibition of intimal hyperplasia by perivascular delivery of paclitaxel in balloon-injured rat carotid arteries. J Vasc Intervent Radiol 2001; 12(1): 79–88.

22. Schwartz RS, van der Giessen WJ, Holmes Jr DR. Biomimicry, vascular restenosis and coronary stents. Semin Intervent Cardiol 1998; 3(3–4): 151–6.

23. Ratner B. The blood compatibility catastrophe. J Biomed Mater Res 1993; 27: 283–7.

24. Christen T et al. Cultured porcine coronary artery smooth muscle cells. A new model with advanced differentiation. Circ Res 1999; 85(1): 99–107.

25. Schwartz R, Holmes DJ. Pigs, dogs, baboons, and man: lessons for stenting from animal studies. J Intervent Cardiol 1994; 7: 355–68.

26. Barker SG et al. The adventitia and atherogenesis: removal initiates intimal proliferation in the rabbit which regresses on generation of a 'neoadventitia'. Atherosclerosis 1994; 105(2): 131–44.

27. Caplice NM. Biologic alternatives to stents and grafts. Curr Cardiol Rep 2001; 3(1): 17–21.

28. Panetta CJ et al. A tissue-engineered stent for cell-based vascular gene transfer. Hum Gene Ther 2002; 13(3): 433–41.

29. Asahara T et al. Bone marrow origin of endothelial progenitor cells responsible for postnatal vasculogenesis in physiological and pathological neovascularization. Circ Res 1999; 85(3): 221–8.

30. Bittner RE et al. Recruitment of bone marrow derived cells by skeletal and cardiac muscle in adult dystrophic mdx mice. Anat Embryol (Berl) 1999; 199(5): 391–6.

31. Campbell JH et al. Blood vessels from bone marrow. Ann NY Acad Sci 2000; 902: 224–9.

32. Campbell JH, Han CL, Campbell GR. Neointimal formation by circulating bone marrow cells. Ann NY Acad Sci 2001; 947: 18–24: discussion 24–5.

33. Fogt F et al. Recipient-derived hepatocytes in liver transplants: a rare event in sex-mismatched transplants. Hepatology 2002; 36(1): 173–6.

34. Goodell MA et al. Stem cell plasticity in muscle and bone marrow. Ann NY Acad Sci 2001; 938: 208–18; discussion 218–20.

35. Han CI, Campbell GR, Campbell JH. Circulating bone marrow cells can contribute to neointimal formation. J Vasc Res 2001; 38(2): 113–19.

36. Hess DC et al. Bone marrow as a source of endothelial cells and NeuN-expressing cells after stroke. Stroke 2002; 33(5): 1362–8.

29. ENDOLUMINAL TRANSPLANTATION OF ENDOTHELIAL CELLS

Nicholas Kipshidze, Michael H Keelan, Mykola Tsapenko, Martin B Leon, Christian Haudenschild and Jeffrey Moses

Introduction

Percutaneous transluminal coronary angioplasty (PTCA) has become a well-established therapy in the management of coronary artery disease. The Bypass Angioplasty Revascularization Investigation (BARI) reported an equivalent 7-year survival rate for PTCA and bypass surgery in patients with multivessel coronary artery disease.[1] However, PTCA causes vessel injury, initiating a healing response, which is mainly due to negative vessel remodeling and neointima proliferation and leads to narrowing of the lumen of the vessel wall and hence to a high incidence (30–50%) of restenosis.[1]

With the introduction of stents, the face of interventional cardiology changed. Results of the STRESS (Stent Restenosis Study) and BENESTENT (Belgium–Netherlands Stent) pivotal trials clearly demonstrated the superiority of stent implantation to PTCA alone, with respect to restenosis in de novo coronary lesions.[2–5] However, it was also evident that neointimal proliferation is not affected by stenting technique.

Further extensive use of coronary stents to prevent restenosis has produced a new disease: in-stent restenosis. With increased use of stent implantation, the frequency of in-stent restenosis also increased. This is particularly true in patients with diabetes, and in some lesion subsets, such as bifurcated lesions and long diffuse lesions, and/or in small vessels, where the restenosis rate remains high, at 30–60%.[6,7] Unfortunately, this complication continues to be difficult to prevent, and regardless of the treatment strategy (plain PTCA, rotational atherectomy, laser angioplasty, cutting balloon angioplasty or repeat stenting), the restenosis rate in cases of in-stent restenosis is still unacceptably high (20–80%), depending on vessel and patient bias.[2–6] Therefore, the development of effective methods to treat and prevent restenosis became a main target of contemporary interventional cardiology.

Role of endothelium in restenosis

The mechanisms of post-angioplasty restenosis have been extensively studied.[8-27]

It is known that one of the most important mechanisms contributing to restenosis is the denudation of the endothelial cell (EC) lining of the arterial wall at the time of intervention.[28] Endothelial denudation is considered as a primary injury event following balloon angioplasty and/or stent implantation. Although ECs are firmly attached to each other and to their basement membrane, forming a monolayer throughout the vascular tree, balloon injury denudes these cells from the vessel wall. ECs, when in confluent monolayer, cease replication. Disruption of cell contact inhibition results in rapid EC replication from the proximal and distal non-traumatized segments. Overlying ECs probably play an important role in controlling SMC proliferation via secretion of heparin and other growth-inhibitory factors (EFRFs), and there is some evidence that neointimal proliferation ceases when ECs regenerate. ECs might themselves maintain the mitogenic quiescence of smooth muscle cells (SMCs) by the growth-inhibitory effect of nitric oxide.[29]

Besides modulating local hemostasis and thrombolysis, producing vasoactive compounds and providing a non-permeable barrier protecting SMCs against circulating growth-promoting factors, ECs themselves synthesize at least three growth factors (fibroblast growth factor (FGF), platelet-derived growth factor (PDGF) and transforming growth factor-ß (TGF-ß)) that are important in SMC proliferation. Moreover, ECs produce a significant number of components of EC basement membrane (BM): types IV and V collagen, laminin, proteoglycans and extracellular matrix (fibronectin). EC denudation leads thus not only to endothelial dysfunction but also to exposure of thrombogenic and adhesive subendothelial layers to platelets and leukocytes, with concomitant release of growth factors.[30] These factors may initiate the activation of SMCs, which proliferate and migrate to the de-endothelialized vessel surface, where they continue to proliferate and secrete extracellular matrix proteins.[31] In many instances the resultant neointima can lead to vessel stenosis.

With denudation of a small area of endothelial surface, little or no intimal hyperplasia is observed.[28,32,33] When larger areas are denuded, there is a greater degree of intimal thickening.[28,34] Haudenschild and Schwartz[35] have demonstrated that SMCs appear in the intima only in areas that are not re-endothelialized 7 days after injury. In theory, early confluent re-endothelialization by EC seeding may reduce SMC proliferation, migration or both.[36] Influences that lead to increased intracellular cAMP may promote re-endothelization and attenuate fibromuscular proliferation.[37]

Until recently, neointimal hyperplasia was believed to be the principal mechanism of restenosis.[8–11,16–20] However, intravascular ultrasound studies have demonstrated that constrictive vessel remodeling is the major cause of restenosis after angioplasty, with neointimal hyperplasia representing a secondary pathologic process that contributes to luminal narrowing.[9,11–14]

Coronary stents provide rigid luminal scaffolding that virtually eliminates elastic recoil and negative remodeling. Stents, however, do not decrease neointimal hyperplasia and in fact lead to an increase in the proliferative component of restenosis.[2,6,21,22]

A wound-healing response elicited by endothelial denudation often leads to luminal narrowing and restenosis. The restenotic process progresses through four distinct phases: thrombosis, inflammation, proliferation and matrix deposition/vessel remodeling.[22–24] Focal fibrin deposition with thrombus formation is universally observed within the first 3 days of stent implantation and is proportional to the depth and extent of injury to the artery wall. Inflammation accompanies vessel injury and attracts a host of cell types, including platelets and leukocytes that release growth factors and cytokines. These growth factors in turn induce SMC migration and proliferation. Transformed SMCs then secrete extracellular matrix that leads to the neointimal tissue formation.[22,25]

By using scanning electron microscopy (SEM) Grewe et al[38] studied the pathomorphologic characteristics of the vessel wall after stent insertion. On the basis of their results, they divided the stent integration process with intraindividual differences into three phases. In the acute phase (<6 weeks), the border between the vascular lumen and the arterial wall is composed of a thin, multilayered thrombus. During the time course of integration, increasing amounts of SMCs and extracellular matrix can be detected. No ECs can be found in the implantation zone. In the intermediate phase (6–12 weeks), the neointima consists of extracellular matrix and increasing numbers of SMCs. The borderline between lumen and neointima is generated by SMCs and extracellular matrix. Increasing amounts of ECs are found on the luminal surface of the stent neointima. Complete re-endothelization is first noted in the chronic phase 3 months after stenting. Matrix structures are increasing, whereas the number of SMCs decreases. In all phases of stent incorporation, the alloplastic stent material is covered by a thin (few nanometer) proteinaceous layer. Thus, re-endothelization of an injured vessel takes a long period of time, and this could contribute substantially to restenosis formation.

Nakatani et al[39] observed that restenosis after balloon injury consisted of arterial remodeling and neointimal hyperplasia, whereas that after stenting consisted mostly of neointimal hyperplasia and lasted longer. They also concluded that continuous inflammation may be an important factor in the restenosis of stenting.

There is also experimental evidence that the degree of inflammation and subsequent neointima formation is proportional to the degree of penetration of the vessel wall by the stent struts.[40] Furthermore, in some individuals, contact allergy to certain metallic ions present in stainless steel stents (e.g. nickel, chrome and molybdenum) may potentially trigger intimal growth.[27]

Up to now, pharmacologic interventions directed against platelet activation, thrombus formation and smooth muscle proliferation have not reduced the incidence of restenosis.[32,33] Inhibitors directed against PDGF and FGF have also been ineffective in preventing restenosis.[41] The practical application of antiproliferative agents is under further investigation by realizing that control of vascular SMC proliferation and growth is complex and involves the participation of multiple cellular and systemic mediators.[42] Indeed, the current studies explored the potential of antiproliferative drugs in the treatment and prevention of in-stent restenosis. With regard to evaluation of these drugs concerning their release kinetics, effective dosage, safety in clinical practice and benefit, several studies have been published or are still ongoing: SCORE (paclitaxel derivative), TAXUS I, II, III and IV (paclitaxel), ELUTE and ASPECT (paclitaxel), RAVEL and SIRIUS (sirolimus), ACTION (actinomycin), and EVIDENT and PRESENT (tacrolimus).

Interventions on endothelium

Local delivery of growth factors

Enhancement of endothelial regeneration has been addressed with a number of techniques, including local delivery of growth factors[41] and EC seeding.[43-48] Studies on the local delivery of growth factors to accelerate endothelialization have yielded very interesting and controversial results.

Callow et al[41] used vascular permeability factor (VPF), which is a naturally occurring growth factor, to stimulate EC proliferation in a rabbit model. They found that VPF stimulated rabbit EC proliferation in vitro at concentrations of 100 ng/ml. However, VPF had no effect on SMC proliferation at concentrations up to 500 ng/ml. Eight weeks of VPF administration resulted in 88.1 ±3.1% re-endothelialization compared to controls (44.7 ±3.8%). Hence, VPF appears to be a specific mitogen for endothelial regeneration.

Recently, Van Belle et al[49] demonstrated that local delivery of vascular endothelial growth factor (VEGF) accelerated stent endothelialization and reduced stent thrombosis in a rabbit model. However, while growth factors increase the rate of endothelial repair, many of them are also potent mitogens for vascular SMCs.[41,49] Indeed, Moulton et al[50] observed that prolonged treatment with the angiogenesis inhibitors endostatin or TNP-470 reduced plaque growth in mice. At the same time, several experimental and human studies[49,51–55] involving direct application of VEGF protein or/and naked DNA to the injured arteries demonstrated no evidence of accelerated atherosclerosis.

Thus, accelerated endothelialization through local delivery of endothelial-specific growth factors significantly reduces in-stent intimal formation in animal experiments and could constitute an attractive alternative to direct antiproliferative strategies.

Endothelial cell seeding

Previous attempts to reseed ECs using a variety of devices for delivery to the vascular wall have been hampered by rapid loss of the seeded cells[43–48] and also because of the difficulty in maintaining cell adherence when bloodflow is restored.[56–64]

At the same time, although transplantation of ECs during or after coronary intervention is an attractive concept, three major limitations are: (1) prolonged seeding time; (2) optimal delivery device; and (3) adhesion of a functional EC to the area of vascular injury. In studies on swine femoral arteries, Nabel et al[44] achieved 2–11% adherence of cells to the denuded arterial wall following 30 min of reseeding. Thompson et al[45] have achieved 36% EC attachment to damaged human saphenous veins in vitro. The same group demonstrated 17% cell retention after 100 min of bloodflow in previously angioplastied external iliac arteries of rabbits.[46]

Nugent et al[65] used EC implants grown in polymer matrices to control vascular repair in a porcine model of arterial injury. Porcine and bovine EC implants significantly reduced experimental restenosis 3 months after angioplasty compared to controls by 56% and 31%, respectively. No implanted cells or focal inflammatory reactions were detected histologically at any of the implant sites at 90 days. They also observed significant increases in titers of serum antibodies to endothelium in animals with bovine (xenogenic) endothelial implants in comparison to animals with porcine (allogenic) implants. These data suggest that tissue-engineered EC implants may provide long-term control of vascular repair after injury, rather than simply delaying lesion formation, and that allogeneic implants are able to provide a greater benefit than xenogeneic implants.

Conte et al[47,66] have shown that autologous venous cells can be genetically modified and returned to the surface of a balloon-injured rabbit femoral artery. In their experiments, vessels examined at 4–7 days after seeding displayed 40–90% coverage with transduced cells, even when seeded at subconfluent density, and an intact EC monolayer, as evidenced by SEM

403

studies. However, their method required surgical exposure of the vessels and complete interruption of bloodflow for 30 min. Another approach has been demonstrated by Kutryk et al.[67] They proposed seeding of intravascular stents by the xenotransplantation of genetically modified ECs, which were capable of modifying the pathophysiologic response to vessel wall damage and providing controllable levels of active compounds. Animal studies have shown the feasibility and great potency of this method. There are also preliminary data suggesting that endoluminal seeding of syngeneic SMCs can be effective in reducing intimal hyperplasia both in a de-endothelialization animal model and in arterial allografts.[68]

Recently, modified autologous cryoprecipitate has become an important reagent in the ongoing attempts to line the luminal surface of vascular prostheses with autologous ECs.[61,69,70] We hypothesized that this fibrin matrix may improve the efficacy of endoluminal EC seeding and reduce restenosis after PTCA.

Rationale for fibrin matrix as a vehicle for endothelial cell delivery

It has been shown that ECs are able to grow faster on surfaces pretreated with plasma proteins, especially those involved in coagulation.[43,71,72] Fibronectin, fibrinogen and vitronectin contained in our autologous cryoprecipitated preparations have specific binding sites for ECs.[43] Our preliminary studies have confirmed that ECs remain attached to the fibrin meshwork and are viable in the three-dimensional glue matrix (unpublished data). The non-cytotoxic fibrin matrix meshwork, in addition, is flexible and compliant, may be easily adapted to a circumferential contour wall and is timely resorbed to leave a completely healed tissue. Areas occupied by adherent ECs and cell-free areas that may serve as a depot for drug delivery characterize the structure. In the cryoprecipitated plasma, the three-dimensional fibrin matrix structure (Figure 29.1) undergoes covalent cross-linking by the formation of glutamyl–lysyl isopeptide bonds, which develop between the protein chains.[43,61,69,70,71]

Utilization of the endothelial cell–fibrin matrix

We applied an alternative technique for EC seeding using fibrin matrix and assessed the impact of this improved endothelial reseeding on restenosis 8 weeks following balloon angioplasty in iliac arteries of atherosclerotic rabbits.

Histologic examination demonstrated the ability of this method to reattach the EC–fibrin matrix circumferentially to $68.0 \pm 6.7\%$ of the denuded arterial wall segment in comparison to $13.5 \pm 3.9\%$ reattachment following seeding with ECs without fibrin matrix (Figures 29.2 and 29.3).

The attachment efficiency of ECs calculated from the intensity of PKM-26 was significantly higher in arteries subjected to matrix/cell reconstruction

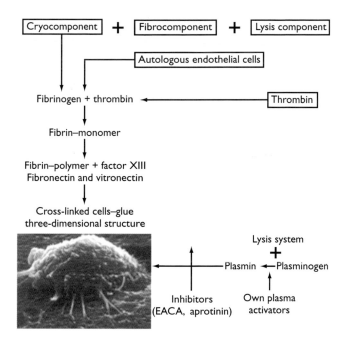

Figure 29.1 *Cell–fibrin three-dimensional structure formation.*

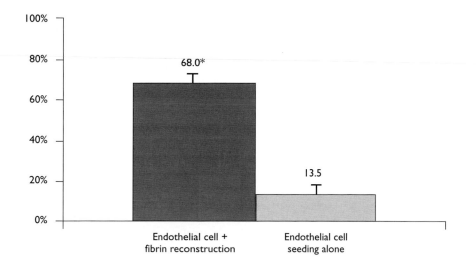

Figure 29.2 *Percentage of cells attached to the vessel wall following EC–fibrin application and exposure to bloodflow (Evans blue).*

405

Figure 29.3 *Fluorescent micrograph of fluorescent-labeled transplanted ECs 4 h after vascular reconstruction. Longitudinal view of cell–glue layer.*

(75.3 ± 13.4%, $P < 0.0003$) in comparison to the arteries subjected to EC seeding alone (10.1 ± 8.8%). SEM also confirmed these results.

Our study also shows that EC–fibrin matrix has a greater effect on restenosis than do ECs alone, and minimal luminal diameter was significantly increased in the EC–matrix group when angiography was performed 60 days later (Figure 29.4).

Late loss in the lumen of control arteries seeded with ECs was 1.12 ± 0.31 mm. In the animals in which endothelial reconstruction was done with fibrin matrix only, the late loss was 1.17 ± 0.28 mm, whereas in the arteries subjected to endoluminal cell–fibrin matrix reconstruction, late loss was significantly reduced to 0.69 ± 0.21 mm (Figure 29.5). Histology demonstrated that all vessels undergoing reconstruction remained patent and appeared grossly free of thrombosis. This was in agreement with previous studies showing that EC seeding also reduces platelet deposition in a canine endarterectomy model at 5 h, 1, 2, 3 and 4 days and 4 weeks.[73] Control segments demonstrate significant fibrocellular hyperplasia with focal macrophage/foam cell accumulation in the core. The internal elastic lamina was not disrupted and the original tunica media was not thinned. In contrast, arterial sections treated with EC–fibrin matrix presented minimal fibrocellular hyperplasia with little variation in thickness, mostly due to the previous neointima (Figure 29.6). There was near complete endothelialization in treated arteries (Figure 29.7).

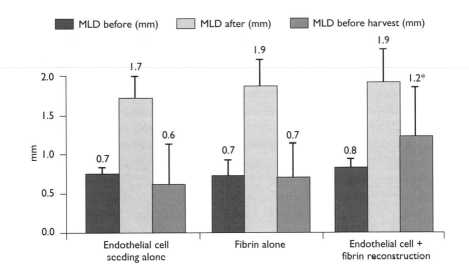

Figure 29.4 *Quantitative angiography. MLD, minimal luminal diameter.*
*p<0.001 comparison between EC/fibrin and EC seeding alone.

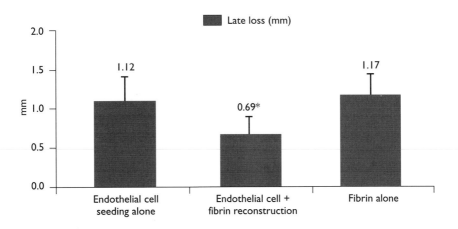

Figure 29.5 *Late loss at 60 days. *p<0.004 comparison between EC/fibrin and*
EC seeding alone.

Morphometric analysis showed that the lumen area was significantly greater in the EC–matrix group ($1.23 \pm 0.35 \, mm^2$) than with EC seeding alone ($0.65 \pm 0.09 \, mm^2$) and with fibrin matrix alone ($0.72 \pm 0.41 \, mm^2$), which was almost entirely accounted for by the statistically significant difference in the intimal area ($0.76 \pm 0.18 \, mm^2$ versus $1.25 + 0.26 \, mm^2$ and $1.01 \pm 0.53 \, mm^2$, respectively) (Figure 29.8).

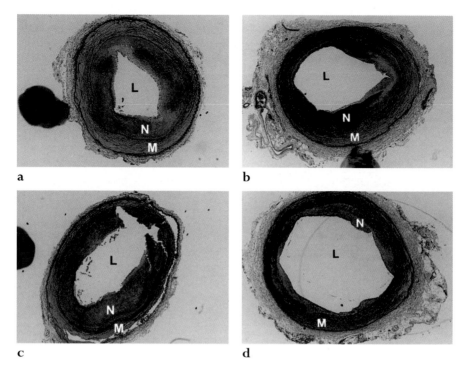

Figure 29.6 *Movat's stain. L, lumen; M, media; and N, neointima. (a) Iliac artery of cholesterol-fed rabbit, 60 days after balloon injury and local saline (control) application via Wolinsky catheter. Cross-section shows representative fibrocellular hyperplasia with focal macrophage/foam cell accumulation in the core. The internal elastic lamina is not disrupted and the original tunica media is not thinned. The waviness of both remaining internal and external laminae is suggestive of a remodeling process leading to shrinkage. (b) Contralateral iliac artery of the same artery as shown in (a), 60 days after balloon injury and local application of glue only via Wolinsky catheter. The cross-section shows representative fibrocellular hyperplasia without significant foam cell accumulation. The internal elastic lamina is less disrupted than in (a), but the tunica media is also thinned, indicating a lesser but comparable initial mechanical injury at this site. Little inflammation and no angiogenesis are seen, but the tunica adventitia displays some reinforcing collagenous thickening in the upper left quadrant. (c,d) Iliac arteries from another cholesterol-fed animal 60 days after the procedure. On both sides there is neointima around the entire circumference, but the internal elastic lamina is intact, and the original tunica media shows intimal cell loss and little compression, indicating that in these positions the initial injuries were present, symmetric and comparable in terms of the same, relatively mild degree. (c) The EC-treated control segment shows a concentric lesion with the fibrocellular intimal hyperplasia. (d) Local treatment with glue–cell results in minimal fibrocellular hyperplasia with little variation in thickness, mostly due to the previous neointima. (a–d) Movat stain, all taken with a digital camera at the same magnification and further processed with photofinish 4.*

Our results show very significant circumferential attachment of the fibrin–EC matrix to the denuded arterial wall when compared to seeding with ECs alone. In this experiment, the addition of fibrin matrix to the ECs also decreased myointimal thickness, and the luminal area was also significantly greater in the EC–fibrin matrix group than in the EC-seeding

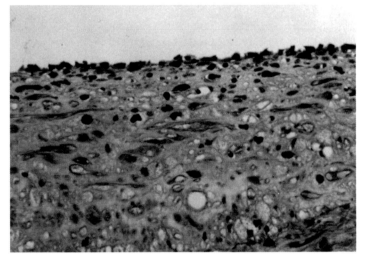

Figure 29.7 *Impact of reconstruction of arterial wall upon re-endothelization in an atherosclerotic rabbit model. Note near complete endothelialization at 8 weeks following balloon angioplasty; EC–glue reconstruction was indicated by visualization of endothelial nuclei on the intima.*

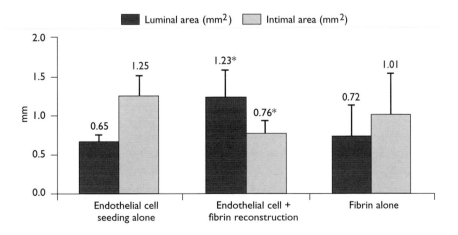

Figure 29.8 *Morphometry at 60 days after treatment. *p<0.001 comparison between EC/fibrin and EC seeding alone.*

group. Recently, it was shown that EC seeding of fibrin-coated stents is less thrombogenic.[74] In addition, the ECs from the border of the denuded area then preferentially migrate into this three-dimensional structure.[71]

Furthermore, as an endpoint of thrombosis, the new fibrin layer may help to limit new thrombosis and fibrin deposition. Indeed, we previously demonstrated[74] that fibrin coating of stents resulted in reduced platelet adhesion in vitro and prevented stent thrombosis in an animal model. However, a study performed by Byer et al[75] has demonstrated that fibrin sealant-coated stents were not detrimental to the vascular wall and did not produce much more stenosis than non-coated stents at 30 days.

The results of our present studies failed to demonstrate a favorable influence of fibrin reconstruction without ECs upon restenosis.

In the clinical setting, this process would require the use of the patient as the autologous donor for the ECs and reagents for the biological matrix. Thus the method has the advantage of avoiding potential immunologic/rejection problems. These data indicate that related plasma proteins are able to perform some of the functions of the extracellular matrix in anchoring ECs to the vessel wall.

One limitation of this technique is that the presence of side-branches within the site of intervention limits the efficacy of the seeding and also potentially may cause their loss. Second, the Wolinsky infusion balloon used in our studies is not optimal for matrix/cell delivery.[76] The limitation of this catheter is pressure-driven local delivery, which causes additional vessel damage and also relatively low efficacy of local delivery. Catheters providing better, less traumatic, local drug delivery (Clearway irrigation system) may increase the efficacy of EC transplantation.[77] Perhaps the construction of a new delivery catheter with two separate channels for delivery, one for thrombin solution and another for fibrinogen loaded with ECs, will help in the delivery of the glue–cell matrix more precisely. This design will also allow matrix to polymerize directly on the surface of the arterial segment and will eliminate possible occlusion of the delivery holes of the catheter, which will make the delivery more homogeneous and may also help to prevent possible distal thrombosis.

One of the limitations of the present study is the animal model. The main disadvantages of the atherosclerotic rabbit model include morphologic differences from human lesions. Another limitation of the study is that the function of transplanted ECs is unknown, and additional studies are needed to address this issue. Finally, it is difficult to differentiate the effect of EC–fibrin matrix transplantation upon the integrity of the new endothelial layer from the independent effect of fibrin matrix. However, the concept of reconstruction of the arterial wall with EC–fibrin matrix to prevent restenosis remains appealing.

Conclusion

The prevention and/or effective treatment of restenosis remains a main obstacle in interventional cardiology. One approach to overcoming this problem is the promotion and acceleration of re-endothelialization in the injured vessel. Along with utilizing growth factors (VEGF, FGF) to enhance endothelial regeneration, vascular EC reconstruction using autologous EC–fibrin matrix appears to have substantial potential in the prevention of restenosis. Autologous EC–fibrin matrix implants are substantially more efficient than EC seeding alone for re-endothelialization and do not cause occlusive thrombus formation in this animal model. Further exploration into the control mechanisms of endothelial implants, their function and their interaction with fibrin matrix and surrounding tissues, as well as clinical trials, would provide additional insight and support for this novel approach in the treatment of restenosis. Despite the major advances made, there remain significant hurdles to overcome before this technique can move to widespread clinical application.

References

1. Nobuyoshi M, Kimura T, Nosaka H et al. Restenosis after successful percutaneous transluminal coronary angioplasty: serial angiographic follow-up of 229 patients. J Am Coll Cardiol 1988; 12: 616–23.

2. Topol EJ, Serruys PW. Frontiers in interventional cardiology. Circulation 1998; 98: 1802–20.

3. Topol EJ. Coronary-artery stents – gauging, gorging, and gouging. N Engl J Med 1998; 339: 1702–4.

4. Serruys PW, Foley DP, Suttorp M-J et al. A randomized comparison of the value of additional stenting after optimal balloon angioplasty for long coronary lesions. JACC 2002; 39: 393–9.

5. Van den Brand M, Rensing J, Morel MM et al. The effect of completeness of revascularization on event-free survival at one-year in the ARTS trial. JACC 2002; 39: 559–64.

6. El-Omar MM, Dangas G, Iakovou I et al. Update on in-stent Restenosis. Curr Intervent Cardiol Rep 2001; 3: 296–305.

7. Faries PL, Rohan DI, Takahara H et al. Human vascular smooth muscle cells of diabetic origin exhibit increased proliferation, adhesion, and migration. J Vasc Surg 2001; 33(3): 601–7.

8. Wilentz JR, Sanborn TA, Haudenschild CC et al. Platelet accumulation in experimental angioplasty: time course and relation to vascular injury. Circulation 1987; 3: 636–42.

9. Wilensky RI, March KL, Gradus-Pizlo I et al. Vascular injury, repair, and restenosis after percutaneous transluminal angioplasty in the atherosclerotic rabbit. Circulation 1995; 92(10): 2995–3005.

10. Stoltenberg RL, Geraghty J, Steele DM et al. Inhibition of intimal hyperplasia in rat aortic allografts with cyclosporine. Transplantation 1995; 60(9): 993–8.

11. Glagov S. Intimal hyperplasia, vascular modeling, and the restenosis problem. Circulation 1994; 89: 2888–91.

12. Schwartz R, Holmes D, Topol E. The restenosis paradigm revisited: an alternative proposal for cellular mechanisms. J Am Coll Cardiol 1992; 20: 1284–93.

13. Schwartz RS, Murphy JG, Edwards WD et al. Restenosis after balloon angioplasty: a practical proliferative model in porcine coronary arteries. Circulation 1990; 82: 2190–200.

14. Ross R, Wight TN, Strandness E et al. Human atherosclerosis. I. Cell constitution and characteristics of advanced lesions of the superficial femoral artery. Am J Pathol 1984; 114: 79–93.

15. Moses PRL, Campbell GR, Wang ZL et al. Smooth muscle phenotypic expression in human carotid arteries. Lab Invest 1985; 53: 556–62.

16. Austin GE, Ratliff NB, Hollman J et al. Intimal proliferation of smooth muscle cells as an explanation for recurrent coronary artery stenosis after percutaneous transluminal coronary angioplasty. J Am Coll Cardiol 1985; 6: 369–75.

17. Clowes AW, Reidy MA, Clowes MM. Kinetics of cellular proliferation after arterial injury. Lab Invest 1983; 49: 327–33.

18. Schwartz SM, deBlois D, O'Brien ERM. The intima: soil for atherosclerosis and restenosis. Circ Res 1995; 77: 445–465.

19. Morishita R, Gibbons GH, Ellison KE et al. Single intraluminal delivery of antisense cdc2 kinase and proliferating-cell nuclear antigen oligonucleotides results in chronic inhibition of neointimal hyperplasia. Proc Natl Acad Sci USA 1993; 90: 8474–8.

20. Sirois MG, Simons M, Edelman BR et al. Platelet release of platelet derived growth factor is required for intimal hyperplasia in rat vascular injury model. Circulation 1994; 90(suppl 1): I-511 (abstract).

21. Mintz GS, Popma JJ, Hong MK et al. Intravascular ultrasound to discern device-specific effects and mechanisms of restenosis. Am J Cardiol 1996; 78: 18–22.

22. Edelman ER, Rogers C. Pathobiologic responses to stenting. Am J Cardiol 1998; 81: 4E–6E.

23. Komatsu R, Ueda M, Naruko T et al. Neointimal tissue response at sites of coronary stenting in humans: macroscopic, histological, and immunohistochemical analyses. Circulation 1998; 98: 224–33.

24. Kornowski R, Hong MK, Tio FO et al. In-stent restenosis: contributions of inflammatory responses and arterial injury to neointimal hyperplasia. J Am Coll Cardiol 1998; 31: 224–30.

25. Jawien A, Bowen-Pope DF, Lindner V et al. Platelet-derived growth factor promotes smooth muscle migration and intimal thickening in a rat model of balloon angioplasty. J Clin Invest 1992; 89: 507–11.

26. Sriram V, Patterson C. Cell cycle in vasculoproliferative diseases – potential interventions and routes of delivery. Circulation 2001; 103: 2414–19.

27. Koster R, Vieluf D, Kiehn M et al. Nickel and molybdenum contact allergies in patients with coronary in-stent restenosis. Lancet 2000; 356: 1895–7.

28. Doornekamp F, Borst C, Post MJ. Endothelial cell recovery and intimal hyperplasia after endothelium removal with or without smooth muscle cell necrosis in the rabbit carotid artery. J Vasc Res 1966; 33: 146–55.

29. Garg UC, Hasssid A. Nitric oxide-generating vasodilators and 8-bromo-cyclic-guanosine monophosphate inhibit mitogenesis and proliferation of cultured rat vascular smooth muscle cells. J Clin Invest 1989; 83: 1774–7.

30. McBride W, Lange RA, Hillis LD. Restenosis after successful coronary angioplasty. Pathophysology and prevention. N Engl J Med 1988; 318: 1734–7.

31. Liu MW, Roubin GS, King III SB. Restenosis after coronary angioplasty. Potential biologic determinants and role of intimal hyperplasia. Circulation 1989; 79: 1374–87.

32. Shirotani M, Yui Y, Kawai C. Restenosis after coronary angioplasty: pathogenesis of neointimal thickening initiated by endothelial loss. Endothelium 1993; 1: 5–22.

33. Reidy MA, Schwarz SM. Endothelial regeneration: III. Time course of intima changes after small defined injury of rat aortic endothelium. Lab Invest 1981; 44: 301–8.

34. Bjokerud S, Bonjers G. Arterial repair and atherosclerosis after mechanical injury: Part 5. Tissue response after introduction of a large superficial transverse injury. Atherosclerosis 1973; 18: 235–55.

35. Haudenschild CC, Schwartz SM. Endothelial regeneration: II. Restitution of endothelial continuity. Lab Invest 1979; 41: 407–18.

36. Clowes AW, Kohler TR. Anatomy, physiology and pharmacology of the vascular wall. In: Moore WS, ed. Vascular surgery. Philadelphia: WB Saunders, 1993.

37. Fantidis P, Fernandez-Ortiz A, Aragoncillo P et al. Effect of cAMP on the function of endothelial cells and fibromuscular proliferation after the injury of

413

the carotid and coronary arteries in a porcine model. Rev Esp Cardiol 2001; 54(8): 981–9.

38. Grewe PH, Deneke T, Holt SK et al. Scanning electron microscopic analysis of vessel wall reactions after coronary stenting. Z Kardiol 2000; 89(1): 21–7.

39. Nakatani M, Takeyama Y, Shibata M et al. Mechanisms of restenosis after coronary intervention. Difference between plain old balloon angioplasty and stenting. Cardiovasc Pathol 2003; 12(1): 40–8.

40. Herdeg C, Oberhoff M, Baumbach A et al. Local paclitaxel delivery for the prevention of restenosis: biological effects and efficacy in vivo. J Am Coll Cardiol 2000; 35(7): 1969–76.

41. Callow AD, Choi ET, Trachtenberg JD et al. Vascular permeability factor accelerates endothelial regrowth following balloon angioplasty. Growth Factors 1994; 10: 223–8.

42. deBono DP, Pittilo M, Pringle S et al. Endothelial–smooth muscle interactions in vitro: effects of high pH, flowing medium, and extracellular matrix. Br J Exp Pathol 1988; 69: 209–20.

43. Schneider PA, Hanson SR, Price TM et al. Confluent durable endothelialization of endarterectomised baboon aorta by early attachment of cultured endothelial cells. J Vasc Surg 1990; 11: 365–72.

44. Nabel EG, Plautz G, Boyce FM et al. Recombinant gene expression in vivo within endothelial cells on the arterial wall. Science 1989; 249: 1342–3.

45. Thompson MM, Budd JS, Eady SL et al. Endothelial cell seeding of damaged native vascular surfaces: prostacyclin production. Eur J Vasc Surg 1992; 6: 487–93.

46. Thompson MM, Budd JS, Eady SL et al. A method of transluminally seeding angioplasty sites with endothelial cells using a double balloon catheter. Eur J Vasc Surg 1993; 7: 113–21.

47. Conte MS, Birinyi LK, Miyata T et al. Efficient repopulation of denuded rabbit arteries with autologous genetically modified endothelial cells. Circulation 1994; 89: 2161–9.

48. Sterpetti AV, Schults RD, Baily RT. Endothelial cell seeding after carotid endarterectomy in a canine model reduces platelet uptake. Eur J Vasc Surg 1992; 6: 390–4.

49. Van Belle E, Tio F, Couffinhal T et al. Stent endothelialization. Time course, impact of local catheter delivery, feasibility of recombinant protein administration, and response to cytokine expedition. Circulation 1997; 438–48.

50. Moulton KS, Heller E, Konerding MA et al. Angiogenesis inhibitors endostatin and TNP-470 reduce intimal neovascularization and plaque growth in apolipoprotein-E deficient mice. Circulation 1999; 99: 1726–32.

414

51. Van Belle E, Tio FO, Chen D et al. Passivation of metallic stents folowing arterial gene transfer of ph VEGF$_{165}$ inhibits thrombus formation and intimal thickening. J Am Coll Cardiol 1997; 29: 1371–9.

52. Asahara T, Bauters C, Pastore CJ et al. Local delivery of vascular endothelial growth factor accelerates reendothelialization and attenuates intimal hyperplasia in balloon injury rat carotid artery. Circulation 1995; 91: 2793–801.

53. Asahara TC, Tsurumi Y, Kearney M et al. Accelerated restitution of endothelial integrity and endothelium dependent function following rh VEGF$_{165}$ gene transfer. Circulation 1996; 94: 3291–302.

54. Isner JM, Baumgartner I, Rauh G et al. Treatment of thromboangiitis obliterans by intramuscular gene transfer of vascular endothelial growth factor; preliminary clinical results. J Vasc Surg 1998; 28: 964–75.

55. Vale PR, Wuesch DI, Rauh GF et al. Arterial gene therapy for inhibiting restenosis in patients with claudication undergoing superficial femoral artery angioplasty. Circulation 1998; 98(suppl I): 1–66 (abstract).

56. Herring M, Gardner A, Glover J. A single staged technique for seeding vascular grafts with autogenous endothelium. Surgery 1978; 84: 498–504.

57. Graham LM, Burkel WE, Ford JW et al. Immediate seeding of enzymatically derived endothelium in Dacron vascular grafts. Arch Surg 1980; 115: 1289–94.

58. Zilla P, Fasol RD, Deutsch M. Endothelialization of vascular grafts. 1st European Workshop on Advances in Vascular Surgery. Basel: Karger, 1987.

59. Herring M, Gardner A, Glovert J. A single-staged technique for seeding vascular grafts with autogenous endothelium. Surgery 1978; 84: 498–504.

60. Herring M, Baughman S, Glover J et al. Endothelial seeding of Dacron and polytetrafluoroethylene grafts: the cellular events of healing. Surgery 1984; 96: 745–54.

61. Zilla P, Fasol R, Preiss P et al. Use of fibrin glue as a substrate for in vitro endothelialization of PTFE vascular grafts. Surgery 1989; 105: 515–22.

62. Zilla P, Fasol R, Dudec U et al. In situ cannulation, microgrig follow-up and low-density plating provide first passage endothelial cell mass cultures for in vitro lining. J Vasc Surg 1990; 12: 180–9.

63. Greisler HP. Endothelial cell transplantation onto synthetic vascular grafts: panacea, poison or placebo. In: Greisler HP, Austin RG, eds. New biologic and synthetic prostheses. Landes Comp., 1991: 47–64.

64. Greisler MP, Cziperle DJ, Kim DU. Enhanced endothelialization of expanded polytetrafluoroethylene grafts by fibroblast growth factor type 1 pretreatment. Surgery 1992; 112: 244–55.

65. Nugent HM, Edelman ER. Endothelial implants provide long-term control of vascular repair in a porcine model of arterial injury. J Surg Res 2001; 99(2): 228–34.

66. Conte MS, VanMeter GA, Akst LM et al. Endothelial cell seeding influences lesion development following arterial injury in the cholesterol-fed rabbit. Cardiovasc Res 2002; 53(2): 502–11.

67. Kutryk MJ, van Dortmont LM, de Crom RP et al. Seeding of intravascular stents by the xenotransplantation of genetically modified endothelial cells. Semin Intervent Cardiol 1998; 3(3–4): 217–20.

68. Gomes D, Louedec L, Plissonnier D et al. Endoluminal smooth muscle cell seeding limits intimal hyperplasia. J Vasc Surg 2001; 34(4): 707–15.

69 Kang S, Gosselin C, Ren D et al. Selective stimulation of endothelial cell proliferation with inhibition of smooth muscle cell proliferation by FGF-1 plus heparin delivered from fibrin glue suspensions. Surgery 1995; 118: 280–7.

70. Gosselin C, Ren D, Ellinger J et al. In vivo platelet deposition on polytetrafluoroethylene coated with fibrin glue containing fibroblast growth factor 1 and heparin in a canine model. Am J Surg 1995; 170: 126–30.

71. Nikolaychik VV, Samet MM, Lelkes PI. A new cryoprecipitate based coating for improved endothelial cell attachment and growth on medical grade artificial surfaces. ASAIO J 1994; 40: M846–52.

72. Warren JB. The endothelium: an introduction to current research. New York: Wiley-Liss, 1990.

73. Sterpetti AV, Schults RD, Bailey RT. Endothelial cell seeding after carotid endarterectomy in a canine model reduces platelet uptake. Eur J Vasc Surg 1992; 170: 126–30.

74. Baker JE, Horn JB, Nikolaychik VV, Kipshidze N. Fibrin coated stents. In: Sigwart U, Endovascular stenting. ed. WB Saunders, Philadelphia: 1996: 94–101.

75. Byer A, Peters S, Settepani F et al. Fibrin sealant coated stents compared with non-coated stents in a porcine carotid artery model. Preliminary study report. J Cardiovasc Surg (Torino) 2001; 42(4): 543–9.

76. Wolinsky H. Local delivery: let's keep our eyes on the wall. J Am Coll Cardiol 1994: 24: 825–7.

77. Lincoff AM, Topol EJ, Ellis SG. Local drug delivery for prevention of restenosis. Fact, fancy, fiction. Circulation 1994; 90: 2070–84.

INDEX

417

418

peripheral blood endothelial precursors
  blood volume required 306
   phenotypic characterization 153–4
   transplantation 171–3
perivascular endothelial cell tissue
  engineering 347–67
  delivery devices 349–50
PKM-26 404
placenta cells, trophoblasts 143–4
platelet endothelial cell adhesion molecule
  (PECAM-CD31) 374
platelet-derived growth factor (PDGF) 77,
  184, 281
polymer-based controlled drug delivery
  systems 349–50
polymeric scaffolds
  examples 371–2
  neointimal thickening stimulation 385
polymeric surfaces (Gelfoam) 355
  transplantation of endothelial cells 350–3
porcine–human heterokaryons 241, 247
proteins, angiogenic, intramyocardial delivery
  via coronary venous system 331–3

radiolabeling
  metabolic activity 102
  SPECT-sestamibi scan analysis 268, 284
rapamycin-eluting stents 384–5

saphenous vein endothelial cells (SVECs)
  156, 158
satellite cells
  activation and production of MPCs 123
  humans 243
  implantation 96–8
  labeling of cultured cells 93–6
  myocardial regeneration 98–102
  properties 91–3, 243–4
  rats 243
  side-population (SP) cells 93
  transplantation 91–105
   clinical observations 102
  see also myoblasts
scar tissue (heart), properties 107
side-population (SP) cells 93
single-fiber (SF) system
  mechanisms 126, 140
  numbers implanted 124–5

preparation of myoblasts 124
sirolimus, clinical trials 402
skeletal muscle-derived progenitor cells see
  muscle-derived stem cells (MDSCs);
  myoblast(s)
small vessel grafts (tissue engineering)
  369–81
  basic stages **370**
  bioreactors 376
  comparison of methods used for in vivo
   evaluation **373**
  endothelial cells 373–5
  evaluation 376–8
  graft design 370–3
  signaling 375–6
smooth muscle cells 374–5, 400–2
  see also myoblast(s); myocardial; muscle
SPECT-sestamibi scan analysis 268, 284
stem cells see bone marrow; embryonic stem
  (ES) cells
stents
  antiproliferative drugs, and restenosis,
   clinical trials 402
  biomimicry concept, testing 393–5
  cell-based implantable 383–97
  drug-eluting stents 384–5
  endothelium role in restenosis 400–2
   vs balloon injury 401
  seeding with genetically modified ECs
   404
systemic administration
  cell implantation 176, 267
  see also administration routes

tacrolimus, clinical trials 402
TaqMan PCR, Sry gene 61–2
target lesion revascularization (TLR) 384
thrombospondin-1, release from cardiac
  fibroblasts 77
tissue engineering
  perivascular endothelial cells 347–67
  small vessel grafts 369–81
tissue inhibitors of MMPs (TIMPs) 377
TNP-470, inhibition of angiogenesis 403
transcription factors
  cardiac-specific 47
  see also GATA
transforming growth factor (TGF-beta)